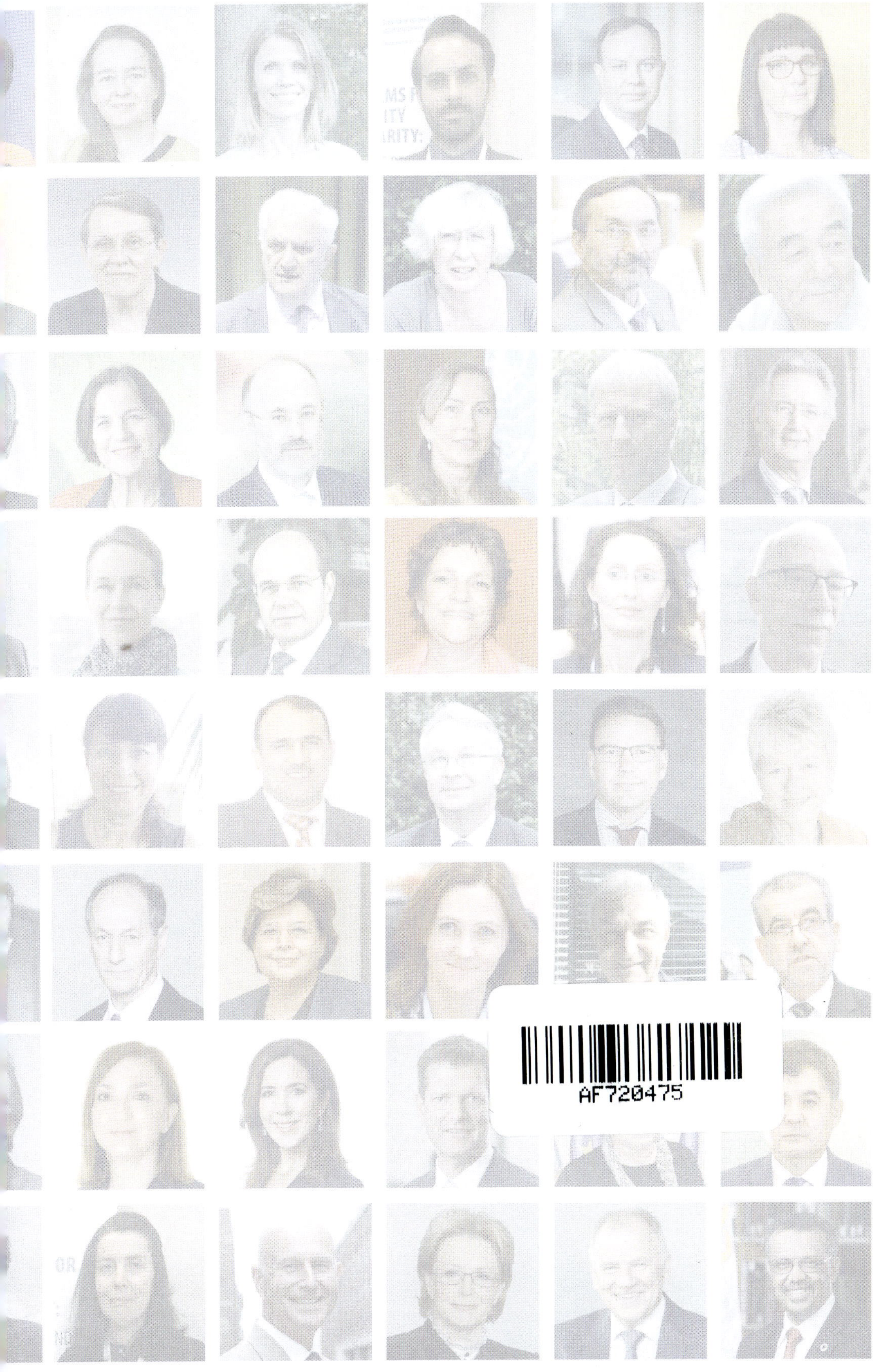

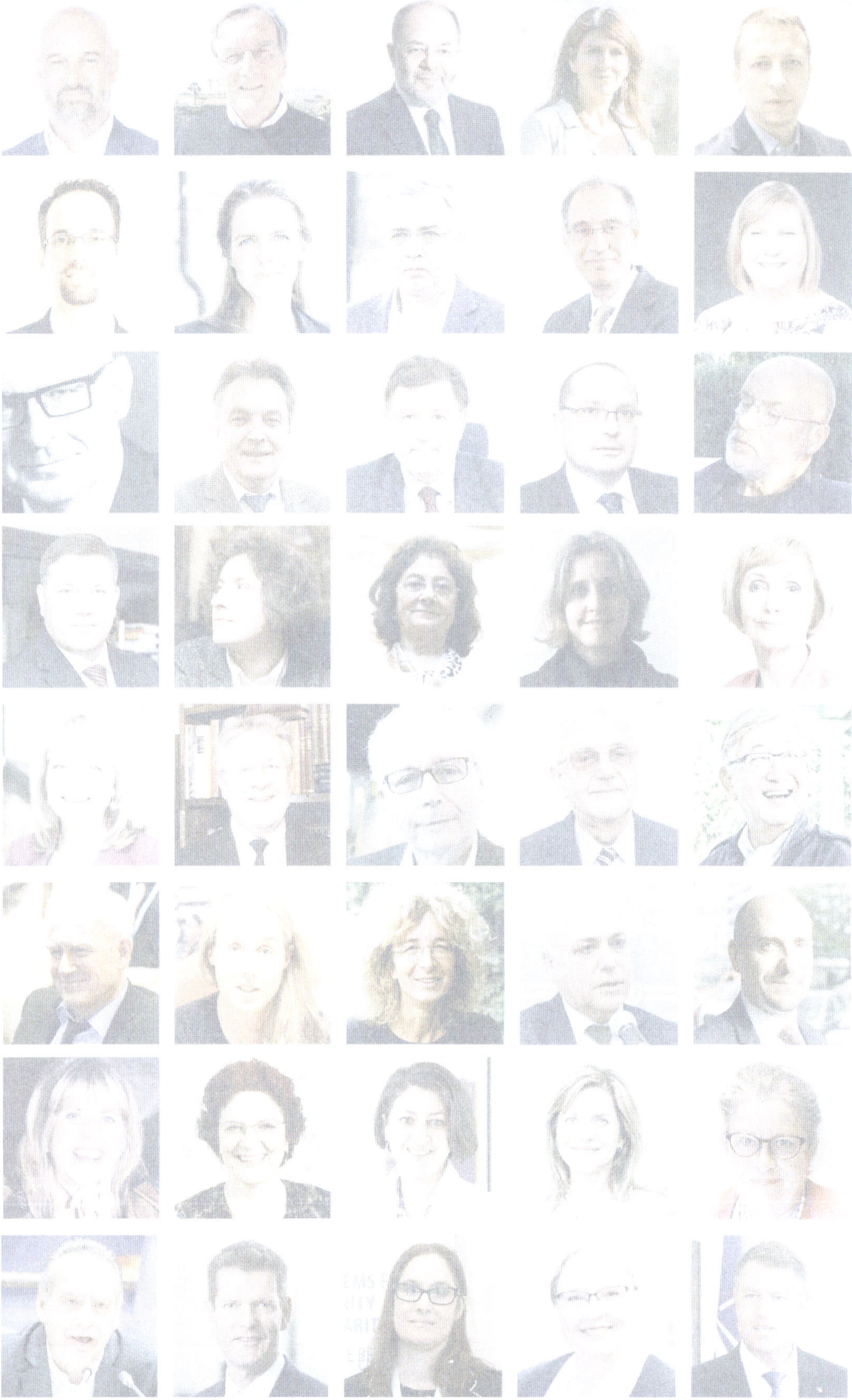

Better Health for Europe:
more equitable and sustainable

Transformational Reflections

2010–2020

World Health Organization

REGIONAL OFFICE FOR Europe

Better Health for Europe: more equitable and sustainable

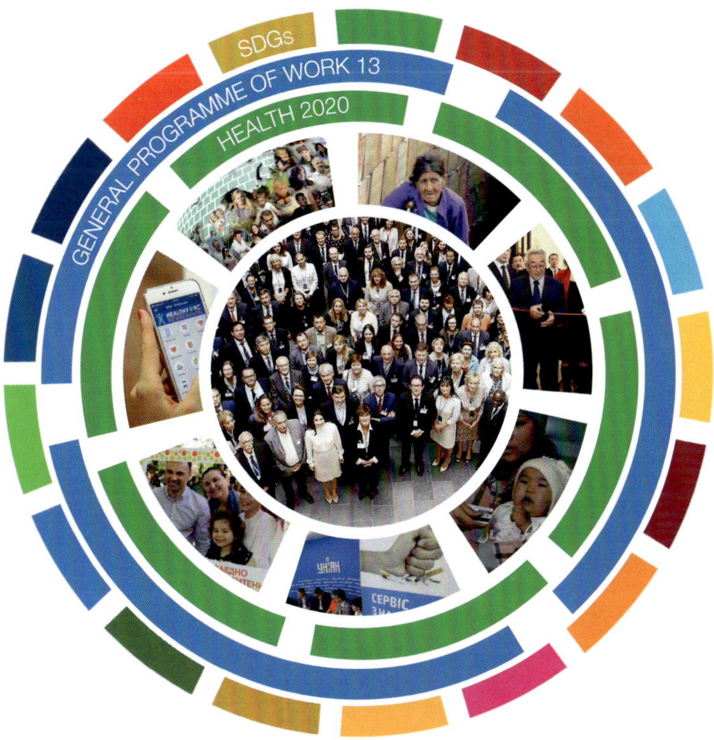

Transformational Reflections

2010–2020

September 2019

Abstract

Better Health for Europe: more equitable and sustainable, tells the story of how people working for WHO in the European Region have sought to make a reality of this goal over the last ten years. Zsuzsanna Jakab, WHO Regional Director for Europe from 2010 until 2020, narrates the story on behalf of all staff and describes the vision, strategic thinking and processes followed, as well as the impact achieved. Political leaders, public health managers and health practitioners and advocates from across the WHO European Region and beyond were invited to reflect upon the relevance and utility of the work of the Regional Office. Extracts from interviews with these 'witnesses' are presented throughout the book to enrich the narrative.

This book is divided into three parts. Part I – Better Health for Europe: the seven strategic action priorities, presents the systematic process the Regional Office has followed in developing the policy frameworks, evidence base, capacities, relationships, partnerships, networks and skills needed to transform and enhance action for better, more equitable and sustainable health and well-being in Europe and beyond. Part II – Better Health for Europe: achievements, describes outcomes and the impacts of Regional Office work on the two objectives and four priority actions of the Health 2020 European policy framework. Part III – Better Health for Europe: conclusions and messages, summarizes reflections and looks at challenges beyond 2020.

ISBN 9789289054225

Address requests about publications of the WHO Regional Office for Europe to:
Publications

WHO Regional Office for Europe
UN City Marmorvej
51 DK-2100 Copenhagen Ø, Denmark

Alternatively, complete an online request form for documentation, health information, or for permission to quote or translate, on the Regional Office website (http://www.euro.who.int/pubrequest).

Suggested citation. Better Health for Europe: More Equitable and Sustainable. Copenhagen: WHO Regional Office for Europe; 2019. Copenhagen: WHO Regional Office for Europe. License: CC BY-NC-SA 3.0 IGO.

Cataloguing-in-Publication (CIP) data. CIP data are available at http://apps.who.int/iris.

Contents

Acknowledgements

First, I want to thank all the 'witnesses' for their contributions, timely reviews and encouragement. I am very grateful to all for sharing different points of view, insights, anecdotes and remembrances and helping to make this story a more entertaining, memorable and understandable way of communicating the complexity of this 10-year history of the WHO Regional Office for Europe. Taken as a whole, this collection of stories helps to capture the wonderful diversity of scientific, cultural and social human experience that underpins the resilience and strength of our amazing Region. The 'witnesses' are all listed in Annex 1.

Second, I want to thank the writing team who have helped tell this story. The team included Richard Alderslade, who worked on the narrative text, and Franklin Apfel and Sabrina Cecconi of World Health Communication Associates who managed the process, interviewed the 'witnesses' and devised the extracts for the book. They all contributed to the editing and editorial processes. Their consistent and persistent enthusiasm, calm devotion, flexible approaches and skilful story-telling capacities made this ambitious project feasible.

Third, I want to thank all WHO staff in the Regional Office as well as other regions and headquarters; United Nations, European Union, civil society and other partner agencies; and network, initiative and coalition collaborators who supported this project as informants, reviewers, managers and logistic coordinators. In particular I want to thank Olga Safronova and Lucia Dell'Amura for their ongoing administrative coordination of the book project. My deep appreciation and gratitude goes to all, including: Susan Marla Rosen Ahrenst; Svetlana Akslerod; Nurlan Algashov; Tomas Allen; Sophie Amet; Maja Holm Andreasen; Aziza Askarova; Metin Balci Cagil; Laurence Ballieux; Jozef Bartovic; David Barrett; Sussan Bassiri; Batyr Berdyklychev; Nail Berengere; Antonella Biasiotto; Bianca Bortot; Christine Elisabeth Brown; Kerstin Carlsson; Snezhana Chichevalieva; Masoud Dara; Siddhartha Sankar Datta; Joan Devlin; Jasna Džemić; Nedret Emiroglu; Mirona Eriksen; Gauden Galea; Arlene Garcia-Esplana; Jose Garnica; Maria Greenblat; Svenja Herrmann; Helena Holland; Palmira Immordino; Assel Jabassova; Gyongyver Jakab; Melitta Jakab; Nataliya Jorgensen; Bahtygul Karriyeva; Nana Kavtaradze; Hans Kluge; Tatiana Kolpakova; Monika Kosinska; Rudiger Krech; Giorgi Kuchukhidze; Kanti Kumar Bit; Tessa Latrez; Lucianne Licari; Amela Lolic; Anne Mccusker; Bettina Menne; Leen Meulenbergs; Bente Mikkelsen; Oskonbek Moldokulov; Halima Mohamed; Rodica Munteanu; Liuba Negru; Holly Nielsen; Dorit Nitzan; Piroska Östlin; Diana Loreta Paun; Christine Pii Hansen; Francesca Racioppi; Anna Roepstorff; Joao Joaquim Rodrigues Da Silva Breda; Jean-Isaias Rodriguez; Debra Romaniuk-Mahoney; Amy Rowland; Cristiana Salvi; Caroline Scott; Darina Sedlakova; Santino Severoni; Nino Sharashidze; Almaz Sharman; Belkania Sopo; Claudia Stein; Eyup Tamdogan; Juan Eduardo Tello; Simone Renée Tetz;

Dubravka Trivic; Marie Villemin; Faith Kilford Vorting; Anne Marie Worning; Liza Zorman; Ingrida Zurlyte.

Finally, I want to thank the main editor, Mike Jempson, and designer, Tuuli Sauren, for their excellent, creative, rapid, flexible and supportive work. Thanks also go to journalism students at the University of the West of England, Bristol, who helped with transcriptions: Clara Bullock; Niamh Butler-Walton; Adam Davies; Hugo Docking; Rosa Eaton; Carys Evans; Alice Homewood; Gabriella Petty; and Phil Sansom.

Zsuzsanna Jakab, WHO Regional Director for Europe 2010–2020
WHO Deputy Director-General

Acronyms and Abbreviations

AMR	Antimicrobial resistance
APN	European Alcohol Policy Network
ASPHER	Association of Schools of Public Health in the European Region
BCA	Biennial collaborative agreement
BRIDGE	Bridging Information and Data Generation for Evidence-based Health Policy and Research
CARINFONET	Central Asian Republics Information Network
CAESAR	Central Asian and Eastern European Surveillance of Antimicrobial Resistance network
CCA	Common Country Assessment
CCS	Country cooperation strategy
CoP	Coalition of Partners
EAEU	Eurasian Economic Union
EAP-PHS	European Action Plan for Strengthening Public Health Capacities and Services
ECDC	European Centre for Disease Prevention and Control
EEC	Eurasian Economic Commission
ECEH	European Centre for Environment and Health
EEA	European Environment Agency
EHII	European Health Information Initiative
EMT	Emergency Medical Team
EPHOs	Essential Public Health Operations
ERC	Emergency risk communication
EU	European Union
EUPHA	European Public Health Association
EVIPNet	WHO Evidence-informed Policy Network
FAO	Food and Agriculture Organization of the United Nations
FENSA	Framework for Engagement with non-state actors
FCTC	Framework Convention on Tobacco Control
GDOs	Geographically Dispersed Offices
GDP	Gross Domestic Product
GLASS	Global Antimicrobial Resistance Surveillance System
GOARN	Global Outbreak Alert and Response Network

GPW13	Thirteenth General Programme of Work
GPG	Global Policy Group
HBSC	Health Behaviour in School-aged Children
HBV	Hepatitis B virus
HCV	Hepatitis C virus
HEN	Health Evidence Network
HESRi	Health Equity Status Report initiative
IANPHI	The International Association of National Public Health Institutes
IBC-Health	The UN Issue based Coalition for Health and Well-being for All at All Ages
ICPD	International Conference on Population and Development
ICP	Intercountry programme
ICRC	International Committee of Red Cross
ICT	Information and Communications Technology
IFRC	International Federation of Red Cross and Red Crescent Societies (Red Cross)
IHR	International Health Regulations (2005)
ILO	International Labour Organization
IOM	International Organization for Migration
IPA CIS	Interparliamentary Assembly of Member Nations of the Commonwealth of Independent States
JEE	Joint External Evaluation
JMF	Joint Monitoring Framework
MAPS	Mainstreaming, Acceleration and Policy Support
MDR-TB	Multidrug-resistant tuberculosis
MEPUs	Mobile emergency primary health care units
MOOC	Massive open online course
NCD	Noncommunicable disease
NGO	Nongovernmental organization
NHP	National Health Policy
NIS	Newly independent states
OECD	Organisation for Economic Co-operation and Development
PAS	The Centre for Health Policies and Studies

PHAME	Public Health Aspects of Migration in Europe (now the Migration and Health programme)
PHC	Primary health care
PIP	Pandemic Influenza Preparedness
PTSD	Post-traumatic stress disorder
RCM	Regional Coordination Mechanism
RIVM	National Institute for Public Health and the Environment, Netherlands
RO	Regional Office (WHO)
SAGE	Scientific Advisory Expert Group
SAR	Search and rescue
SCHIN	Small Countries Health Information Network
SCRC	Standing Committee of the Regional Committee
SDG	Sustainable Development Goal
SEEHN	South-eastern Europe Health Network
SG	Secretary General
SOPs	Standard operating procedures
SSI	Social science interventions
SRC	Strategic Relations with Countries unit
STI	Sexually transmitted infection
TB	Tuberculosis
TB-REP	TB Regional Eastern Europe and Central Asia Project
THE PEP	Transport, Health and Environment Pan-European Programme
TRIPS	Trade-Related Aspects of Intellectual Property Rights
UHC	Universal Health Coverage
UNDAFs	United Nations Development Assistance Frameworks
UNDG	(Regional) United Nations Development Group
UNECE	The United Nations Economic Commission for Europe
UNFPA	The United Nations Population Fund
UNHCR	Office of the United Nations High Commissioner for Refugees
UNICEF	United Nations Children's Fund
UNRRA	United Nations Relief and Rehabilitation Administration
URCS	Ukrainian Red Cross Society
USSR	Union of Soviet Socialist Republics

WAAW	World Antibiotic Awareness Week
WaSH	Water, Sanitation and Hygiene
WCO	WHO country office
WHO	World Health Organization
WPRO	Regional Office for the Western Pacific
WR	WHO representative

Foreword

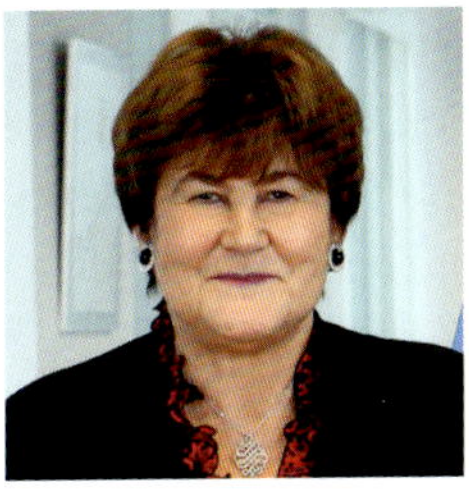

It is my pleasure to welcome you to *Better health for Europe: more equitable and sustainable*. It has been my privilege to serve as the WHO Regional Director for Europe from 2010–2020.

In 2010 we selected 'Better health for Europe' as the goal of the WHO Regional Office for Europe. It was a goal that we knew most policy-makers, public health leaders, managers, workers and advocates could support. However, when we started to develop plans to help our Member States move further towards this goal, many issues and questions arose. How do we achieve it? How do we measure it? Do we know enough? Do we have the right policies? Do we work enough across sectors and organizational borders? And how do we implement policies to ensure that everyone is included?

This book tells the story of how all of us working in the Regional Office in Copenhagen, the geographically dispersed offices (GDOs) and the country offices of the WHO European Region over the last 10 years have sought to answer these questions and make a reality of our goal. We have built on the achievements of the Regional Office under the leadership of my predecessors. Several of them have published similar books describing public health challenges and achievements in the European Region during their tenures *(1, 2)*. As my term of office as Regional Director comes to an end, I too want to reflect on our decade of work to share our learning.

Each generation of WHO staff works to preserve and advance the Organization's values, approaches and impact, and then deliver these into the hands of their successors to further develop. When our turn came in 2010, the Health 2020 – A European policy framework and strategy for the 21st century became the platform for our contribution.

It turned out to be the right set of ideas at the right time. Introduced in 2010 and adopted by the WHO Regional Committee for Europe in 2012, Health 2020 anticipated two key changes in global thinking.

The first relates to the changed global development narrative, as expressed in the United Nations 2030 Agenda for Sustainable Development and the Sustainable Development Goals. These include a wider set of development outcomes than solely economic gain. Health 2020 presented an early example of this thinking and prepared European Member States to take leadership roles in maintaining health at the centre of the development agenda and advocating for universal health coverage.

The second change relates to people and public health leadership. The tools, skills and competencies needed to champion 21st century public health within the new global development narrative shifted to focus more on identifying and implementing effective system-wide responses to todays' many determinants of health. The voice and work of existing and future public health leaders in all 53 Member States of the European Region have been strengthened by our collaborative work and collective experience in developing and implementing Health 2020 and the European Action Plan for Strengthening Public Health Capacities and Services, as well as many other relevant strategies and action plans.

The vision, strategic thinking and processes we followed in relation to these achievements and others – our contribution to WHO's ongoing mission – form the substance of the story we tell in this book.

The book is divided into three parts. Part I – Better Health for Europe: the seven strategic action priorities, presents the systematic process the Regional Office has followed in developing the policies, plans, evidence base, capacities, relationships, partnerships, networks and skills necessary to transform and enhance our work for better, more equitable and sustainable health and well-being in Europe and beyond. Part II – Better Health for Europe: achievements, describes the specific outcomes and impacts of our work on the two objectives and four priority actions of Health 2020. Part III – Better Health for Europe: conclusions and messages, summarizes reflections and looks at challenges beyond 2020.

I am narrating this story on behalf of our Regional Office. However, the central characters and protagonists are all our leadership, technical and administrative staff, as well as our extended public health family of partners and associates across the WHO European Region and beyond. I am proud and very grateful to have had the chance to work alongside these very talented and dedicated people.

I have also invited political leaders, public health decision-makers, health workers and advocates from across and beyond the European Region to help us tell our story. These 'witnesses' were asked to reflect on the relevance and utility of the work of the Regional Office to their work on developing and implementing of global, regional, national and local public health policies and programmes. They were also asked to share stories and anecdotes about practical ways they have worked with the Regional Office and the lessons learned in addressing their own public health challenges. Their responses help to describe and analyse the broad range of our collaborative activities; including, policy and programme development, evidence generation, tool creation, partnerships, networks, communications, advocacy and values promotion. Extracts from these witness interviews are used throughout the text to enhance and enrich the narrative.

All our work and passion have been fuelled, of course, because we are part of WHO. For myself it has been an abiding privilege and honour to work in such a value-driven, evidence-informed and consensus-based Organization.

I believe that the processes we followed and the lessons we have learned over these last 10 years give important pointers to help shape current and future public health strategies and responses at all levels. I welcome you to read and reflect on our story presented here, and I look forward to a continuing dialogue that will bring about more equitable and sustainable health for Europe and beyond.

Zsuzsanna Jakab, WHO Regional Director for Europe 2010–2020
WHO Deputy Director-General

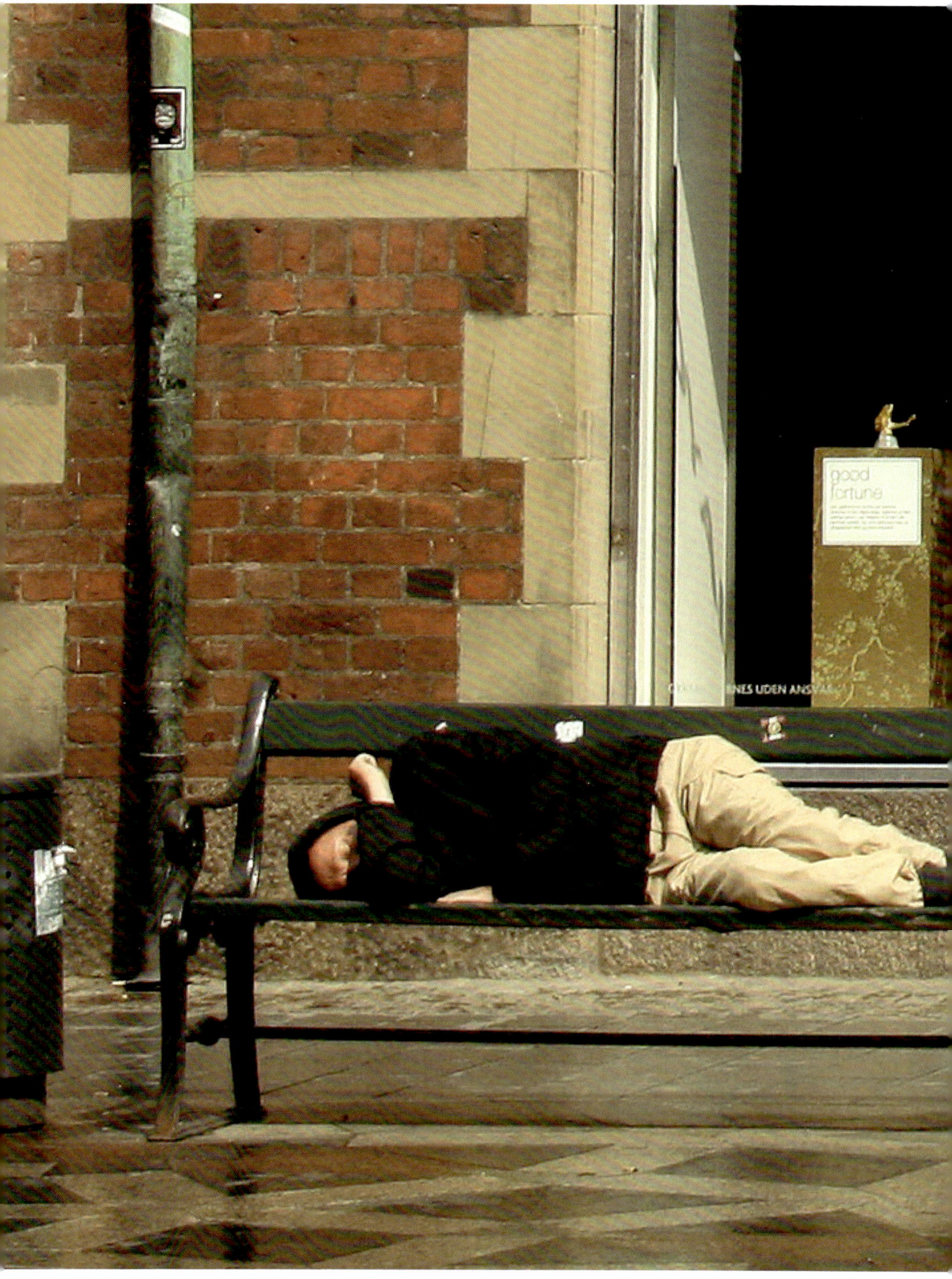
good
fortune

Part I – Better Health for Europe: the seven strategic action priorities

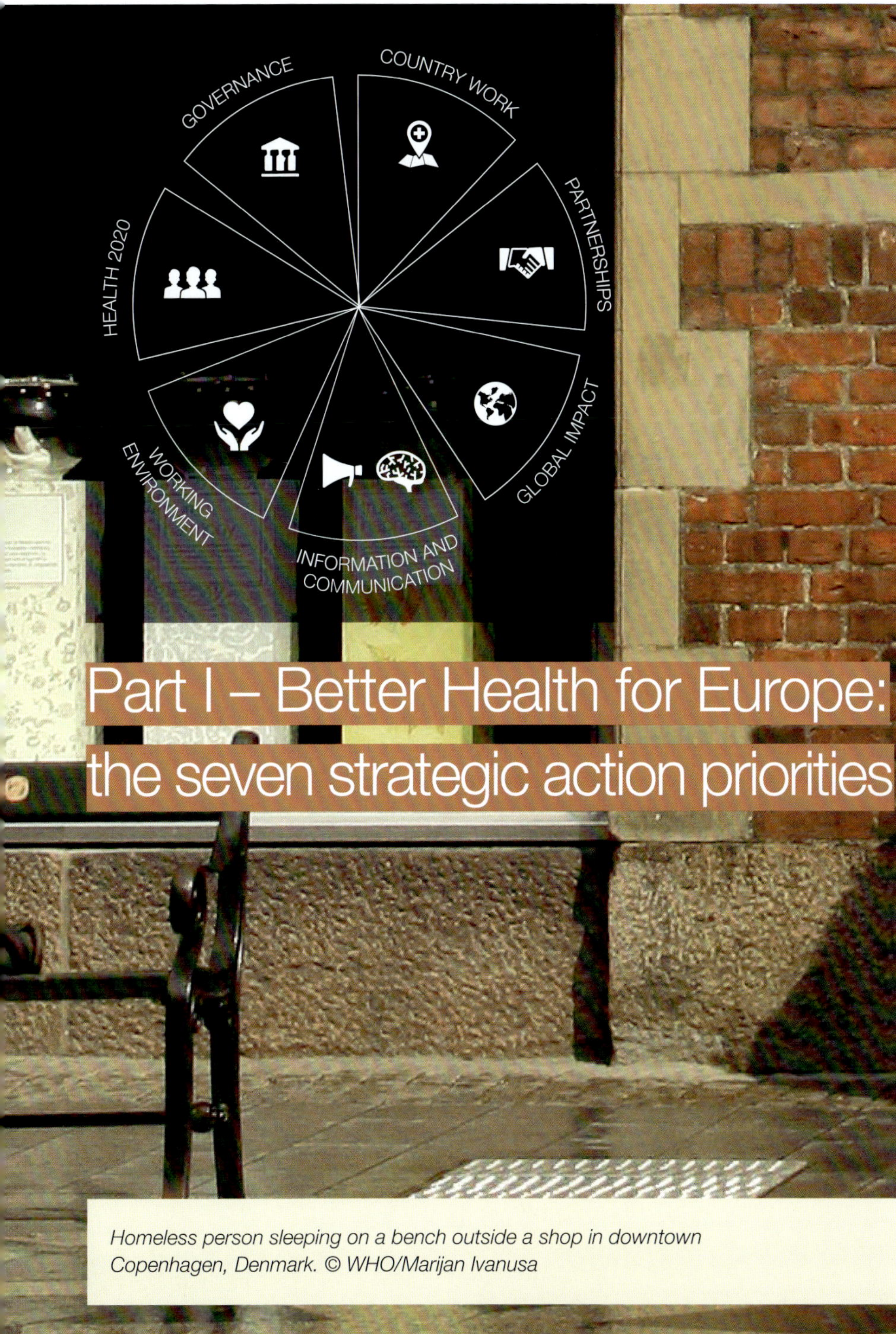

Homeless person sleeping on a bench outside a shop in downtown Copenhagen, Denmark. © WHO/Marijan Ivanusa

Prologue – Voices from across the European Region and beyond

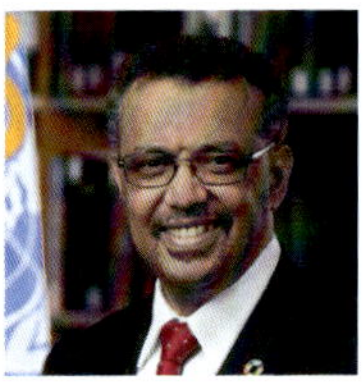

The Regional Office for Europe has been in the forefront of WHO reform globally. It has been a major innovator for processes and policies and a leader of several important global initiatives.

Tedros Adhanom Ghebreyesus, WHO Director-General

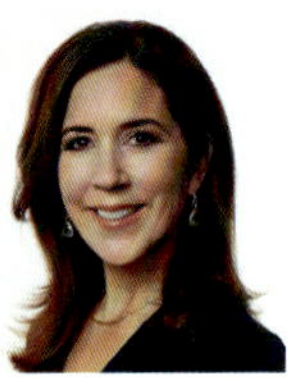

© Daniel Stjerne

In my time as Patron it has been rewarding to be part of the work to achieve the mission of the Regional Office. I have experienced first-hand its approach to addressing health challenges, always based on sound values, evidence and practice. It has also been impressive to see the growth and development of the Office, under strong leadership, in touch with the time we live in. There is no doubt that the WHO Regional Office for Europe has created a very strong platform together and in partnership with the Member States in work towards achieving health for all.

HRH Crown Princess Mary, Patron of WHO/Regional Office for Europe

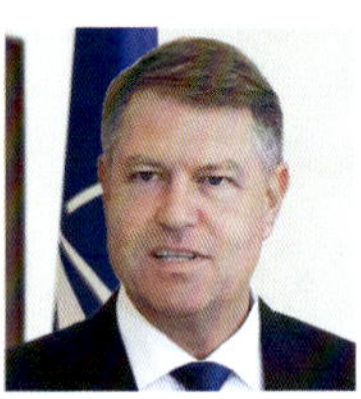

Threats to public health are increasing and beyond solving the problems we are already facing, we must have the ability to anticipate and be prepared to face new challenges, in order to ensure healthy lives and well-being for all citizens, regardless of age. For this reason, it is important that health becomes a priority for any governance. That is why we so value our shared commitment to the development of a fair, sustainable and responsible health, in accordance with the guidance contained in the Health 2020 policy framework of the European Region of the World Health Organization.

Klaus Iohannis, President, Romania

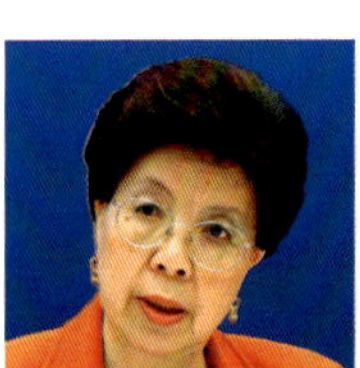

The Health 2020 policy framework and its development process in the European Region has raised awareness of health as a political choice and strongly bolstered all our efforts to position health in the centre of development. Importantly, it has also foreshadowed the SDG agenda.

Margaret Chan, WHO Director-General, 2006–2017

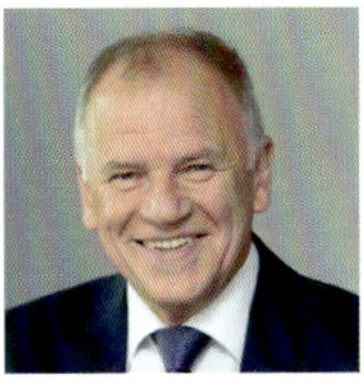

The European Commission and the WHO share the same agenda, and as strong and mutually supporting partners, we are achieving concrete impact in the countries and improving the health and well-being of people.

Vytenis P. Andriukaitis, EU Commissioner for Health and Food Safety

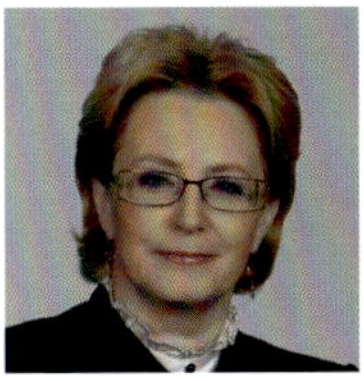

The WHO Regional Office for Europe has strengthened its emphasis on intersectoral collaboration and has created new standards for health interventions, meetings and events. Now we have the added presence of various sectors; for example, environment and finance, and can shape political decisions for health more effectively together.

Veronika Skvortsova, Minister of Health, Russian Federation

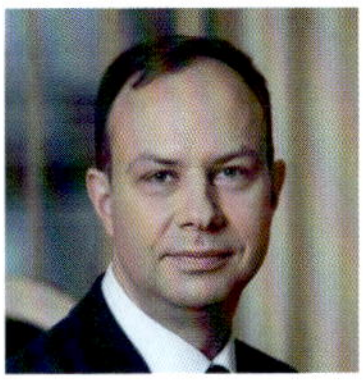

I never get a negative answer when we ask for something from WHO. If we need an expert, for example, to change our hospital network and system, we get a quick promise to bring an expert to the country to help us. Not to tell what should be done, but mainly to get the insights into what other countries have done, to learn from their experiences, because it is very sensitive issue. It is an issue that kills ministers. Even the discussions usually create a lot of political opposition. So, it is very good to have an independent evidence-based WHO expert informing the debates.

Aurelijus Veryga, Minister of Health, Lithuania

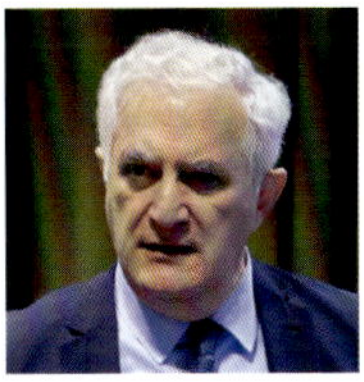

WHO is the source of the most qualified and evidence-based advising in the health care field and its guide is valuable. The WHO Regional Office for Europe assists governments in developing their national health policies and strengthening health systems; provides appropriate technical assistance as needed; helps improve preparedness and response mechanisms for emergency situations; promotes enhanced standards of education and training; and, provides evidence-based expertise and information in the health sector.

Amiran Gamkrelidze, Director General of the National Center for Disease Control and Public Health, Georgia

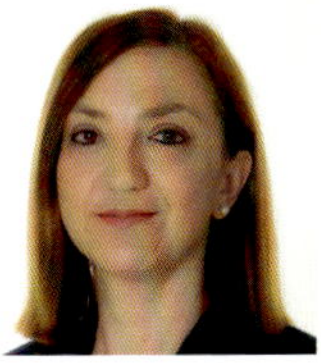

© Brian Cassar

Today we are at a stage where it is very important that we have the leadership WHO is exhibiting at the European level…not only for its 53 countries but also as a source of support and inspiration that can help develop ideas and action in the other WHO Regions.

Natasha Azzopardi Muscat, President of the European Public Health Association (EUPHA), Malta

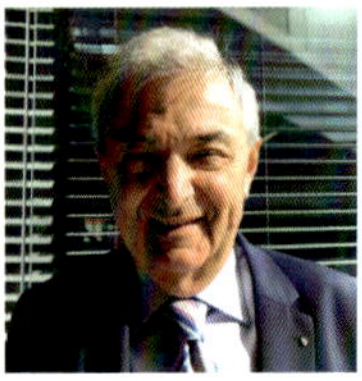

The WHO European Office has been consistently able to 'catch the moment'- 'the windows of opportunity' over these 10 years, to quickly recognize public health needs and take leadership in catalysing and facilitating action by Member States and the global community on critical issues like austerity, UHC, migrant health and men's health.

Mihály Kökény, Former Minister of Health, Hungary

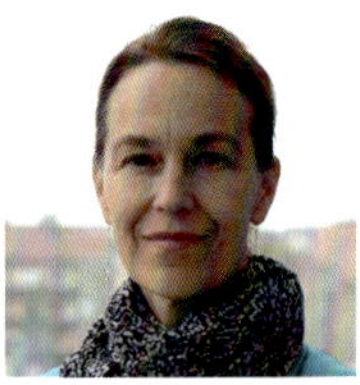

The WHO Regional Office for Europe is a professional, open and knowledge-based organization which is always ready to discuss with and assist Member States in their work, nudge them forward if needed and celebrate their success when called for. It is always a pleasure to work with them.

Olivia Wigzell, Director General, National Board for Health and Welfare, Sweden

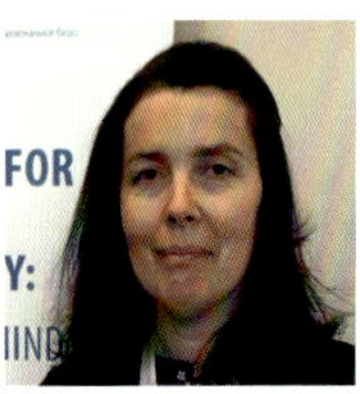

The last ten years for the WHO Regional Office for Europe have been a wonderful period of development and growth in qualitative and quantitative terms.

The European Region has become a Region with visible expertise and good cooperation between the Regional Office, country offices and Member States.

Elena Jablonicka, WHO national counterpart, Ministry of Health, Slovakia

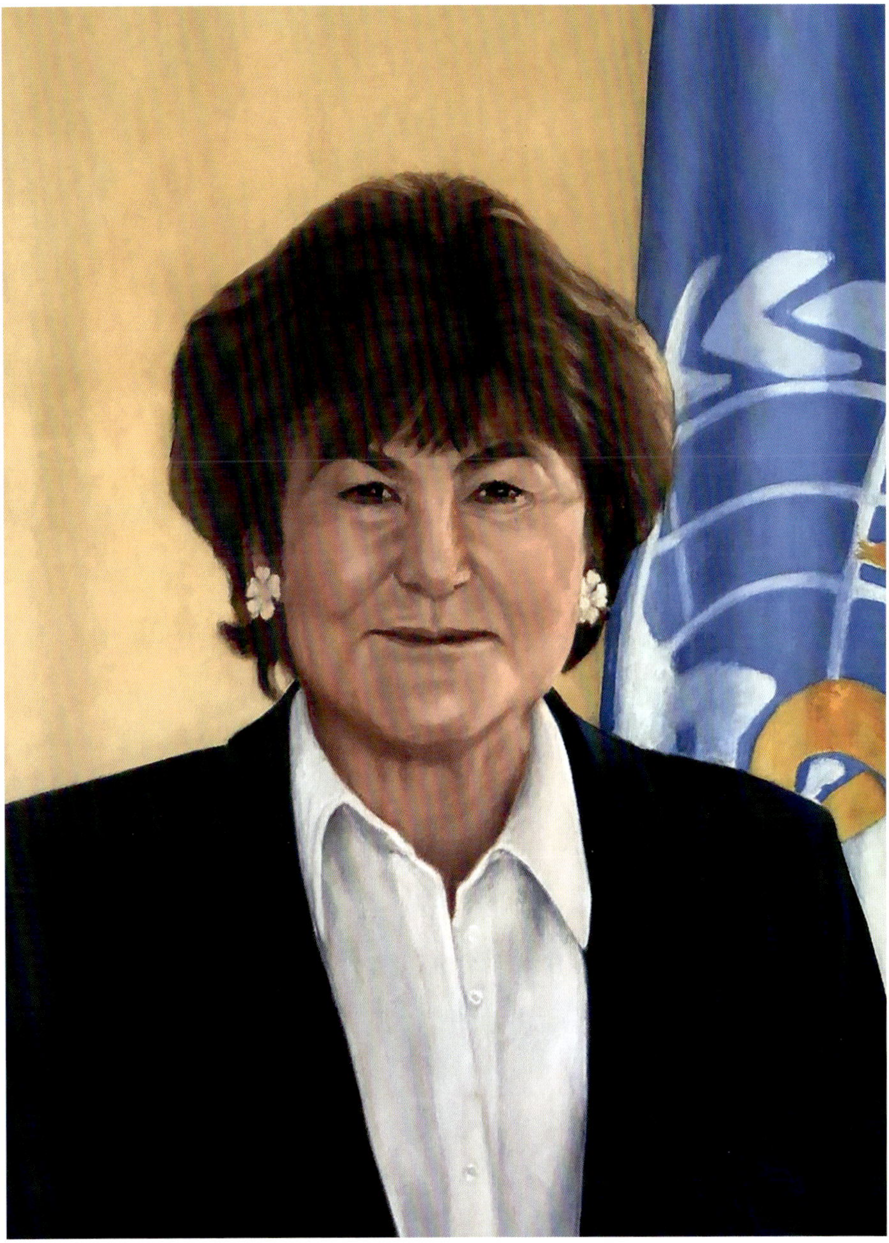

Zsuzsanna Jakab, WHO Regional Director for Europe and Deputy Director-General narrates this story on behalf of the people who have worked in the Regional Office in Copenhagen, the geographically dispersed offices (GDOs) and the country offices of the WHO European Region between 2010–2020. Official portrait painted by Moira Cutajar, 2019

PART 1

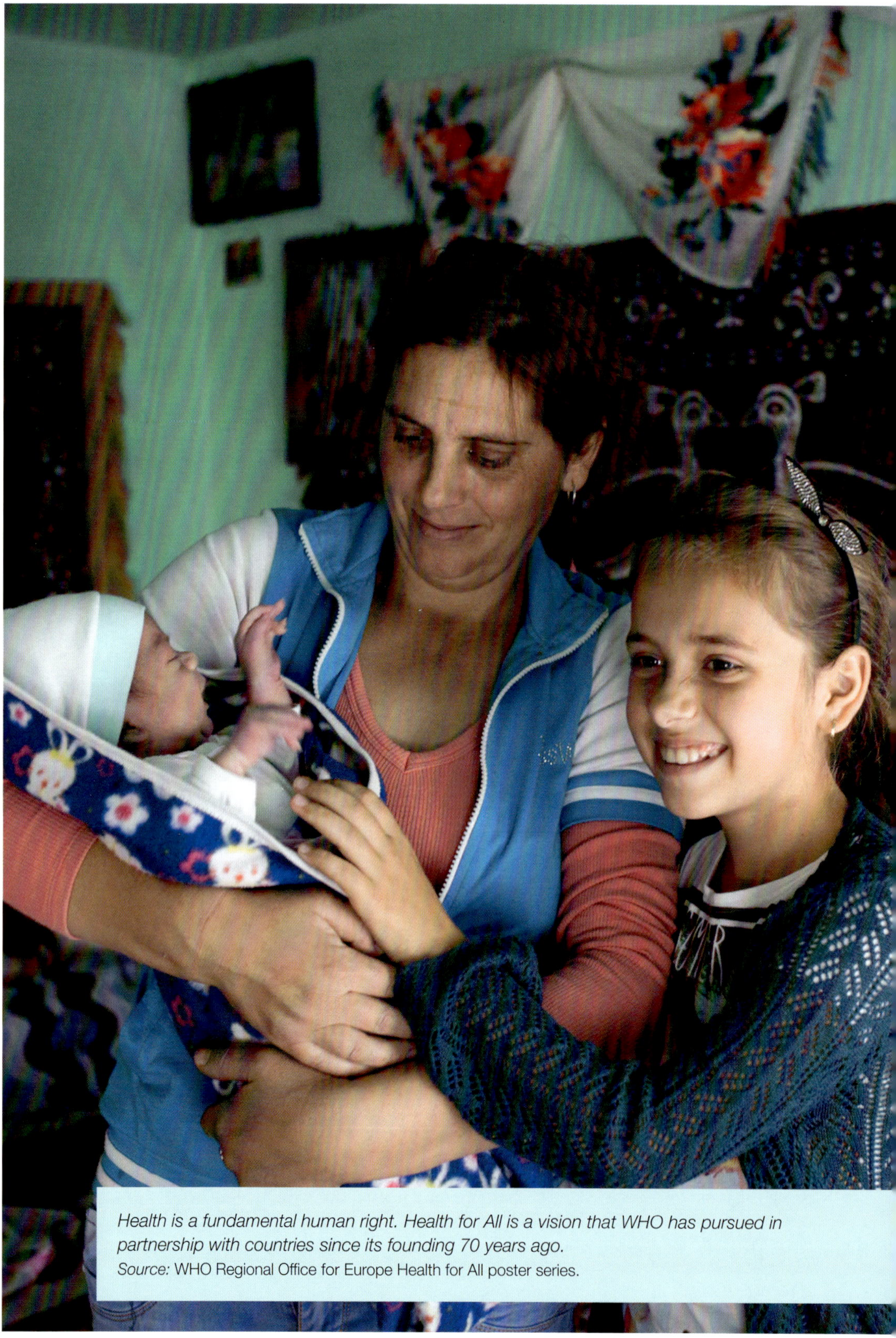

Health is a fundamental human right. Health for All is a vision that WHO has pursued in partnership with countries since its founding 70 years ago.
Source: WHO Regional Office for Europe Health for All poster series.

1. The vision and the context

There are nearly a billion people in the 53 countries that make up the WHO European Region, stretching from Iceland in the west to the Pacific coast of the Russian Federation in the east; and from Svalbard, Norway and Franz Josef Land, Russian Federation in the north to Greece and Israel in the South.

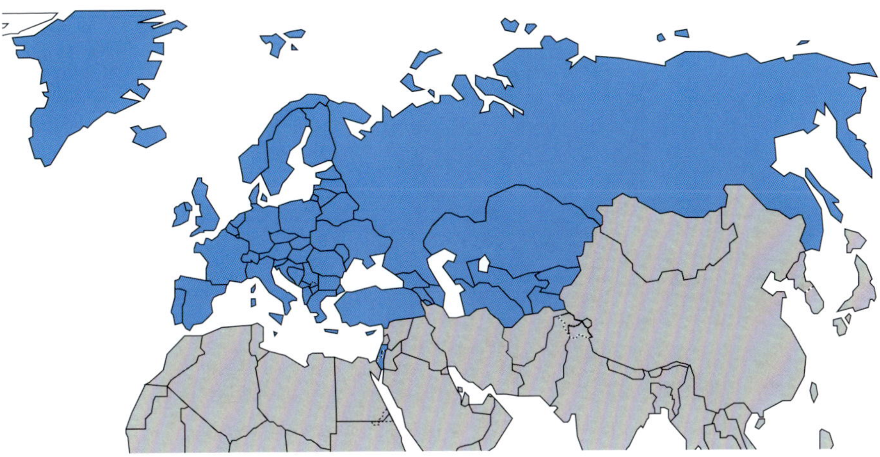

The boundaries and names shown and the designations used on this map do not imply the expression of any opinion whatsoever on the part of the World Health Organization concerning the legal status of any country, territory, city or area or of its authorities, or concerning the delimitation of its frontiers or boundaries. Dotted and dashed lines on maps represent approximate border lines for which there may not yet be full agreement.

Data Source: World Health Organization
Map Production: Health Statistics and Information Systems (HSI)
World Health Organization

PART 1

Fig. 1. WHO European Region.

Across these 53 countries health has certainly been improving. Life expectancy is longer, avoidable premature mortality is reducing, and maternal and infant health and under five mortality are improving. But these improvements are not yet uniform. There remain wide variations in health and well-being, both between and within countries. Persistent health-related inequalities stratify populations in various ways, including ethnicity, gender, socioeconomic status, educational status and geographical area.

Improving health and well-being, and resolving these inequities, remain our great challenge, as has been the case since the start of WHO in 1948. WHO has always worked towards fulfilling the core commitment made by all our Member States in the WHO Constitution (1948) that the highest possible state of health and well-being should be ensured for all. It is this human goal that has motivated and continues to motivate us. WHO's current General Programme of Work (GPW13), under our Director-General Dr Tedros Adhanom Ghebreyesus, has reaffirmed and reinvigorated this commitment, and aims to enhance healthy life expectancy for all by acting to achieve the 'triple billion' targets: 1 billion more people benefiting from UHC, 1 billion better protected from health emergencies, and 1 billion enjoying better health and well-being primarily through multisectoral policy, advocacy, and regulation.

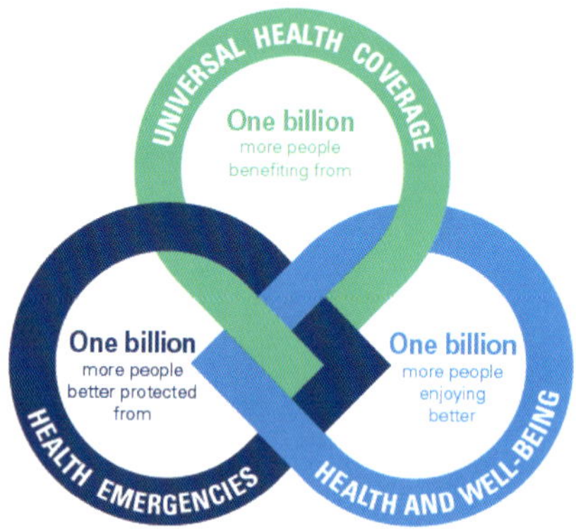

Fig. 2. Thirteenth General Programme of Work (GPW13) Targets.
Source: WHO *(221)*

We believe that health is a human right from which no one should be excluded. While health in Europe is 'better' for most people compared with elsewhere in the world, and compared with the past, that is not good enough. Improvement should affect everyone. Better health for Europe means, to us, equitable and sustainable improvement of health and well-being for all.

This vision and these ideas motivated me during my campaign for the position of Regional Director for WHO Regional Office for Europe in 2009–2010, as I worked to develop my strategic plan about the way forward. They have also been the driving force behind all our work at the Regional Office over the last ten years.

I thought hard about how to put into practice these ideas and principles. I was determined to identify ways for the Regional Office to:

1. further develop its strengths as a respected evidence-based 'European centre of public health excellence and innovation';
2. develop and promote its leadership in health policy and public health in Europe; and,
3. be able to more effectively anticipate, understand, support and meet the needs of its Member States in their efforts to enhance the health and well-being of all their peoples.

In 2009, I had the privilege to visit many countries and meet with politicians and public health workers from all our 53 Member States. I talked with many people, from presidents, prime ministers and ministers of health to public health and community health workers and discussed public health needs, challenges and assets. I asked them to share their ideas about how the Regional Office could better serve them. I went to listen and 'test' some of my ideas about possible strategic approaches.

Country visit

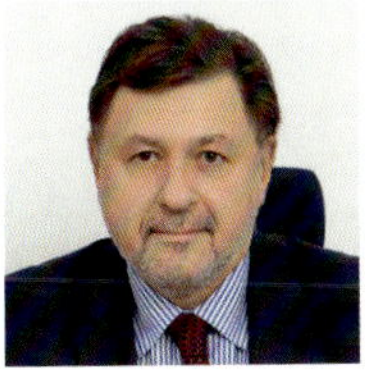

Zsuzsanna Jakab visited Romania in 2009 to present her ideas for the development of the WHO Regional Office for Europe to the Romanian Minister of Health. We had a very open and frank discussion. As we explored our potential Member State and institutional relations with the Regional Office, we had a chance to appreciate her vision and leadership capacities. We felt that her strategic ideas provided real solutions for helping and giving advice to Member States. We saw her as a person who quickly finds answers and solutions, not someone who spends months or years dealing with a problem while nothing happens. Things happen with Zsuzsanna, so Romania supported her election.

Alexandru Rafila, Ministerial Adviser, Romania

Our discussions ranged widely across the demographic, economic, political and social shifts affecting people's right to health across the WHO European Region. A long list of issues and concerns were identified, including: ageing and the greater longevity of populations; globalization; changing living, working and consumption patterns; the negative impact of the 2008–2009 financial crisis and austerity programmes on health and equity; unplanned urbanization; increasing migration; rising health care costs; outbreaks of infectious diseases; the increasing threat of antibiotic resistance; climate change; and, the mounting challenge of NCDs.

As we talked, I realized just how great these challenges were. Many that I spoke with made it clear that public health institutions and services, across the WHO European Region, were not in great shape to respond, and needed to be reinvigorated and promoted. The need to enhance primary health care services with much greater emphasis on health promotion and disease prevention was also expressed. Concerns were raised about Regional Office governance, and the need to strengthen the relevance of our work, as well as to improve collaboration with Member States and partners. I was very pleased to see that Member States were very open and clear on the directions they wanted.

Relevance

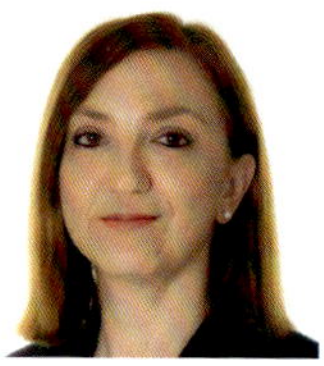

© Brian Cassar

In the late 1990's, there was a feeling that the WHO Regional Office for Europe was becoming less relevant in the western part of the Region. The European Union had acquired a new mandate in public health through the Maastricht Treaty, and they had strong leadership. They seemed to be doing all the right things.

Natasha Azzopardi Muscat, President of the European Public Health Association (EUPHA), Malta

Practical advice

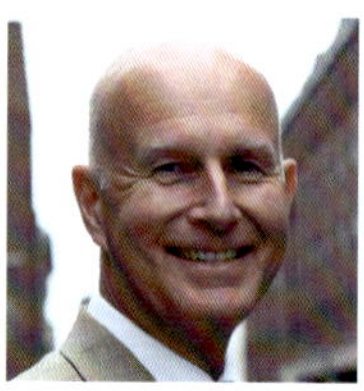

Before 2010, I found the material that the WHO Regional Office for Europe developed quite useful in many respects but often it was more useful for elaborating on issues, presenting context and content, than as practical advice.

Bjørn Dagfinn Guldvog, Director General of Health and Chief Medical Officer, Norway

Coordination

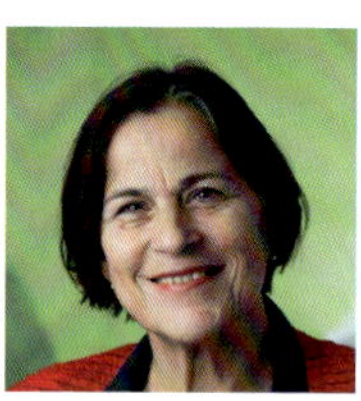

In the 1990s and early 2000s, I was puzzled about what was the WHO's role and what was the Council of Europe's or European Union's part. I was a bit surprised that the same things were done in the different organizations. There was competition between them and a tendency not to coordinate.

Annemiek Van Bolhuis, Director of Public Health and Health Services, National Institute of Public Health and the Environment (RIVM), Netherlands

Debate and inclusiveness

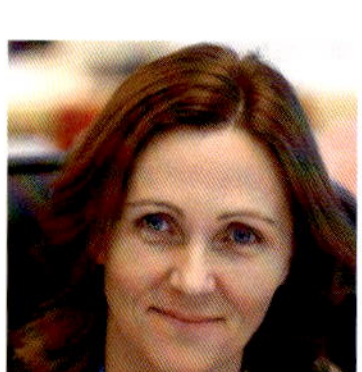

In 2009 we began having reform debates in Geneva at the Executive Board and World Health Assembly. It was clear that Member States really looked for more inclusiveness and more actual exchange of opinion and debate... not just convening at Regional Committees and Assemblies and opting everything that is put forward.

Maris Jesse, Director of Estonian National Institute for Health Development, Estonia

All these concerns emphasized to me the need to develop a strategic plan for health improvement. I wanted this to be a shared and collaborative vision built around universally supported values. It would not just exist on paper but be a plan which would be crafted and implemented through practical mechanisms, with Member States and WHO working together to achieve our goals.

Countries didn't want WHO to just identify and describe problems. They wanted more than 'what to do' messages and information. They wanted to know 'how to' (for example):

1. implement well-researched policies, knowledge and approaches;
2. navigate, manage and influence the many social, political and economic factors that determined both health and health equity; and,
3. better make the case for investment in health.

Building on these discussions, I carefully considered ways to proceed. It was important to be realistic. WHO has a considerable influence in countries, yet it is not in charge of the governments and the resources of countries. It is not responsible for organizing and funding health systems. So, to develop a strategic approach the Regional Office had to work closely with Member States and encourage their participation and commitment.

I was confident that through discussion and debate, and building consensus and ownership, we could proceed in convincing and effective ways. I knew that to accomplish this we would need to play our role in the best possible way. We could not just sit back and rely on countries to participate or not; to implement or not. We would need to actively inform and debate with countries, work with them, encourage them, and convince them to consider and implement ideas and policies within their own contexts, priorities, and administrative and legal frameworks.

Some have criticized WHO for its limited use of legal frameworks and its reliance on consensus and Member State ownership of resolutions and decisions. Some look for more authoritative interventions on global health matters, with WHO being more assertive as a 'directing and coordinating' authority. There may be an argument here, but I would not agree that such legally binding instruments are always necessarily more effective. I believe that WHO has many other means of influence. Perhaps most important are our roles in providing evidence-based technical knowledge and experience, as well as strategic directions and guidelines, and normative standard setting. These contributions reinforce our power and credibility to convince and influence as part of our ongoing support to countries.

Having worked with WHO throughout most of my professional life, I have come to understand the profound influence that the Organization's normative and convening power can have. WHO has a unique capacity, strength and power to bring people together and create 'safe' environments for exchange and learning. Whether it is in meeting rooms or 'front line' settings, WHO has a distinctive ability to provide independent, authoritative and scientifically well-informed guidance and advice, not only to public health leaders and practitioners but also to all those people whose work influences health. Ultimately WHO can help the entire public health related community to find, adapt, and implement effective solutions to the many challenges they confront in their daily work.

Non-threatening, supportive and helpful

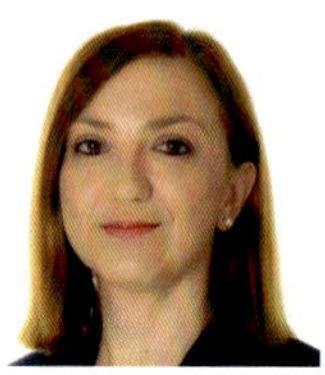
© Brian Cassar

What distinguished bilateral support from the WHO Regional Office for Europe, different to the European Union, was that it was always non-threatening, not compulsory, very normative but not prescriptive, and therefore allowed the country and people in senior executive positions to open up…because they are not afraid of sharing information about their weaknesses and fearful that they will be taken to task for them, but knowing that in WHO they are going to find the support of partners. They knew this was going to help them address weaknesses and gaps.

Natasha Azzopardi Muscat, President of the European Public Health Association (EUPHA), Malta

By 2009–2010 the time seemed right to further develop and use WHO's essentially 'soft power' to help bring about the transformational changes needed if Member States were to effectively address the many health challenges we had identified together.

Knowledge was working on our side, with an increasing understanding of the complexity of human health and the role it plays in development. There was much more scientific knowledge, awareness and interest about the many determinants of health beyond the health system, including social, economic, political, behavioural, environmental, commercial and cultural determinants.

There was exciting new evidence about how health was affected by genetic, epigenetic and intrauterine legacies, environmental exposures, family and social relationships, behaviours, political and cultural contexts, social norms and opportunities, gender roles and health system interventions. Much more was known about how all these factors operate across the life-course and are carried into future generations. It was also clear that these factors are shaped or modified by policies, environments, opportunities and norms created by society.

The implications of this knowledge were profound. We needed to think much more broadly than before and find ways to consider all the determinants of health as a spectrum across the whole of society. We had both the knowledge and the opportunity to help countries move beyond their historically normal 'business as usual' strategic focus on strengthening health systems. Health systems do indeed have a major impact on health, yet we now know that their impact is one among many. Our message therefore could not be simply that more should be spent on health systems, desirable though this may be.

We needed a whole new strategic approach to improving health as part of development: one which dealt with all the determinants of health at once, within a framework of thinking and informed by values. And one which reflected the new scientific understandings. Crucially, such an approach would involve all sectors of governments and societies, as well as health systems. It would focus on health promotion and disease prevention as well as treatment. It would advance universal and affordable access to what health systems could offer.

While our growing awareness and knowledge about how health was affected by all sectors and segments in society were very exciting, it was clear that we still had a lot to learn about how to engage effectively with all these other non-health system contributors to, and shapers of health. In my view, the time was right to respond to this new knowledge and rise to these challenges.

By 2009–2010 most of these ideas were already supported by a substantial literature and experience. What did not exist at that point, however, was a common European action framework – with a clear political commitment – that linked existing knowledge, filled knowledge gaps, for example, in areas of social determinants and governance for health, and provided concrete action options to put the ideas into practice. An adequate cadre of public health workers with the skills, competencies and financial support needed to act was also missing.

Once I took up office as WHO Regional Director for Europe in 2010, together with my colleagues I set about creating such a framework. I was confident that our staff had the knowledge and experience needed to succeed. Our multinational staff of public health, scientific and technical experts is based in the main office in Copenhagen, Denmark, in 5 technical centres of excellence and in country offices in 29 Member States. They are all intimately aware of the challenges and opportunities affecting our search for better health and well-being. They understand that the scope for action is often limited by a shortage of human, material and financial resources, weak institutions and limitations in powers and competence, yet, they are all dedicated to using their individual and collective talents and knowledge to help Member States move forward and improve public health.

We also wanted to (re)invigorate the governing bodies of the WHO Regional Office for Europe and involve them actively within a Region-wide debate about the development of a new coherent European health policy framework. We all hoped that a new political commitment would emerge in order to achieve shared health goals. In addition to continued and even increasing support to health services, we also knew that this would need the development of comprehensive national health policies, strategies and plans, re-energized and enhanced public health capacities and services, and strengthened investment in disease prevention and health promotion.

These ideas were brought together in my vision document for the next ten years entitled: 'Better Health for Europe'. It contained seven strategic action priorities (Box 1), which I presented to the 2010 Regional Committee for discussion and adoption.

Box 1. The seven strategic action priorities of Better Health for Europe

1. Developing a European health policy framework as a coherent framework for equitable improvements in health and well-being;
2. Improving governance in the WHO European Region and in the Regional Office;
3. Further strengthening of collaboration with Member States;
4. Engaging in strategic partnerships with other stakeholders to jointly improve health and policy coherence in Europe;
5. Strengthening the European contribution to global health;
6. Reaching out through an information and communication strategy; and,
7. Promoting the Regional Office as an organization with a positive working environment and sustainable funding for its work.

These seven strategic action priorities were adopted unanimously and have guided all the work of the Regional Office over the last 10 years.

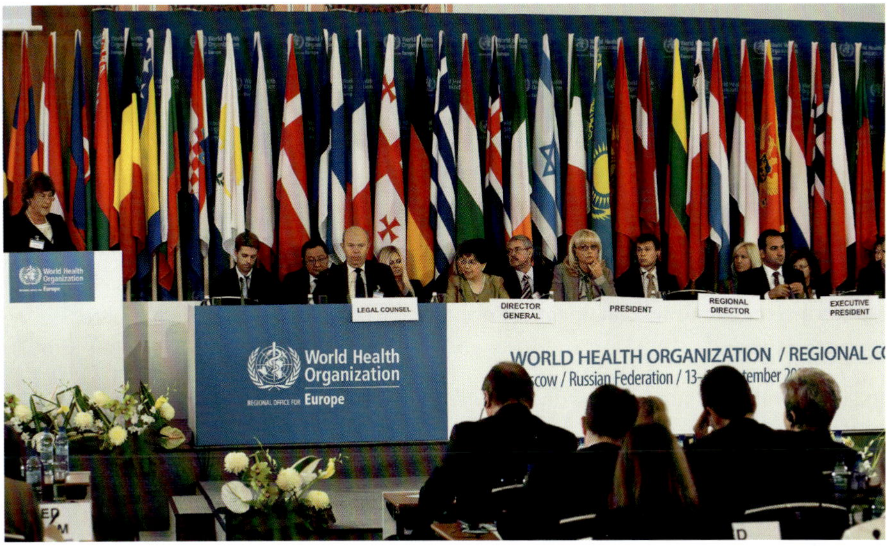

Zsuzsanna Jakab giving her opening address to the delegates at the 60th session of the WHO Regional Committee for Europe, Moscow, Russian Federation, 13–16 September, 2010. © Ministry of Health, Russian Federation.

Summary reflection

The seven strategic action priorities and narrative

The seven strategic action priorities reflect our joint understanding that a cross-sectoral integrated policy framework would be useful to all Member States. These priorities identify the need for actively promoting improved governance, collaborative working, partnerships, information and communication systems to support implementation of policies. The importance of an improved working environment across the WHO European Region at all levels is also acknowledged.

Through the development and implementation of these seven strategic action priorities, our goal was to position the WHO European Region at the centre of the global public health development process. We knew we would need to be proactive to help ourselves and others adopt the new behaviours, policies and approaches needed to implement these seven strategic action priorities, as well as earn recognition for our leadership.

We now turn to reflect further on key health challenges and assets that have shaped the context of our work.

1.1 Global and Regional health context

I believe that the context for health improvement in this second decade of the 21st century in the WHO European Region has been influenced by five key factors. These have shaped the needs of countries for advice and technical assistance and consequently the way the Regional Office has responded. First is the ever-increasing scale and complexity of today's health challenges. Second is the relative wealth and health of our Region. Third is the persistence of health inequities between and within countries. Fourth is the rapid growth of knowledge and technologies. Fifth is the emergence of a new sustainable development narrative with health in a more central position.

In taking action to support our diverse Member States in responding to these Regional contextual factors, we are, of course, keenly aware that each country, locality and institution approaches policy implementation within the context of their own assets, priorities and cultures. Creating a selection of optional approaches to policy and programme development and implementation that can be tailored and adapted for use at national and local levels has been an ongoing characteristic of our work.

1.1.1 Complex health challenges

Today's health challenges include (inter alia) demographic trends, tackling the social and commercial determinants, globalization, migration, urbanization, new and old infectious disease outbreaks and threats, vaccine hesitancy, antimicrobial resistance (AMR), NCDs, environmental threats including climate change and air pollution, emergencies, gender and equity related issues, as well as health systems strengthening. While each has its own specific set of issues, they are all inherently complex problems, with multiple determinants. They all have non-linear and interrelated causal factors, and are context sensitive. They are frequently characterised as 'wicked' problems because they are not usually amenable to quick single discipline, sector or agency responses. They require collaborative, coherent, whole-of-society and whole-of-government approaches which apply health in all policies. Finding ways to help ourselves and our Member States develop the knowledge, skills, partnerships, networks, relationships and political savvy to address these challenges have been defining features of our transformational work over these last ten years.

As an example, consider the social determinants of health. These are affected by policy decisions across a wide range of sectors. Yet we know that ministries of health may not readily be able to address many of these determinants, as they may lie 'outside' the political mandate of health ministries and certainly beyond the boundaries of the health system.

How do we break down barriers and silos? How can we and Member States develop the whole-of-government, whole-of-society and health-in-all-policies (HiAP) approaches that are needed? How could we demonstrate the dividends for all sectors that could be realized through cooperation and coordination? These were some of the questions we sought to answer by using our convening, normative and networking authority and capacities to:

- find effective evidence-informed behaviours, policies and approaches to these challenges; and, then
- help Member States and ourselves further develop, adapt, adopt and/or scale them up.

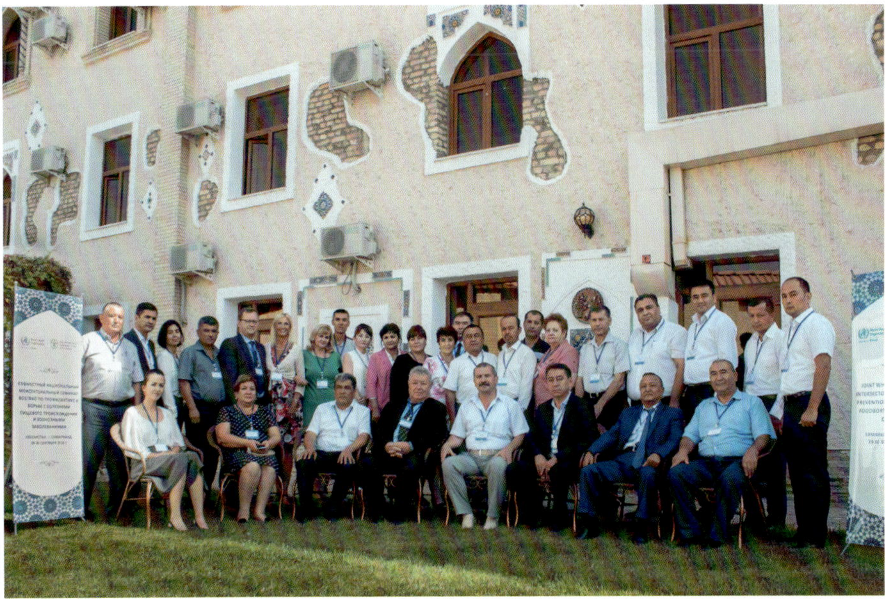

A joint WHO/FAO national intersectoral workshop on prevention and control of foodborne and zoonotic infections was conducted in Samarkand, Uzbekistan 29-30 September 2016. © WHO

1.1.2 The relative wealth and health of the WHO European Region

Since the end of the Second World War the world has become both wealthier and healthier, with global life expectancy increasing from 47 years in 1950 to 72.0 in 2016. This is a dramatic and historically unique improvement. Overall the one billion people living in the WHO European Region have done even better, enjoying life expectancy which has reached 77.9 years for both sexes, according to the latest available figures for 2015 *(3)*.

By 2018, almost all countries in the WHO European Region were classified as low-middle, middle- or high-income countries *(4)*. We knew that with our human and knowledge assets we could do more and do better in promoting health and well-being in all our Member States, and elsewhere. We knew we could not only enhance health improvements in our own Region (see Box 2) but could also help identify new policy options that could set an example for other Regions to make advances. Our achievements in these areas, over the last ten years, are part of the story told in this book.

Box 2. WHO European Region Health Improvements – Highlights 2018 *(3)*

1. Maternal mortality – there has been a decrease in maternal mortality across the European Region, which fell from 13 deaths per 100 000 live births in 2010 to 11 deaths in 2015.
2. Infant mortality – the European Region has also seen a considerable reduction in infant mortality rates, which have fallen from 7.3 infant deaths per 1000 live births in 2010 to 6.8 in 2015.
3. NCDs – only the European Region is on track to achieve the SDG target to reduce premature mortality from the four major NCDs – cardiovascular diseases, cancer, diabetes mellitus and chronic respiratory diseases – by 1.5% annually until 2020. For adults aged 30 to 69, premature deaths due to these diseases fell from 421 per 100 000 in 2010 to 379 per 100 000 in 2014; similar progress was made in all-cause (all ages) mortality rates, which fell from 786 to 715 deaths per 100 000 between 2010 and 2015.
4. Injuries and poisoning – deaths due to external causes of injury and poisoning (all ages) have declined steadily in the European Region, from 82 deaths per 100 000 in 2000, to 57 in 2010, and to 50 in 2015.
5. Communicable diseases – the European Region has seen an increase in treatment success for new cases of pulmonary TB, which rose from 72% in 2012 to 75% in 2016. The Region continues to be declared polio-free and was designated malaria free in 2016.

1.1.3 The persistence of health inequities

We are making progress, yet this positive picture is scarred by persistent inequities in health and well-being within and between countries across the Region. For example, life expectancy varies between 70.0 and 83.1 years as illustrated in Fig. 3, which shows major differences in life expectancies across the 53 Member States of the European Region within three country groupings: the whole WHO European Region; Member States of the European Union; and Member States of the Commonwealth of Independent States.

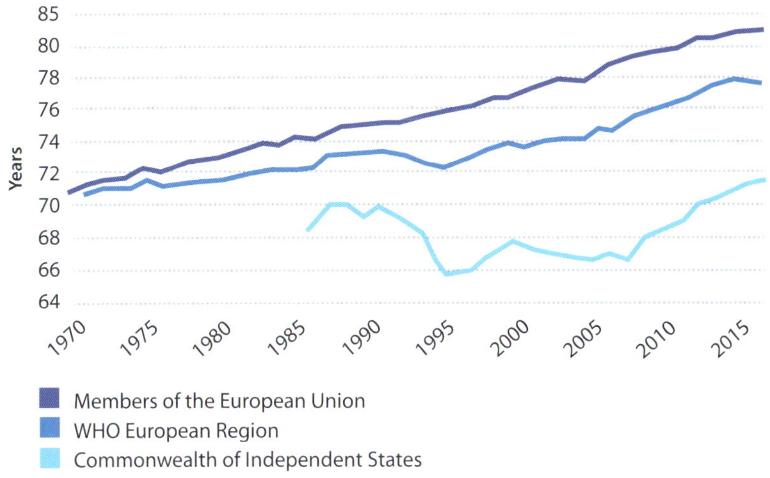

Fig. 3. Life expectancy at birth across the WHO European Region between 1970 and 2015.
Source: European Health Information Gateway *(5)*.

PART 1

Differences in life expectancy also exist between different population groups within countries *(7)*. Here the available information is weaker, and a major innovation and contribution made by our Regional Office has been the development of new metrics to assist countries in measuring, monitoring and addressing health equity within national, regional and local settings (see Section 9.1).

When we look at premature mortality the same picture of Regional variation emerges. Fig. 4 shows overall age-standardized premature mortality rates from 30 to 70 years for the four main NCDs between 2000 and 2015. In terms of deaths per 100 000 population there remains a considerable difference between the maximum and minimum values reported in the Region, although the difference has been reducing.

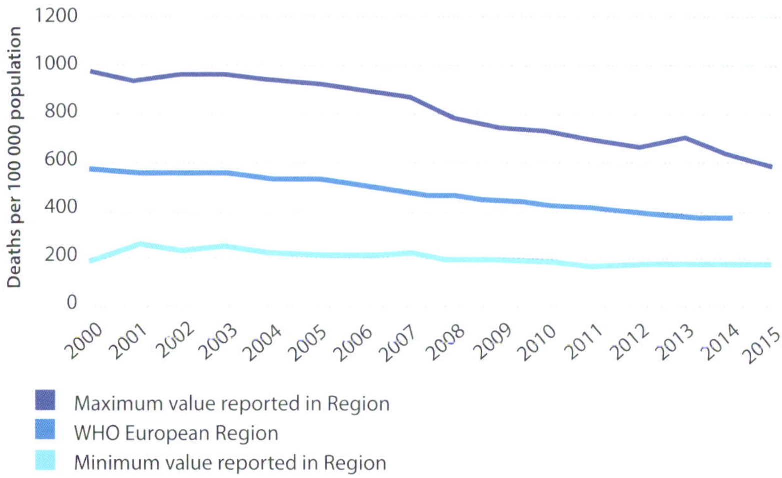

Fig. 4. Age-standardized overall premature mortality rates (from 30 to under 70 years old) for four major NCDs deaths per 100 000 population, showing the yearly trend for the WHO European Region as a whole, and both the maximum and minimum values observed across the Region. The European regional average is calculated for those years when more than 26 countries (50% of 53 Member States) reported in that year.
Source: Health Information Gateway *(6)*.

All available evidence suggests that these inequities are determined by the environment in which people are born, grow up, live, work and age as well as the policies and systems in place to prevent and deal with illness. In addition, interactions between individuals and their environment are not momentary or static but extend across their life-courses and across generations.

The persistence of these health inequities points to the profound need for all Member States to strengthen capacities to understand and address underlying causes of ill health. To help this process, we have commissioned research, convened expert groups, gathered and shared knowledge of why these differences occur, analysed the impact of different policy approaches, and identified 'packages of measures', technologies and interventions which could eliminate many of these unfair and unnecessary deaths, and associated disabilities and suffering (see Table 1 and Developmental reflection 5). We have developed many new tools and programmes with a wide range of partners working on housing, employment, education, income, social capital, human rights, gender and environmental aspects of health equity. We have also worked hard to share this knowledge amongst Member States, and our partner institutions and organizations across the European Region.

Achieving political and policy actions to address the causes of these inequities, and 'leave no one behind', has been central to all our work over the last 10 years. Indeed, current changes in the global political environment towards more divisive and less consensus-based policy thinking make more urgent the need for a countervailing advocacy for health equity and interventions across the Region.

WHO's voice and values

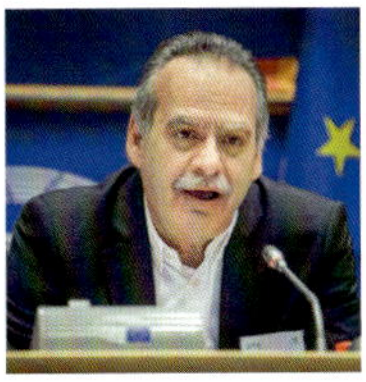

I feel that the direction and focus of the WHO Regional Office for Europe nowadays on universal health coverage, solidarity, and equality is very important and helpful for all our work. Not everybody thinks the same way in Europe, and what WHO Europe says and how it acts about this is very, very, very important. We have to keep going the same way. Even if the political situation in some countries in Europe totally changes, it will be tremendously useful if WHO continues to act this way, and to keep saying what it says now.

Ioannis Baskozos, Secretary General of Public Health, Ministry of Health, Greece

1.1.4 The rapid growth of knowledge and technologies

Public health's increasing knowledge and evidence-based insights are another profoundly important contextual shaping development, along with the growth of innovative technologies that can allow for new and more effective public responses

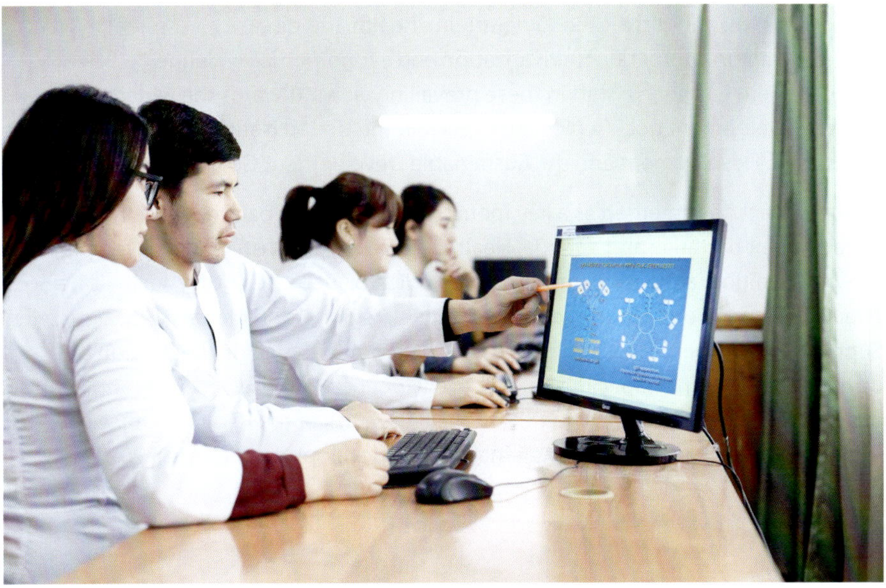

Students at Kazakh National Medical University in Almaty training in telemedicine, 2019. © WHO/Jerome Flayosc

We know so much more about ways, for example, to address all the social, economic, commercial, environmental, cultural and health system related determinants of health *(7)*. We know more about how to conceptualise and implement strategies for governance for health; to encourage whole-of-government, whole-of-society and health-in-all-policies approaches; and to analyse the economic impacts of health-related policies and behaviours.

Just as new diagnostic and treatment technologies have transformed clinical practice, technological breakthroughs in public health – such as digitalization with its analytic, information and communication capacities for predictive epidemiology and disease management, patient empowerment, and personalized prevention, diagnostic and treatment enhancements – offer revolutionizing opportunities.

Knowledge, however, is one thing: practice another. Implementing and applying new knowledge and technologies is an ongoing challenge reported by researchers in Member States across the Region *(8, 9)*. Bridging implementation gaps requires new skills in research and practice, and often the involvement of new sets of players. There are also always political and social considerations. This is an area where we think our advocacy and intergovernmental convening power at WHO can be very helpful. Developing our capacities to serve well as a regional knowledge broker and action facilitator has been a key aspect of our work over these last ten years.

1.1.5 New sustainable development narrative

The models that have dominated global economic and development thinking since the 1990s, and often used to determine health and disease investment, have been focused on competition, privatization and econometrically defined efficiency. Recently there has been a shift in these prevailing views, towards the wider range of human development goals which are explicit in the United Nations 2030 Agenda for Sustainable Development and the Sustainable Development Goals (SDGs).

Health impact has emerged as a key metric, driver, lens and barometer of this new development narrative and agenda. Health is necessary to sustainable development, as a precondition, as an outcome and as an indicator. Because of this, health is being effectively repositioned in the centre of national, regional and global political debates. Supporting Member States and public health communities across the Region to develop the skills and capacities to effectively function in these new roles and arenas has been a central thread running through all the work of the Regional Office over the last 10 years. It was also a key element in the development of Health 2020 (see discussion Section 2.1).

1.1.6 Twenty-first century public health challenges across the WHO European Region

Let us now consider briefly twelve of our Region's specific complex challenges. Links are identified to later sections in the book where more information can be found about responses that the Regional Office with Member States and other partners are developing.

1. **Demographic shifts.** One very significant change is the rapid ageing and greater longevity of the population, which creates opportunities and challenges. For example, the proportion of people aged 65 years and older is expected to reach 25% by 2050 (see Section 9.3.1.2). These demographic changes have increased the occurrence, complexity and costs of multiple disease patterns. Better predictive risk assessment and disease management may be able to help address some of these problems (see Section 9.3.4.8).

2. **Globalization.** This complex issue arouses strong feelings, both positive and negative. While it may increase access to more and better services, social opportunities, goods and technologies it may also give greater prominence to the interests of powerful transnational entities, have a disproportionate impact on the poor, and increase inequities (see Section 9.3.2.2).

3. **Economic crisis.** The financial crisis and the austerity measures taken in response to the economic crisis of 2008–2009 put further strains on health and health equity, as well as on the capacity of health systems. Regional Office actions addressing the economic crisis and austerity can be found in Section 9.3.4.3.

4. **Urbanization.** In the WHO European Region, 70% of the population now lives in urban areas. Urbanization is associated with many health challenges and opportunities – infectious diseases and NCDs, including cancer and heart disease – as well as unhealthy life choices such as tobacco use and alcohol abuse. At the same time, cities are increasingly serving as laboratories for new forms of governance for health, including whole-of-government and whole-of-society approaches (see Section 5.5).

5. **Environmental threats and climate change.** The environment is a major determinant of health, estimated to account for at least 15% of all deaths in the WHO European Region. For example, one year of life expectancy is lost for every person in the WHO European Region due to exposure to air-borne particulate matter (PM), mainly because of the increased risk of cardiovascular and respiratory diseases and lung cancer *(10)*. One of our key priorities has been to work in partnership with Member States, United Nations, European Union, and other agencies to raise and maintain awareness, and protect population health, from the present and future environmental threats, e.g., climate change and air pollution (see Section 9.3.5.1).

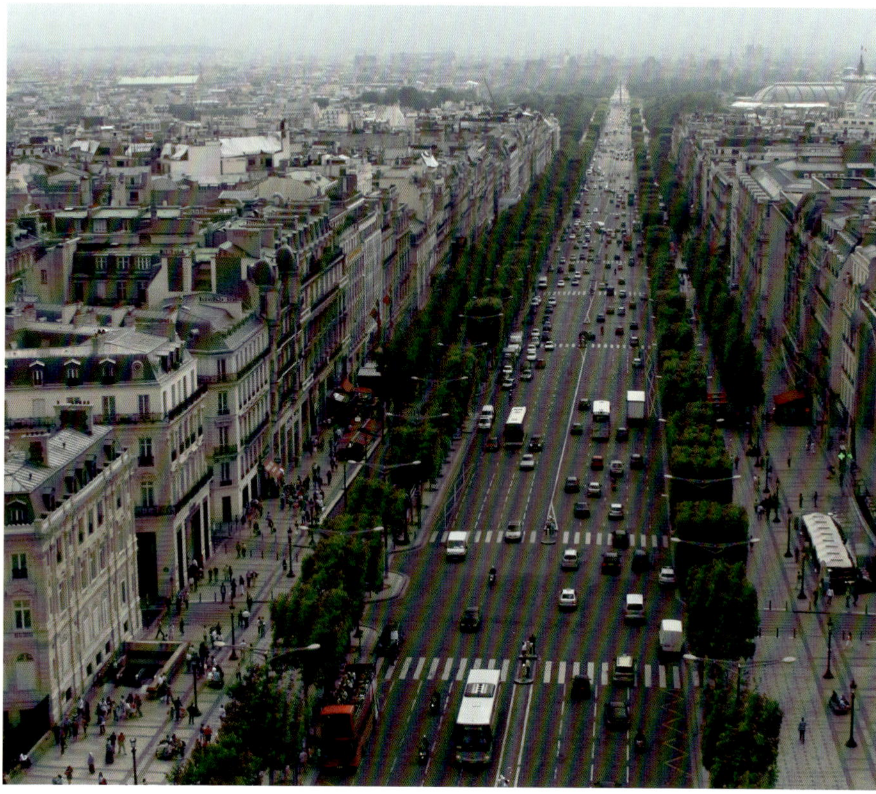

Overhead view of traffic on a busy street in Paris. © WHO/Marijan Ivanusa

6. **NCDs, lifestyles and behavioural health determinants.** Historically increased wealth, taken together with improved nutrition, sanitary standards, housing and living conditions have contributed to the declining impact of communicable diseases in the overall burden of disease. The disease burden in all countries has now shifted towards NCDs. These diseases contributed an estimated 89% of deaths (all ages) and 86% of years lived with disability in 2015 *(11)*. In spite of inexpensive and effective prevention and treatment being available, the four main NCDs –cardiovascular disease (CVD), diabetes mellitus, cancers and chronic respiratory diseases – are responsible for two thirds of premature death (30–69 years) in the WHO European Region *(12)*.

   The factors or determinants causing NCDs are complex and need multi-faceted responses. Behavioural determinants e.g. tobacco, alcohol, diet, sugar and salt, physical inactivity, and substance abuse, are shaped by the political, social, environmental and commercial determinants of health. For example, the opportunity for healthy behaviours is powerfully affected by social determinants such as poverty and education, as well as by environmental conditions and circumstances.

Coronary heart disease and lung cancer provide good examples here. The scientific evidence that smoking is the major risk factor for these diseases is irrefutable and long-standing. Yet, smoking is still promoted by large and powerful transnational corporations that produce and market tobacco products and which operate in political, economic and cultural environments that may be more, or less, sympathetic to their activities.

Regional Office actions addressing NCDs determinants and policies can be found in Section 9.3.2.

7. **Gender as a health determinant.** Women and men differ in biology, the roles and responsibilities that society assigns them, and their positions in the family and community. These differences affect health risk, the management of disease and ill health, efforts towards health improvement, and how the health system responds to their needs. Discriminatory gender-based values, and social and cultural norms and stereotypes, may also translate into practices that affect health and well-being. Discussion of the Regional Office initiatives on gender and health can be found in Section 2.6.

8. **Mental disorders.** Mental disorders have now become the largest contributor to chronic conditions. The estimated prevalence of mental disorders in the WHO European Region in 2015 was 110 million, equivalent to 12% of the entire population at any one time *(13)*. In addition, eleven countries in the European Region fall within the top 20 countries with the highest estimated suicide rates globally *(14)*. Regional Office actions addressing mental disorders can be found in Section 9.3.2.5.

9. **Health emergencies.** Over the last ten years WHO has significantly increased its capacity and responsiveness to assist Member States in preparing for, responding to and recovering from health emergencies which may impose serious pressure on health and health services. These emergencies are often linked to international and national security concerns, above and beyond health considerations, and are very high on the political agenda of many Member States (see Section 9.3.4.10).

10. **Increased population movement.** Migration to and within the WHO European Region has been a long-time phenomenon. Overall there are now some 90 million migrants estimated to be living in the WHO European Region, accounting for nearly 10% of the total population *(15)*. I am proud to say that the Member States of the WHO European Region were early and strong responders in identifying and addressing the health needs of these populations, through the development of a *Strategy and action plan for refugee and migrant health in the WHO European Region* which was agreed by the Regional Committee in 2016 (see Section 6.4.1 and Developmental reflection 2) *(16)*.

11. **Communicable diseases, vaccine hesitancy and antimicrobial resistance (AMR).** Communicable diseases continue to pose significant threats to human health and international health security. Socio-economic, environmental and behavioural factors, as well as international travel and vaccine hesitancy issues, may foster and increase the spread of these diseases. AMR threatens the effective prevention and treatment of an ever-increasing range of infections, making control more difficult. The European Region (as are all other WHO Regions) has been addressing these threats by working with Member States to strengthen public health systems and functions that ensure reliable surveillance, high immunization coverage and full transparency and compliance with the International Health Regulations (2005) (see Sections 7.3 and 9.3.3).

12. **Challenges to health systems.** Rapid and accelerating advances in health technologies offer many potential benefits yet pose a challenge as one of the causes of the seemingly ever-rising costs of health care. Other causes include the growing demand for health care and rising expectations.

    A key factor for this cost-inflation is the oft-seen failure to invest in effective primary care as well as effective programmes of health promotion and disease prevention. Another factor is the almost universal failure to integrate health and social care systems. Regional Office actions addressing health systems can be found in Section 9.3.4.

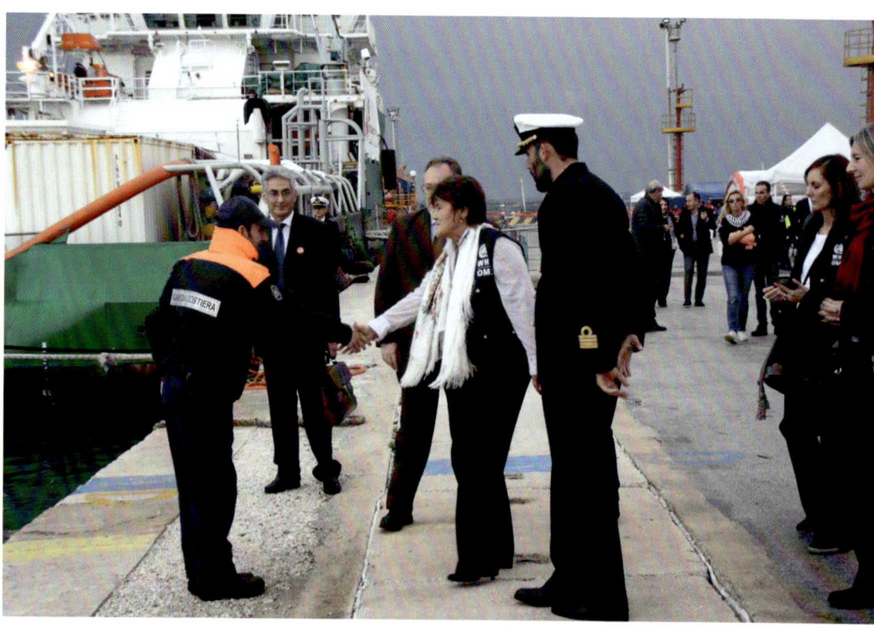

Zsuzsanna Jakab, WHO Regional Director for Europe, meeting Coast Guard and Navy teams at Trapani Harbour, which received approximately 10% of all migrant and refugee arrivals to Italy in 2016. © WHO/Sara Barragán Montes

Summary reflection

Contextual factors

The complex nature of today's health challenges; our Region's relative assets; its persistent health inequities; new knowledge and technological capacities; and the changing role of health in the new sustainable development narrative set the context for the transformational changes we hoped to catalyse with our seven strategic action priorities. How we developed these actions and what they achieved are described in Sections 2–8.

We now turn to take stock of WHO's historical development and some of the social, political and economic factors which have shaped and continue to shape our value- based and evidence-informed responses to both needs and opportunities across the Region.

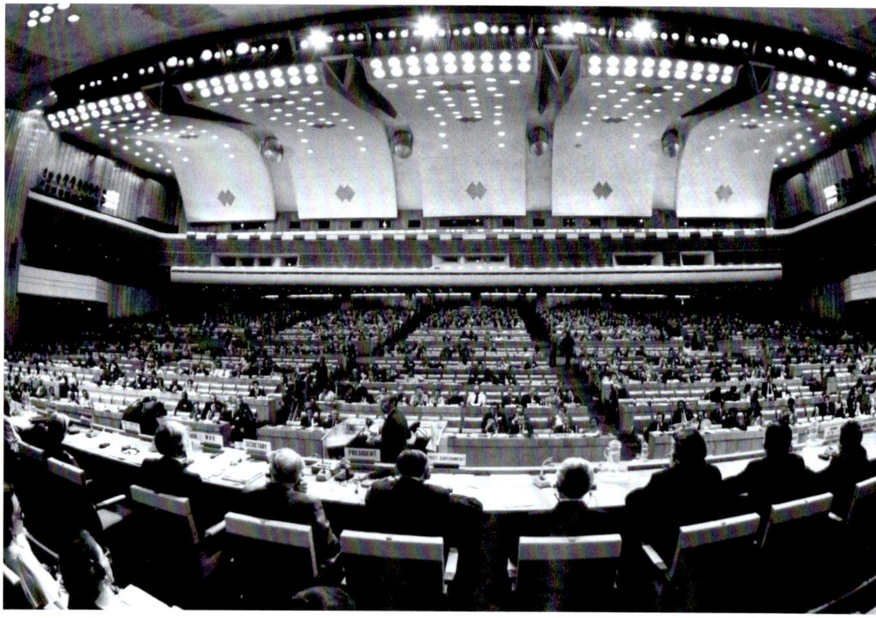

Halfdan Mahler, WHO Director-General 1973–1988 addressing the International Conference on Primary Health Care in Alma-Ata, the then capital of the Kazakh Soviet Socialist Republic, USSR (now Almaty, Kazakhstan), September 1978. © WHO/Novosti

1.2 Historical WHO context

WHO's history reflects a continuous broadening of the main dimensions of public health perspectives: scientific, economic, psychosocial, engineering, logistical, leadership, management, communication, advocacy and, more recently, diplomatic knowledge and skills. We need all these perspectives to work together, with and between the WHO European Region and our Member States, if we are to move closer towards Health for All (HFA). All we have done over the last 10 years has built upon these organizational legacies. I will now consider that history in more detail.

1.2.1 WHO constitution and global structures

WHO was established in 1948 as a specialized agency of the United Nations, to serve as the 'directing and coordinating authority' for international health matters and public health. Throughout its life, WHO has remained committed to one principal objective: the achievement by all peoples of the highest attainable level of health. This commitment is enshrined in the WHO Constitution (see Box 3), which defines 'health [as] a state of complete physical, mental and social well-being and not merely the absence of disease or infirmity'.

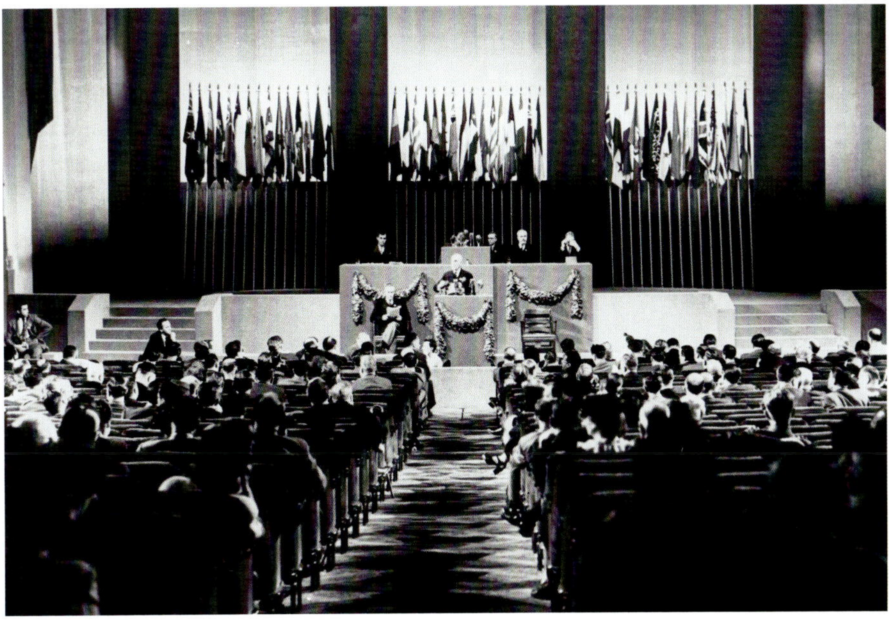

The 1945 United Nations Conference in San Francisco, USA, unanimously approved the establishment of a new autonomous international health organization. © United Nations

PART 1

The Constitution came into force on 7 April 1948 – a date we now celebrate every year as World Health Day. Its prevailing objective has been the guiding principle of WHO and all of those that have worked within it ever since.

You are not just working in any old kind of place

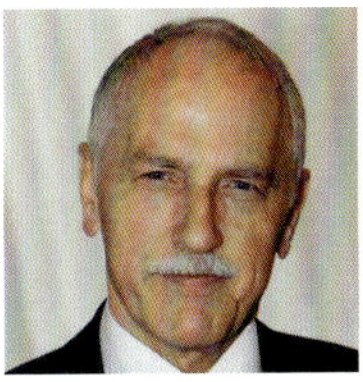

You are working in an organization that was given a global mandate not only to try to lift health, but to do it in a way that reflects a set of ethical principles. This should, of course, be reflected in the conduct of the management of WHO and in the way WHO behaves on the global scene… there was a strong feeling at the end of the Second World War that one had to create a better world and the United Nations was the structure that could do that.

Within the United Nations, WHO was going to be taking on the health sector. So, WHO was not seen just as a technical organization; it was seen to be an important part in a bigger picture that was linked to some of the noblest aspirations of mankind.

Jo Asvall, WHO Regional Director for Europe 1985–2000 *(17)*[1]

---

1 All quotes from Jo Asvall are taken from transcripts of tapes he made for the WHO Oral History project. Extracts of these transcripts were first published in the Jo Eirik Asvall Memorial Guide *(17)*.

Box 3. WHO constitutional commitments and roles *(18)*

WHO is committed to the enjoyment of the highest attainable state of health as one of the fundamental rights of every human being, without distinction of race, religion, political belief, or economic and social condition. It believes that the health of peoples is fundamental to the attainment of peace and security; is dependent on the fullest cooperation of individuals and states; and its achievement in any State is of universal value to all States. Unequal health development on the other hand, is a common danger. Health development, particularly of children, is of basic importance and the ability to live harmoniously in a changing total environment is essential to such development. All peoples should benefit from medical, psychological and related knowledge, which is essential to the fullest attainment of health. People themselves should be informed and cooperate actively in the improvement of health. Lastly, countries have a responsibility for the health of their peoples which can be fulfilled only by the provision of adequate health and social measures.

To implement these key principles WHO is recognized to have specific roles, which are to:

- provide leadership on matters critical to health and engage in partnerships where joint action is needed;
- shape the research agenda and stimulate the generation, translation and dissemination of valuable knowledge;
- set norms and standards and promote and monitor their implementation;
- articulate ethical and evidence-based policy options;
- provide technical support, catalyse change, and build sustainable institutional capacity; and,
- monitor the health situation and assess health trends.

Uniquely, WHO has a primary role to direct and coordinate international health within the UN system and offers the opportunity to put these high global goals into practice. Its tasks are many, including implementing the human right to health; preventing and overcoming threats to health; preparing for future health challenges; and advocating for, and implementing, public health programmes and activities.

WHO works closely with its Member States, supporting countries to develop and sustain country health policies, systems and programmes; coordinating the efforts of governments and partners – including bi- and multi-lateral organizations, international funds and foundations, civil society organizations and the private sector.

Today WHO works with 194 Member States, across six Regions (see Fig. 5), and from more than 150 country offices. It employs more than 7 000 people working in our country-based offices, in six Regional Offices and at the headquarters in Geneva, Switzerland *(205)*. While global policy initiatives are developed and coordinated from Geneva, within this global context each Regional Office develops its own Region-specific dimension focused on contributing both to global health needs and priorities, to the needs of the Region as a whole, and to the more specific needs of the countries it serves.

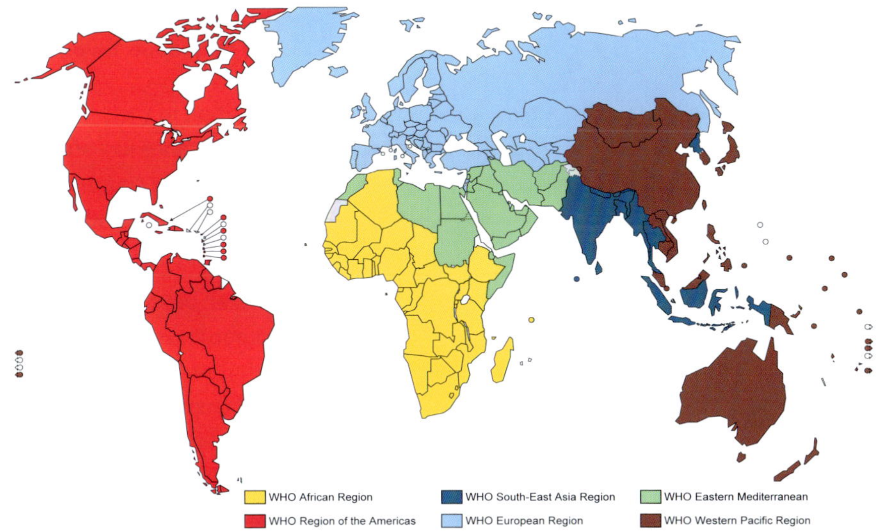

Fig. 5. Map of the six regions of the World Health Organization, showing the European Region (19).

1.2.2 The WHO Regional Office for Europe 1948–2010

The rich history of the WHO Regional Office for Europe has been recently reviewed *(2)*. At the end of the Second World War, a WHO Special Office for Europe was established to take over the work from the United Nations Relief and Rehabilitation Administration (UNRRA). The Special Office opened on 1 January 1949 with Dr Norman Begg of the United Kingdom as Director. It focused its work on communicable disease problems including TB, malaria, and venereal diseases, as well as maternal and child health and environmental sanitation. Damaged health systems also needed to be rebuilt after the Second World War, including in countries where these systems had previously

PART 1

been quite sophisticated. This stimulated the Office to include the rebuilding, reorganization, and modernization of countries' health systems amongst its priorities.

Damaged health systems

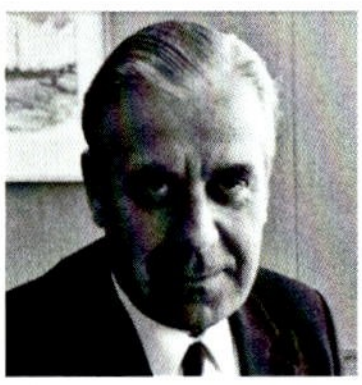

> Health services and infrastructures were severely damaged in the war-devastated countries. Scientific and medical contacts were loosened or broken, the construction of hospitals and other health institutions was at a standstill, and Europe faced increased and serious health problems, including malnutrition and a number of communicable diseases.
>
> **Leo A. Kaprio, WHO Regional Director for Europe 1966–1985** [2]

The Union of Soviet Socialist Republics (USSR) citing their opposition to the dissolution of the UNRRA (which had given them considerable assistance just after the war), withdrew from cooperation and demanded that other socialist countries (Albania, Bulgaria, Czechoslovakia, Hungary, Poland and Romania) withdraw as well.

Despite this withdrawal, under Dr Begg's leadership the Special Office continued its work with the support of the remaining countries. It established an action framework that made cooperation possible throughout the whole of geographic Europe. Dr Begg initiated the 'Travelling Seminars on Public Health Administration' programme,[3] which provided the agency with a practical way to create a network of champions, study health services and exchange experience. This also provided a first evidence base for health system planning. Many of those who featured strongly in the history of the Regional Office started their involvement with these seminars!

The Office moved to Copenhagen in 1957 after a selection process involving several European countries and cities. Sadly, Dr Begg died in office in 1956 and his successor, our second Regional Director, Dr Paul Van de Calseyde from Belgium, opened the Copenhagen office and welcomed back the socialist countries, which had decided to re-join the Region.

The 1960s saw the growing contribution of NCDs to the burden of disease, and accordingly the work of the Office shifted towards health promotion and disease prevention. Several innovative new programmes were started, including environmental pollution, nutrition, accident-prevention, drug use, mental health, epidemiology and health statistics.

Communicable diseases, however, remained important and vaccines needed to be obtained. WHO worked with UNICEF to increase vaccine availability in Europe. WHO

---

2 All quotes from Leo Kaprio are from his book on 40 years of WHO in Europe *(1)*.

3 Between 1951 and 1966, travelling seminars visited 14 countries and brought together 162 health officials to study other countries' health care methods. The seminars usually visited two countries in quick succession to see how their administrative structures in similar domains differed. For example, in 1960 Bulgaria and France hosted two seminars on the administration and organization of health services in rural areas.

also worked with countries to strengthen public health laboratory systems in support of communicable disease management. The global eradication of smallpox was a singular achievement after more than a decade of work. The European Region itself was officially declared smallpox free in 1977. The eradication of a disease which had been a scourge of mankind for centuries is considered one of WHO's greatest global achievements.

Under Dr Leo A. Kaprio, our third Regional Director, new thinking about human rights and the right to health emerged. Innovative philosophical and practical ideas about improving health were discussed. The global Health for All (1977) movement, the Alma-Ata Declaration (1978) and the Ottawa Charter (1986) all gave impetus to these new ideas which would progressively revolutionize the way we think about health and health interventions. It is remarkable that so much that was new in our thinking about health emerged in the difficult Cold War environment.

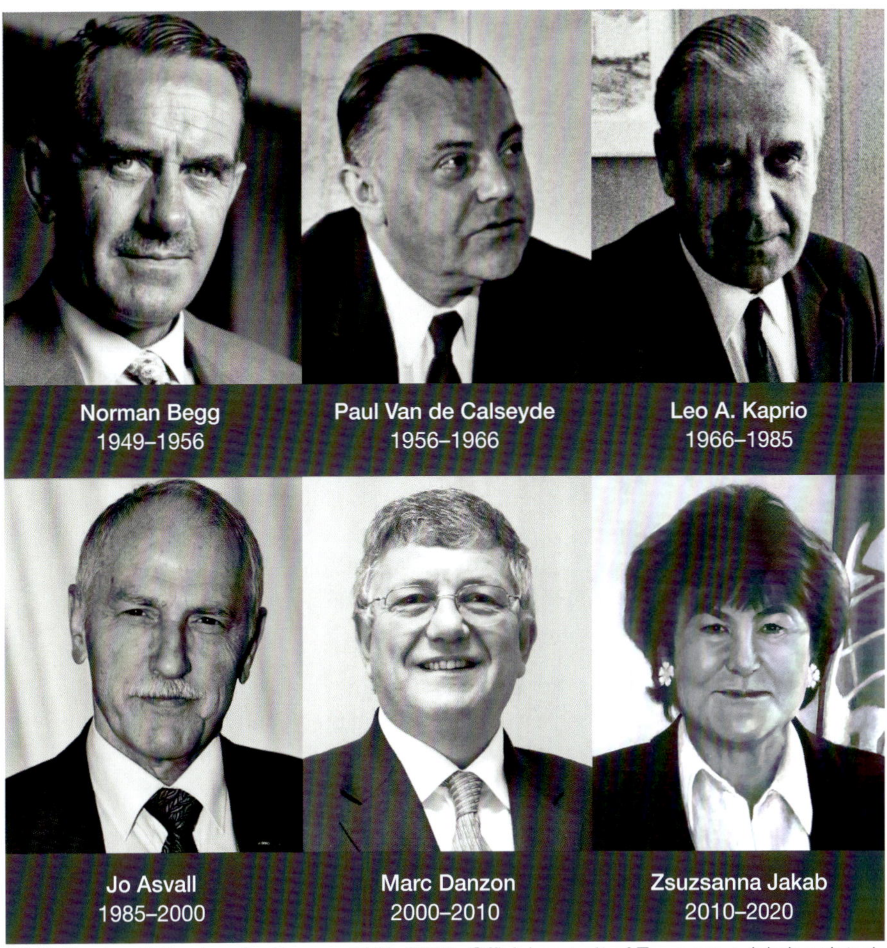

WHO Regional Directors for Europe 1949–2020. Official portrait of Zsuzsanna Jakab painted by Moira Cutajar, 2019 © WHO

Perhaps the most important initiative was the development of the global Health for All policy and movement, which was an initiative of the WHO Director-General Dr Halfdan Mahler and the WHO Executive Board. In the 1970s concerns were raised about deteriorating health conditions in low-income countries and their continuing lack of even basic health services. To address this challenge the World Health Assembly (WHA) passed a resolution that called for Health for All by the year 2000 and initiated a global movement to achieve this aim.

I witnessed first-hand the huge influence this common strategy and vision, with its political legitimacy, made on public health development, practice and impact in the diverse countries of the European Region and beyond. It also helped develop a common language and introduced common values such as equity and solidarity and the right to health for all.

Some people over the years have criticized Health for All by saying that it was clear that by 2000, Health for All would not (and was not) achieved for all. These views have missed the purpose of the strategy and target date. This first designated date was set as an inspirational target to help mobilize global action, and indeed significant progress was made.[4] Health for All was then and continues to be an inspiration for national health authorities and public health practitioners globally. It was and is a goal to aspire towards and to measure progress against. Each successive generation has moved, and hopefully will continue to move, us closer.

Now, for example, in 2019 we have WHO Director-General Dr Tedros' s leadership with the GPW13 Triple Billion Challenge which again has set ambitious targets w ith the aim of catalysing action around the world towards UHC and Health for All. All our Health 2020 actions have also been geared towards developing the evidence, partnerships, and actions needed to move our Member States closer to these goals.

Dr Mahler, who had a long practical experience in TB care in rural Africa, knew the importance of the active engagement of people in building their own health. With UNICEF, WHO launched studies to gather the best evidence on what interventions encouraged such participation most successfully, and jointly organized the International Conference on Primary Health Care in Alma-Ata, in the Kazakh Soviet Socialist Republic, USSR, in September of 1978.

The Alma-Ata Declaration was the key outcome of the conference, and one of the most important policy documents to emerge during the period since the Second World War *(20)*. It was simply a marvellously inspiring Declaration. It reaffirmed global commitment to health in its broad definition and clearly identified health as part of development. Health was acknowledged as a fundamental human right,

---

4 For example, in 1997, 106 countries representing 64% of the global population had an average life expectancy at birth above 60 years; an infant mortality rate below 50 per 1000 live births, and an under-5 mortality below 70 per 1000 live births. In 1975, only 69 countries representing 30% of the global population met these targets *(138)*.

and the Declaration called for political commitment to, and a social contract for, the attainment of the highest possible level of health, as a worldwide social goal.

The Declaration identified the need for action by many other social and economic sectors in addition to the health sector. It brought equity and health equity for the first time to the international agenda. The Conference and Declaration also connected health with well-being, quality of life and world peace.

The Conference called on the world community to consider health as the main social target to enable people to lead economically and socially productive lives. These ideas live on in the SDGs, Health 2020 and the GPW13. All of these policies and programmes incorporate the key principles always associated with Dr Mahler – the involvement and participation of people, individually and collectively, in the planning and delivery of their health care; and the significance to be given primary health care, as an integral part and main focus of the health care system. Primary health care was affirmed as the first level of contact with the health system for individuals, the family and community, as well as contributory to the overall social and economic development of the community.

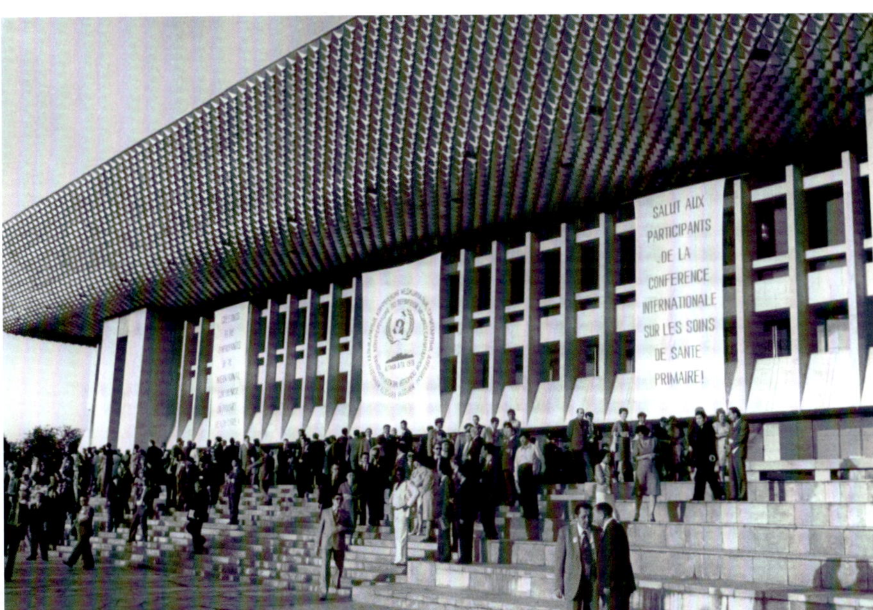

The International Conference on Primary Health Care, convened by WHO and UNICEF, was held at the Palace of Lenin in Alma-Ata, the Kazakh Soviet Socialist Republic, USSR (now Almaty, Kazakhstan) in September 1978. © WHO

This Alma-Ata Conference of 1978 and its Declaration and aftermath achieved a status in history that set a standard to which every subsequent event and policy pronouncement has aspired. Our gratitude goes to all our predecessors who were leading this process: Dr Halfdan Mahler, the charismatic leader of WHO; Henry Labouisse, the Executive Director of UNICEF; Dr Leo A. Kaprio, WHO Regional Director for Europe; Professor Petrovsky, Minister of Health of USSR and Dr Benediktov, his first deputy and Professor Sharmanov, Minister of Health of the the Kazakh Soviet Socialist Republic, USSR – together with ministers of other Republics, like Kyrgyz and Uzbek, who hosted many of the side events of the Conference.

City evidence showed us the way

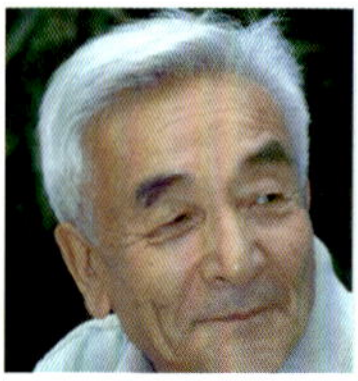

When we were developing the Declaration, we looked at cities around the world and we were able to show that cities like Alma-Ata where they had primary care providers had better health outcomes. We used this as evidence that this was the way we should all go and were able to get agreement of all nations for our Alma-Ata Declaration.

Toregeldy Sharmanov, Minister of Health, Kazakh Soviet Socialist Republic, USSR, 1978

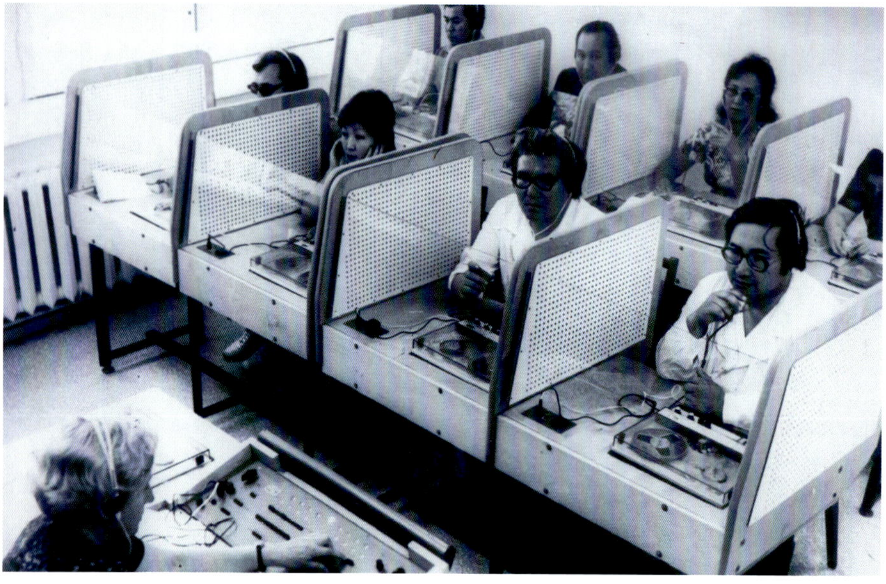

Interpreters at the International Conference on Primary Health Care, Alma-Ata, the Kazakh Soviet Socialist Republic, USSR (now Almaty, Kazakhstan) in September 1978. © KazNMU

Bags, declarations, schools and leaders

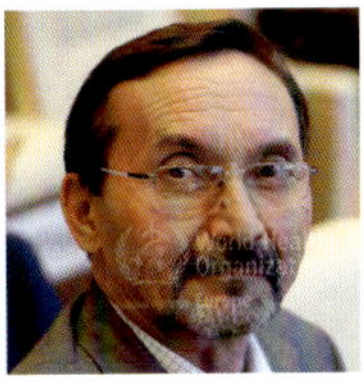

As a junior research worker in our Scientific Research Institute of Epidemiology and Hygiene in the Kazakh Soviet Socialist Republic, USSR, in 1978, I was not admitted to the Alma-Ata conference meeting room. My job was to carry the bags of the international experts arriving at our then very small airport and help them navigate their way to hotels and the conference halls. We were very proud to be part of what we knew was an historic occasion for public health and our nation.

This landmark event which has had a continuing influence on global health, set the stage for our later work in developing the first School of Public Health in Almaty. The school, with the help of WHO and the Association of Schools of Public Health in the European Region (ASPHER), was established in 1996 with the aim of training and retraining specialists in public health and advanced training of heads of public health bodies and institutions on current issues of public health, policies and management in modern society. Our school was the first public health training institution in the 10 post-Soviet Republics in Eurasia. Since its formation it has continued to play a leading role in the field of research advancement and innovation. Our various courses and degree programmes now provide academic and practical skill training for heads of health and health service organizations on all levels, primary health care specialists, and government officials of Kazakhstan and Central Asia.

Maksut Kulzhanov, Professor, Kazakhstan Medical University – Higher School of Public Health (KSPH), Almaty, Kazakhstan

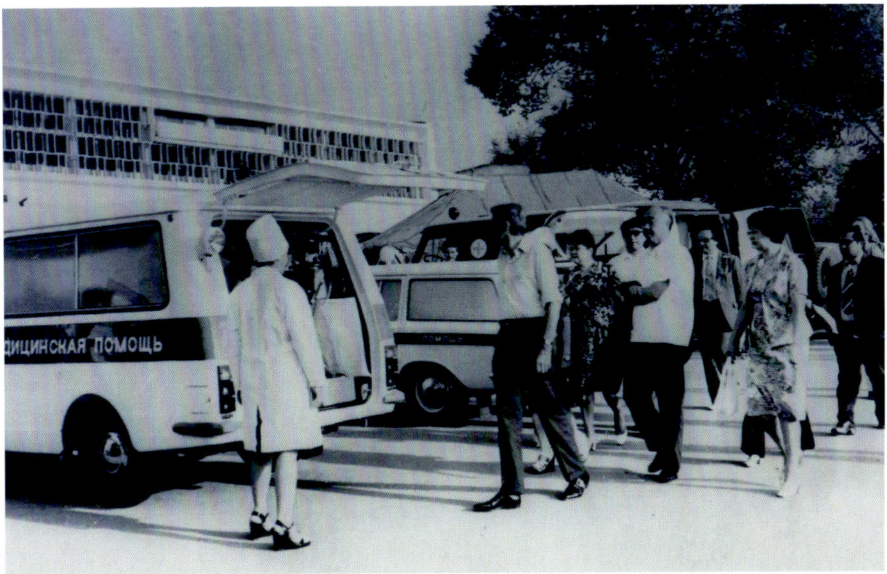

Delegates making field visits to different health institutions before the International Conference on Primary Health Care, Alma-Ata, the Kazakh Soviet Socialist Republic, USSR (now Almaty, Kazakhstan) in September 1978. © WHO

Dr Halfdan Mahler, Alma-Ata and the Cold War

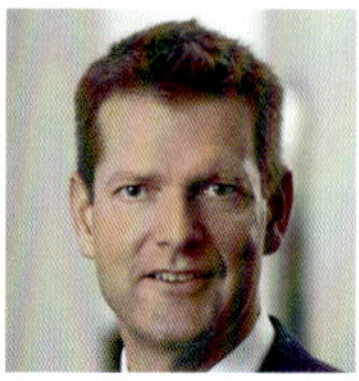

We have a very strong legacy in universal health coverage and in primary health care. And that legacy stems very much from the tenure of Dr Mahler as Director-General of the WHO from 1973 to 1988. He was from my country, Denmark.

He guided WHO in formulating the Health for All 2000 and in its strong focus on primary health care, with the Alma-Ata Declaration of 1978. That was an impressive feat in the midst of the Cold War; to gather people in what was then the Soviet Union, and to reach international agreement with a strong focus on primary health care.

Søren Brostrøm, Director General, Danish Health Authority, Denmark

Dr Mahler called on all Regional Directors to build support for Health for All and the Alma-Ata Declaration. In the European Region, Dr Kaprio gathered opinions from Member States. Both Dr Mahler and Dr Kaprio realized that to persuade the low-income countries to adopt Health for All they would need the industrialized countries to get involved, otherwise Health for All would be seen as 'second-rate'.

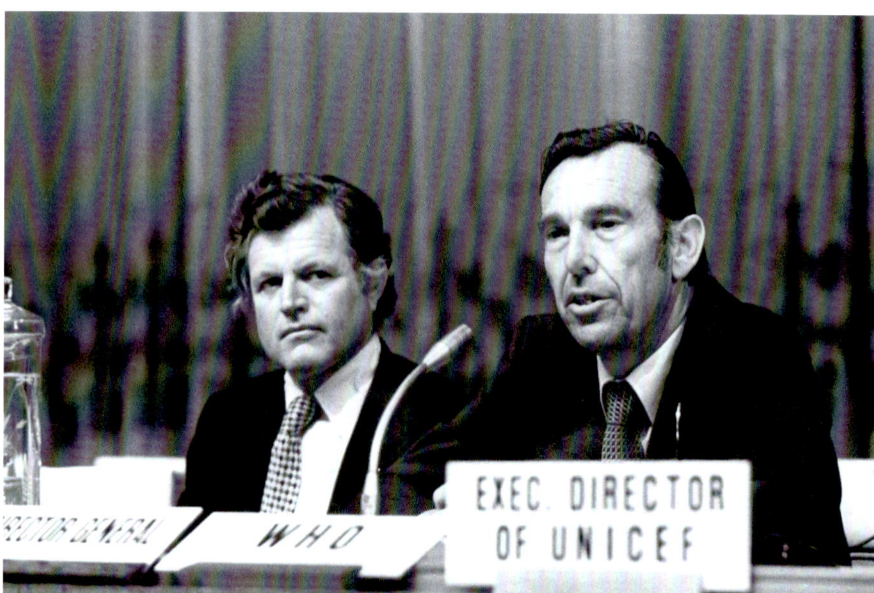

Halfdan Mahler, WHO Director-General sits at the podium of the Lenin Convention Center with US Senator Edward Kennedy at his side at the time of International Conference on Primary Health Care, Alma-Ata, the Kazakh Soviet Socialist Republic, USSR (now Almaty, Kazakhstan) in September 1978. © PAHO/WHO

Health for All and industrialized countries – not our problem

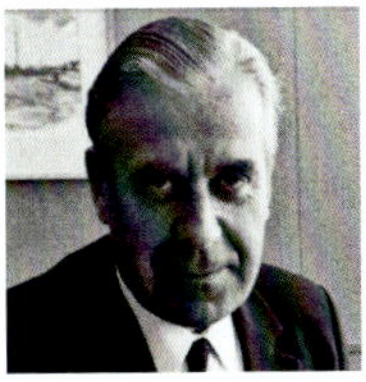

The industrialized countries of the Region took seriously the global resolution on Health for All. They believed, however that it had no relevance to them, except as the new approach required from them to provide more assistance to the third World

Leo A. Kaprio, WHO Regional Director for Europe 1966–1985 *(1)*

Dr Kaprio and his then Deputy Dr Jo Asvall, gathered evidence on the ways Health for All and primary care could help the countries of the European Region and began making the case for a European version of the strategy. There was some initial hesitancy, which they were able to overcome.

Evidence informed reframing

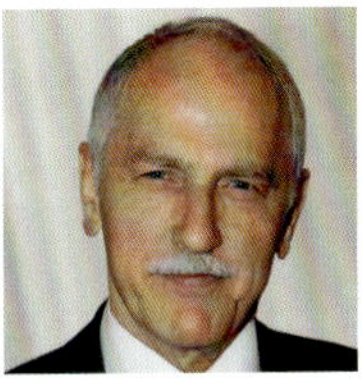

Importantly, we did a major epidemiological review of life expectancy. Dramatically, it showed that middle-aged men in 40% of European Region countries had static or declining life expectancy — in spite of massive increases in investment in hospital beds, physician–patient ratios, intensive care units, premature baby high technology, etc.

Basically, we showed that for a large group of Europe's citizens, ill health and pathology were growing faster than care capacity. In 1980, the WHO Regional Committee meeting was held in Fez, Morocco (it was a Member State in the European Region at that time), the new data were presented and a new European Health for All policy approach was introduced with four strands of action:

- lifestyle and health;
- health services and primary health care;
- environment and health; and
- support activities (training, information systems, multisectoral action, community involvement, etc.).

I remember the moment well. When I finished presenting there was absolute silence in the room. This went on for what seemed like an age. Kaprio leans over to me and says, "Jo, the first to speak will decide the fate of this policy." Then Halter — this rigorous, scientifically conservative Director General for Health from Belgium — gets up. He was known and respected for his sharp-tongued critical analyses.

He said, as best I remember, "Lifestyles and health? What is that? A very vague concept, I think. We know nothing about it. But we have to acknowledge there is a problem here. We cannot close our eyes to what is now a forgotten but clearly important intervention area. We must take action here."

Many other countries, as predicted by Kaprio, followed with positive comments and the resolution passed unanimously.

Jo Asvall, WHO Regional Director for Europe 1985–2000

The strategy that resulted, Health for All in the European Region, launched in 1980, was an enormous achievement at a time when the Cold War and the division of the Region into two competing power blocks was an ever-present background. The Health for All strategy provided an agreed, comprehensive, coherent and consistent long-term approach for the Region as a whole, including objectives and programmes for the promotion of healthy lifestyles; a reduction in preventable conditions; and the provision of adequate and accessible health care for all.

However, as the European Region had already met most of the global targets by 1981, it needed to set its own targets. This was done between 1982 and 1983 and the publication of *Targets for Health for All* provided the foundation for all future WHO activities in the Region *(21)*.

Growing tolerance and intellectual courage

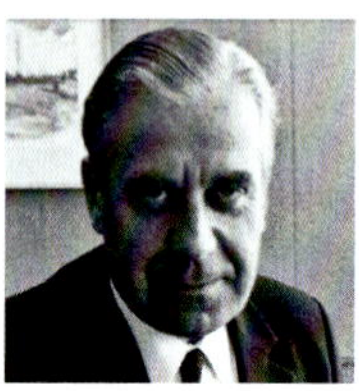

The Health for All Policy and targets in Europe is the story of growing tolerance and intellectual courage in building international health cooperation. Much earlier than political leaders, the health authorities of the Region, under the umbrella of WHO and working in the forum of the Regional Committee for Europe, reached both an understanding of the similarity of their problems and a common solution.

Accordingly, the Regional Committee agreed on a European strategy in 1980 and approved a common health policy in 1984: a blueprint to be applied independently in each country but monitored and reported on jointly.

Leo A. Kaprio, WHO Regional Director for Europe 1966–1985

Not a 'straight jacket'

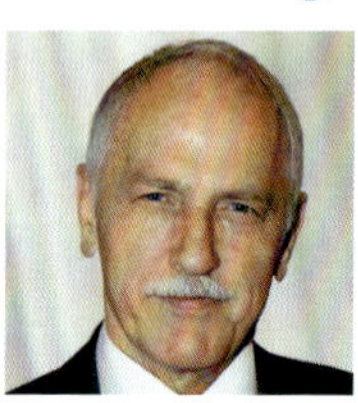

The Health for All policy gave us a clear framework which was quite detailed, enough to say where we were going but open enough to give space to move on how we get there. There was a lot of discussion and possibilities of getting to the thing in different ways; you could therefore exploit your own thinking. You were not in a 'straight jacket'.

Jo Asvall, WHO Regional Director for Europe 1985–2000

Health for All included several elements that we now think of as crucial cornerstones of any health policy. It contained a clear value-based and ethical framework for policy development. There was a pivotal shift in focus away from hospital-oriented health systems towards systems based on improved primary health care. The priorities of the strategy included the prevention of disease, the promotion of healthy lifestyles and the management of the full range of health determinants. Also, at the insistence of Dr Asvall there were clear, achievable yet demanding targets to promote Regional and Member State accountability.

The Health for All policy also emphasized that investment in health is vital to social and economic development. It follows therefore that health policy is also a social and economic policy. This crucial point has been given even more focus and priority across all the subsequent health policy developments over the last 20 years or so.

The first international conference on health promotion, held in Ottawa in November 1986, which resulted in the Ottawa Charter was another seminal event in the development of health policy *(22)*. It focused on the contribution of all determinants to health experience, and the role and contribution of all sectors across society to health policy and the improvement of health and well-being.

It incorporated five key action areas in health promotion:

1. create supportive environments for health;
2. strengthen community action for health;
3. develop personal skills;
4. reorient health services; and,
5. build health promotion strategies – enable, mediate and advocate.

The Charter inspired a widening of thinking about Health for All and promoted later work on movements and settings for health, notably the Healthy Cities and Health Promoting Schools movements.

I participated in this conference and trace my love for and loyalty to WHO to this experience. My position in the Hungarian Ministry of Health at that time, as the manager of our international relations with WHO, enabled me to attend this landmark meeting and to be directly part of the group that created the Ottawa Charter. It was an experience that has made a lasting impact on my thinking and career.

I later had the privilege of representing Hungary at the WHO Executive Board and developed a further understanding of the Organization, its goals and ways of working. I was able to attend WHO meetings, and met and was inspired by Dr Mahler, as were so many others. I also had the opportunity to introduce many WHO programmes in Hungary and help those working in public health in the country to become involved with WHO's work, for example in WHO networks like the Healthy Cities.

The Ottawa Charter

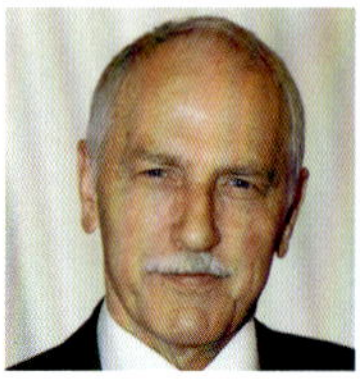

The First International Conference on Health Promotion took place on 21 November 1986 in Ottawa. It had a huge impact on our programme, on WHO and I think actually on the world. It was one of those big events where people came together around a new concept with many interesting ideas.

The movement also helped WHO reframe the way we talked about public health. We had some catch phrases. We knew that lifestyle and health was controversial, and many people felt that it was an infraction of individual choice. So, we said that it was all about making the healthy lifestyle choices the easy ones to choose.

We felt that formulation was good in many ways — it was politically acceptable but it also meant that the emphasis was not just on the individual, although that was part of it, but it was also on the conditions around the individual: economic and social conditions as well as the physical environment to make it easier to have a healthy lifestyle. So that became an important basic philosophy underlying the whole movement and the practical methods we were carrying out. Health promotion was kind of the unifying basic concept.

Jo Asvall, WHO Regional Director for Europe 1985–2000

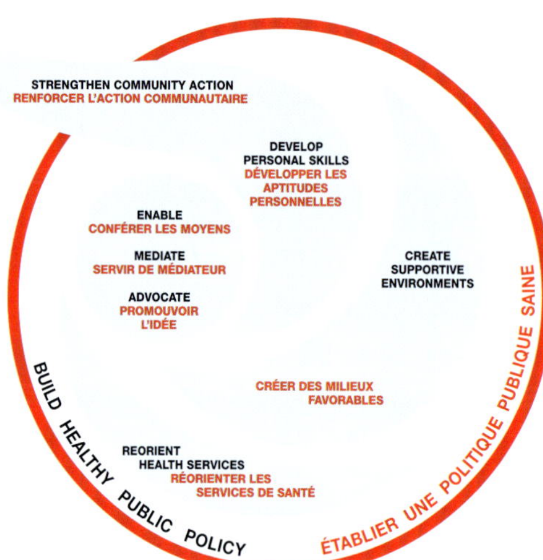

Fig. 6. This logo was created for the First International Conference on Health Promotion held in Ottawa, Canada, in 1986. Since then, WHO kept this symbol as the Health Promotion logo (HP logo), as it stands for the approach to health promotion as outlined in the Ottawa Charter for Health Promotion.

Source: The Ottawa Charter for Health Promotion *(22)*.

In 1986 an unexpected event of profound later significance occurred. The nuclear power plant at Chernobyl, in what is now Ukraine, exploded. This created enormous problems for health, environment and politics. Moreover, it changed the way people looked at environment and health issues and consequently created a demand for action. Several countries declared their interest in convening a joint environment and health ministerial conference in Europe. Germany hosted the first conference of ministers of health and the environment, held in 1989 in Frankfurt, which produced the first European Charter on Environment and Health.

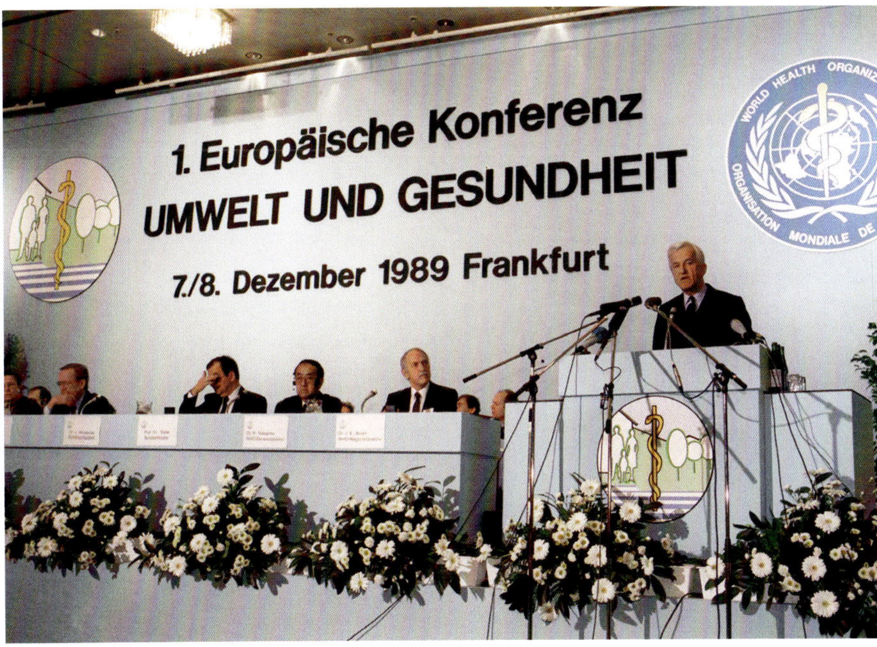

First WHO European Environment and Health Ministerial Conference, Frankfurt, Germany, 1989. © WHO

I attended the Frankfurt conference as part of the Hungarian delegation, and all the Environment and Health Ministerial Conferences afterwards when I became a WHO staff member. I have cherished this heritage and throughout my mandate as WHO Regional Director for Europe I have adopted this intersectoral approach model wherever possible. Before Frankfurt, there was virtually no cooperation between environment and health, as this was not within the spirit of the time. Since the Frankfurt Conference, cooperation between environment and health expanded and such intersectoral collaboration is now seen to be natural and necessary if equitable improvement in health and well-being is to be achieved.

The European Charter on Environment and Health was very progressive for that time. It stipulated that the preferred approach in public policy should be to promote the 'precautionary principle' and called for giving health and the environment precedence over considerations of economy and trade. Moreover, the European Charter on Environment and Health emphasized that one of the principles of public policy should be to pay attention to the protection of health and the environment of biologically vulnerable and socially disadvantaged groups. The European Charter on Environment and Health set out a broad framework for action by all levels of government, by all sectors of society, and at the international level.

Change agent of the Regional Office

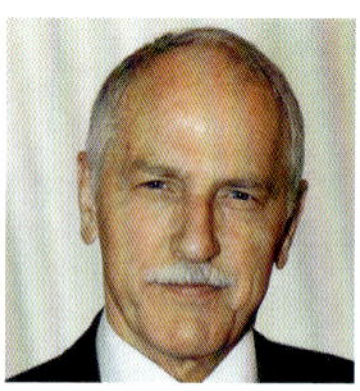

The Environment and Health ministerial conferences dramatically changed public health approaches in general, and the basic nature of the WHO Regional Office for Europe. The conferences helped, for example, to catalyse a shift and a reframing from a technically focused Regional Office, reactive to the emerging needs of Member States, to a change agent Regional Office, proactively advocating, with partners, for public health-oriented policies in all sectors.

Jo Asvall, WHO Regional Director for Europe 1985–2000

On 9 November 1989 another change of profound importance occurred; the fall of the Berlin Wall. This was then followed over the next two years by the collapse of the former USSR and the communist system. The WHO Regional Office for Europe was no longer dealing with the USSR as a monolithic political bloc, but with a group of emerging independent countries within the Commonwealth of Independent States, as well as the countries of central and eastern Europe which were now no longer under Soviet influence. As a result, the Regional Office then (as now) dealt with an expanded number of 53 Member States.

In many of the new Member States there was a profound economic collapse and a marked deterioration in the health situation. The Regional Office moved quickly to develop a special programme, named the EUROHEALTH programme, which created WHO liaison offices central and eastern Europe and in the newly independent states (NIS). These offices, small at first, were established to maintain local links with ministries of health and coordinate relevant public health activities. This was the beginning of what has now developed into an extensive network of country offices, to be described later (see Section 4).

It was the EUROHEALTH programme which first brought me into WHO employment. I had the privilege to direct this programme for the countries of central and eastern Europe from 1991 to 1997 and then work as the Director of Country Health Development between 1997 and 2000.

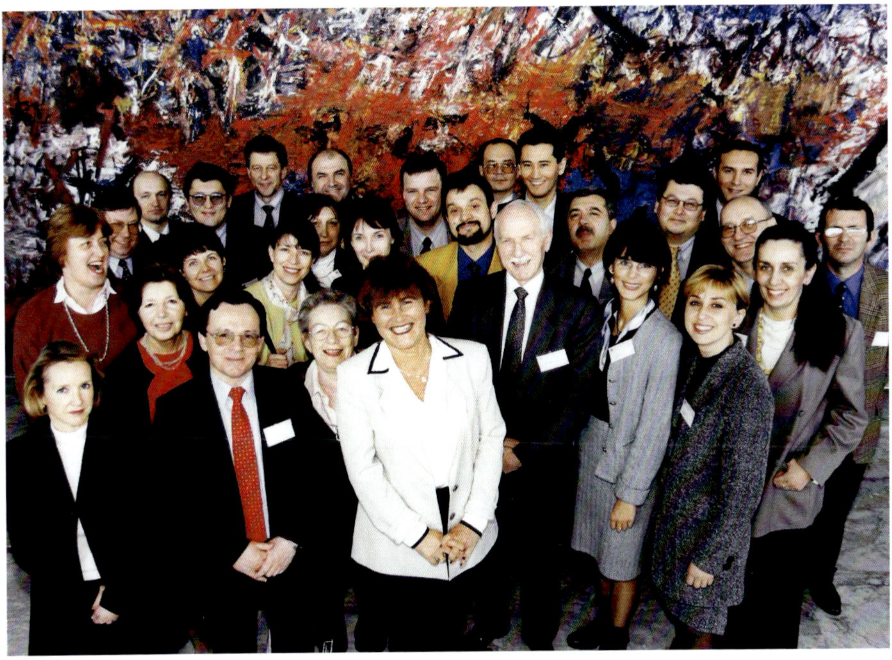

Jo Asvall with Zsuzsanna Jakab and WHO liaison officers and other WHO Regional Office for Europe staff, Paris, France 1995. © WHO

PART 1

There was pressure from some countries to focus narrowly on the immediate health crises, but Dr Asvall, now the fourth Regional Director, was not inclined to focus only on narrow disease-specific issues. The Office adopted a broader approach and tried to help countries, even during the economic crisis, to start to look at the determinants of health and to consider how best to reorganize health and health care services. Accordingly, health policy and health care reform became top priorities.

From Semashko to Free Market

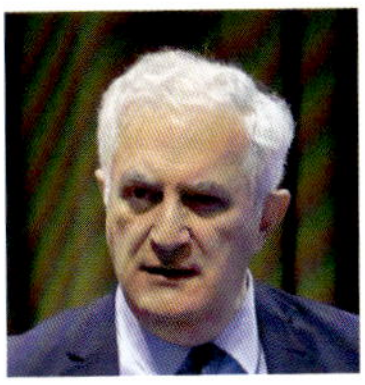

After the collapse of the Soviet Union and the restoration of independence, we had many economic and social challenges. The Semashko model of health care, adopted during the Soviet period (1921–1991) in Georgia as in other Soviet countries, was destroyed and our economy was shifting rapidly to a market system.

Our Ministry of Health in particular was challenged by the task of health care reform and the need to make major changes to adapt health policy and the health system to the new environment.

In this challenging period for the country, assistance and expertise from the WHO Regional Office for Europe was crucial in many different strategic health and health policy areas; such as assisting the government in developing its national health policy and strengthening health systems and decision-making capacities; restoring the immunization chain; and, providing guidance on developing interventions for control of the infectious diseases. This latter assistance was particularly important during our diphtheria outbreak (early 1990's) as well as a polio eradication campaign under MECACAR operation in the Region (from 1995), after which Georgia became free from the wild poliomyelitis virus. WHO also helped us in combatting TB and implementing the directly observed treatment, short-course (DOTS) strategy and in improving maternal and child health.

Georgia received significant technical assistance from WHO and the best expertise to improve the equity, accessibility and affordability of health services.

Amiran Gamkrelidze, Director General of the National Center for Disease Control and Public Health, Georgia

Vital support at time of need and beyond

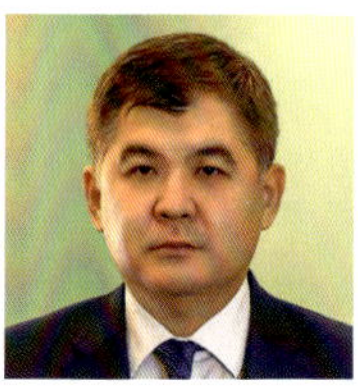

Since our country became independent 28 years ago, the work with WHO was essential to keep our health care system functioning and to further develop it. At the start we had very strong economic difficulties and it was very challenging for us to maintain access to services for our population and quality of care. So, for us the strong support from WHO in basic areas such as primary health care, maternal and child health, fighting against tuberculosis, HIV and overall improving the management of the system, was critical. Thanks to WHO, especially the WHO Regional Office for Europe, we have been quite successful in maintaining and reforming our health care system during these last 28 years.

Yelzhan Birtanov, Minister of Healthcare, Kazakhstan

Another new form of challenge appeared soon afterwards in the early 1990s, with the developing war across former Yugoslavia. This unexpected war close to the centre of Europe posed many public health problems and dilemmas to which the Regional Office needed to respond. We developed experience in providing a new set of immediate humanitarian interventions, working with other parts of the UN system. Field offices were established and staffed across the republics which were emerging from former Yugoslavia, and a series of public health programmes developed and implemented. During the war, my role as Director of Country Health Development, was to supervise the work of the WHO team leading the humanitarian work. After the end of the war with the 1995 Dayton Peace agreement, WHO worked to help guide health system reconstruction and reform efforts in the countries that had suffered.

Should we engage during the war?

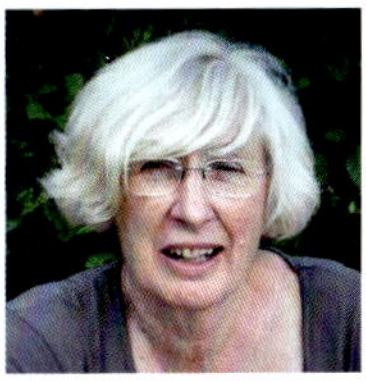

There were huge debates and arguments in the Regional Director's Executive Committee about whether or not we should go into Yugoslavia. Many were very much against it. Jo Asvall's big and deciding argument was, "What will we do after the war if we have not been there with them during the war? How can we move in after the war and tell them how to do this or that? You know, we have to help them now!" And we did *(17)*.

Carolyn Murphy, Former Director of Administration and Finance at the WHO Regional Office for Europe

City to city support

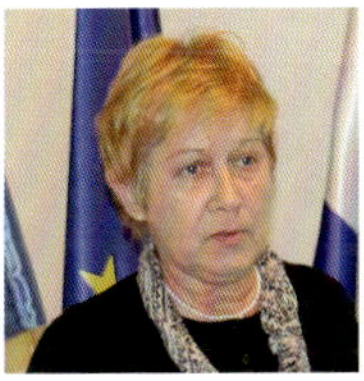

War changed everything. At first, we were trying to prevent the war with our 'Physicians Against the War' and 'Physicians for Peace' groups. But we learned it was inevitable. So, we shifted to preparing communities and health services for the war.

We contacted different WHO Regions and learned about disaster management 'technology' like how to shelter displaced persons and refugees, what is emergency medical kit, etc. Our different Healthy Cities (we already had 11 there by the start of the war) had very different needs. Dubrovnik was under siege, Vinkovci and Osijek were heavily shelled.

In 1991 one of our major concerns was that Croatia was not recognized (by the UN) as a State and therefore we were not able to receive aid as a State. With the help of the Regional Office for Europe Healthy Cities Programme, we decided we would initiate a city-to-city support programme. And this was our main support through 1991 until we were able to get international recognition in 1992.

Our sister healthy cities across the Region were amazing in gathering and transporting materials based on the city-to-city assistance. This, for example, included a complete field hospital from the Danish Red Cross with a surgical suite, beds, etc., that we brought to Vinkovci, where their hospital had been destroyed.

Selma Sogoric, National Network Coordinator Croatian Healthy Cities Network Andrija Stampar School of Public Health, Croatia

The experience of the Regional Office in humanitarian public health work was again needed during and immediately after the war in Kosovo *[1]* between February 1998 and June 1999. There, WHO worked extensively with other UN organizations.

[1] All references to Kosovo in this document should be understood to be in the context of United Nations Security Council resolution 1244 (1999).

Since then support from the Regional Office to the countries of south-eastern Europe has been continuous. This involvement was formalized in early 2001, under the leadership of Marc Danzon, as the fifth Regional Director for Europe. The Regional Office organized a high-level meeting to create a health network of the south-eastern European countries involved in the Stability Pact and to agree a joint action plan featuring 11 principles of cooperation in support of strengthening health services *(23)*.[5]

A health component was added to the Pact's social cohesion initiative, aiming to bring people together across borders to improve health in the whole region. The South-eastern Europe Health Network (SEEHN) was established with political, technical and financial support from partner countries and organizations. Today the SEEHN continues its work to promote peace, dialogue, reconciliation and economic development through its involvement in health systems development with WHO Regional Office and other partners.

An exceptional moment

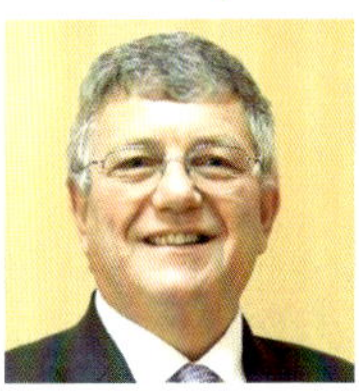

Mrs Gabriella Battaini-Dragoni, Director, Directorate of Social Affairs and Health, Council of Europe, met with me in 2001 to share her concern that health was not included as part of the Stability Pact for South Eastern Europe. We agreed to see how we could use health as a peacemaker.

We organized a high-level meeting to create a transnational health network in the subregion that would facilitate and stimulate dialogue and debate between countries and explore ways that each participating country would take on a health system strengthening project for the benefit of all the other participating countries. It was a fantastic meeting. After nearly a decade of fighting between some of the Stability Pact countries, they agreed to work together on public health strategies targeting the most vulnerable in the region.

In a way it reminded me of the way the European Union began just after the Second World War, an organization aimed at ensuring peace through joint economic and industrial interests – except that in our case, we were sharing health projects! The Dubrovnik meeting was really an exceptional moment.

Marc Danzon, WHO Regional Director for Europe, 2000–2010

5 The Stability Pact for South Eastern Europe was an institution aimed at strengthening peace, democracy, human rights and economy in the countries of south-eastern Europe from 1999 to 2008. It was replaced by the Regional Cooperation Council (RCC) in February 2008.

Health as bridge to peace and reconciliation

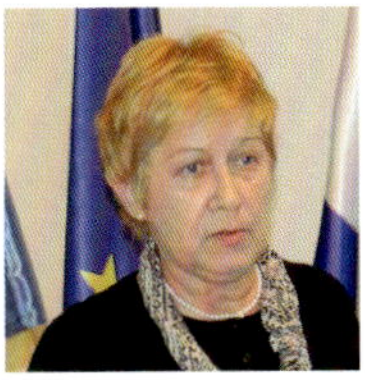

After the Dayton Agreement, it was impressive how cooperation was restarted after the war. Wounds are still open today so you can imagine what it was like in the years just after the war. We decided that the area around which everyone would like to cooperate was health. Throughout the war we kept some of our contacts; we lived in the same country for 70 years and of course we knew each other.

The idea was to have cooperation on a ministerial level under the umbrella of the 1999 Stability Pact. A health component was added to the Stability Pact social cohesion package and we (initially all the countries of former Yugoslavia) identified what were the topics that everyone would like to chip in and work around with others. 'A Dubrovnik pledge' in 2001 formalized the SEEHN. The WHO Regional Office for Europe has played a central role in supporting this network and has helped bring in additional countries. Many donors have now contributed to different health initiatives.

Selma Sogoric, National Network Coordinator Croatian Healthy Cities Network
Andrija Stampar School of Public Health, Croatia

During and after these humanitarian programmes, the Regional Office became more focused and experienced concerning the transition from humanitarian to post-humanitarian development, involving careful attention to the reconstruction, rehabilitation and reform of health systems. This work required the development of intensive collaboration with other UN humanitarian and development actors.

Dr Danzon was committed to responding to, and serving, the needs of Member States, and in 2000, the Regional Committee adopted a new Country Strategy: 'Matching Services to New Needs'. Actively negotiated country-based agreements between the Regional Office and Member States were formalized as biennial collaborative agreements (BCAs) signed between the Regional Office and the Ministry of Health in each country.

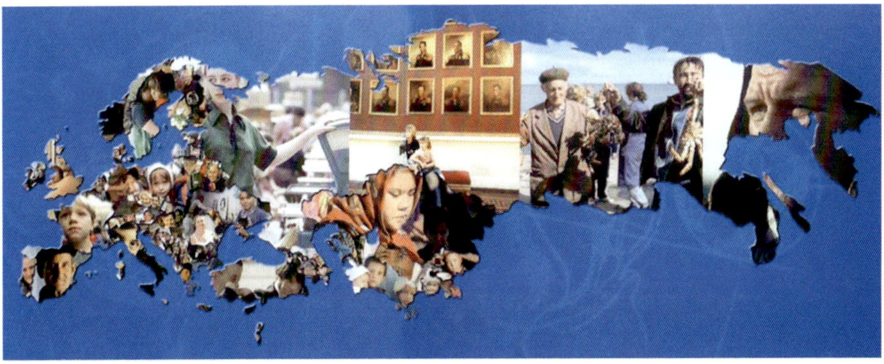

'Matching Services to New Needs' design concept 2002.
© WHO/INSPIRIT Creatives – Tuuli Sauren

A new country focused strategy

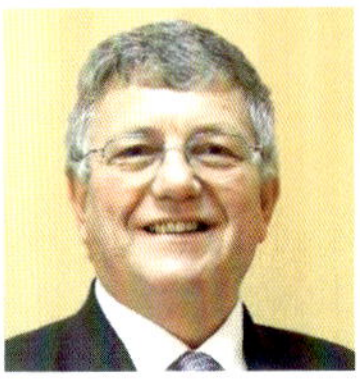

My aim was to ensure that the countries were given the decision-making power, support and resources to set their developmental agenda with the Regional Office.

This Country Strategy gave the Regional Office a new mission to support Member States in developing their own health policies, health systems and public health programmes; preventing and overcoming threats to health; anticipating future challenges; and advocating public health.

Our focus on health systems grew out of this strategy. Countries who were receiving our technical assistance wanted to make sure that it helped strengthen their health systems. There was also a growing research interest in the relationship of health and wealth.

Marc Danzon, WHO Regional Director for Europe, 2000–2010

Another initiative was to explore further the importance of health to the wider development of human societies. The relationship between wealth and health is two-way, wealth contributes to health, but health also contributes to economic growth and therefore to wealth. Health systems form the other arm of what is now seen as a triangular relationship between health, wealth and health systems, with health systems contributing to both wealth and health. The European Observatory on Health Systems and Policies, and other researchers, actively developed and extended the evidence base underpinning these relationships.

To further explore these issues, a major event was held in Tallinn in June 2008. The Health Systems for Health and Wealth Conference remains perhaps the most important legacy of Dr Danzon's period in office. The Conference culminated in the Tallinn Charter which stated clearly that investing in health is investing in human development, social well-being and wealth, and that well-functioning health systems are essential for improving health and saving lives *(24)*. Tallinn made the point strongly that today it is unacceptable that people become poor because of ill health. With these commitments by Member States the Tallinn Charter anticipated UHC with its emphasis on access for all to health promotion, disease prevention, treatment and rehabilitation, without an overwhelming or unmanageable financial burden *(25)*.

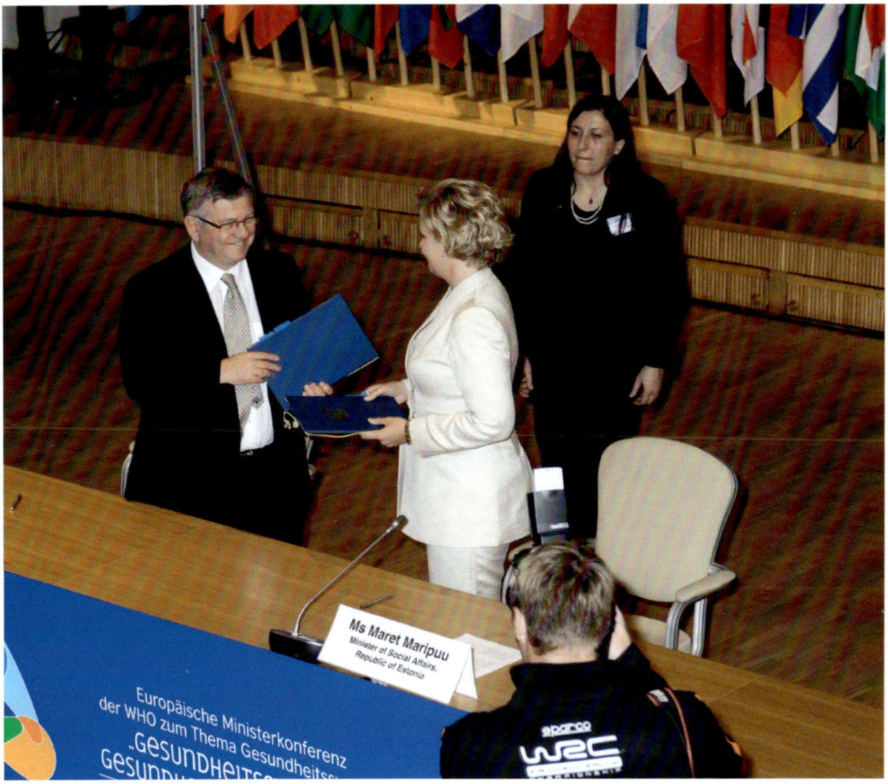

PART 1

Marc Danzon and Maret Maripuu, Minister of Social Affairs Republic of Estonia, signing the European Charter on Health Systems, Tallinn, Estonia, 27 June 2008. © WHO

Summary reflection

WHO Historical Context

Looking back, we can now see that the commitments made by Member States within the Tallinn Charter prepared countries well for their later engagement with both Health 2020 and the SDGs. UHC has now become one of the defining health goals of WHO within the GPW13. Taken all together the ideas define modern approaches to the equitable improvement of health and well-being as a societal and developmental goal, as well as indicating practical approaches towards that goal's achievement.

These ideas within the Tallinn Charter were uppermost in my mind when I considered standing for the post as WHO Regional Director for Europe. Other important issues I felt strongly about were the need to strengthen public health, both as a vision and as a set of institutions and functions, and to give full attention to the social determinants of health.

I had always been drawn to these issues, and of course to the globally fascinating work and inspiring role of WHO. At the time I was just finishing my term as the first director and founder of the European Centre for Disease Prevention and Control (ECDC). My role at ECDC allowed me the unique and very rewarding opportunity of working with EU institutions and Member States in starting a new type of agency. It was a wonderful experience, however, the possibility to return to work at WHO, and this time as WHO Regional Director for Europe, was for me an opportunity of a lifetime.

Especially as in this transformational period we knew so much more about the determinants of health, our long-sought goal of making health a priority political choice seemed more reachable. That is why I stood for the post of WHO Regional Director. I was fortunate enough to be successful and took up my position in February 2010. Since my very first days as Regional Director I wanted to help identify practical institutional mechanisms which would allow health systems to work proactively with other sectors and create policies that would have positive impacts on health determinants and health status. I also wanted to minimize any unintended negative impact.

I knew that this would mean promoting policy coherence while implementing intersectoral action. What I didn't know was what would be the implications for governance, partnerships and ways we would work with countries. What advocacy and communication skills would be needed? These were all questions which my colleagues and I have tried to address in developing and implementing our seven strategic action priorities towards our Better Health for Europe goal.

We felt it was high time to collect all our current and legacy knowledge and experience together into one coherent strategic whole that could guide the Regional Office and countries for the years ahead. We needed a new strategic vision for health and public health, to the development of which the whole WHO European Region could contribute, and which could guide all our policy and programme development.

Hence was developed the idea of what came to be called Health 2020, a health policy framework which could provide a value- and evidence-based umbrella beneath which we could all work. I saw our efforts as the latest instalment in WHO's long history of working towards Health for All. As noted earlier, each generation of WHO staff has worked to preserve and advance its values, approaches and impact and then deliver them into the hands of their successors to build further on what they have done. The early days of the travelling seminars, the focus on needs and responses in countries and the intra-country support required from the Regional Office, the idea of an accountable overall policy for Health for All and the focus on improving public health capacities – all these developments contributed to a coherent story from which we have all been able to benefit.

In 2010 it was our turn. We focused on identifying and implementing more effective system-wide responses to the many determinants of health, and the Health 2020 became our platform for this contribution. The origins of Health 2020, its content and its achievements comprise the main story I wish to tell here, on behalf of all my colleagues and staff who have accompanied, supported and worked with me in this amazing mission and adventure. It is to that story that we now turn.

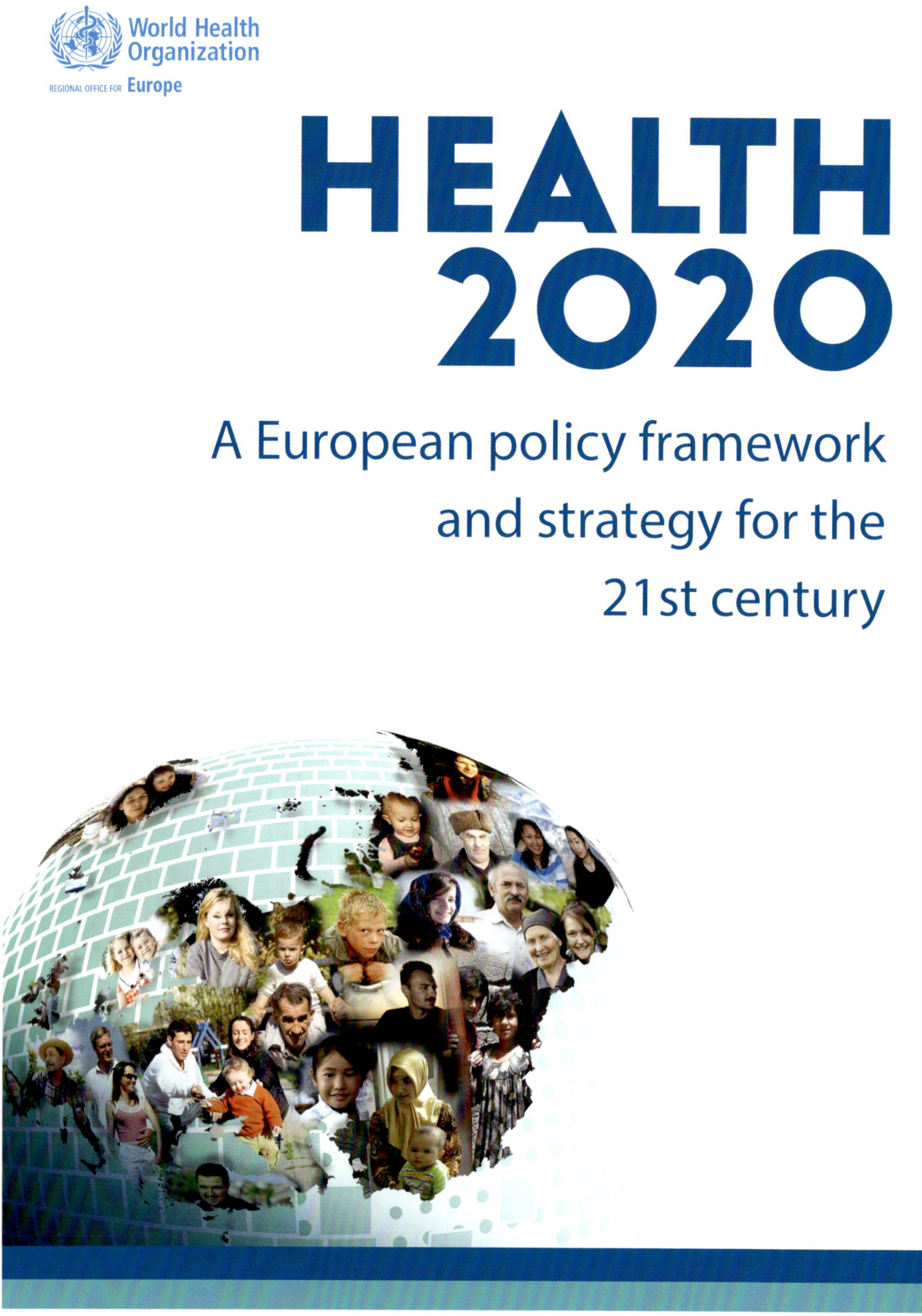

Book cover of Health 2020. A European policy framework and strategy for the 21st century.
Source: Health 2020 *(26)*.

2. Health 2020 – developing the policy and its evidence base

Soon after my election as Regional Director in 2010, work started immediately on the development of Health 2020 – A European policy framework and strategy for the 21st century *(26)*. At the same time, we initiated a process to strengthen public health, by producing a European Action Plan for the Strengthening of Public Health Capacities and Services (EAP-PHS) *(27)*. Throughout this process, I was determined that both Health 2020 and the EAP-PHS, and all our technical work to come, would be infused with our new knowledge about the full range of determinants of health.

We wanted to create tools and resources, adaptable to different countries and contexts, that could support the development and implementation of health policies that would be coherent, value-driven, and evidence informed. It was a good time to act, as the climate of opinion had moved towards regarding health much more seriously on global and national agendas. Health was now increasingly understood as a global public good, as a human right, and as a matter of social justice. Importantly, health was also seen more and more as a vital issue for other sectors such as the economy, trade and security; as an investment sector for human, economic and social development; and as a major economic sector in its own right. Put simply, ours was now a world where health mattered as perhaps never before.

2.1 Co-creation of the European health policy framework

In developing Health 2020 we catalysed and managed an action-learning co-creation process, designed from the start to be a collaborative initiative between WHO, Member States and their health-related institutions, as well as many diverse stakeholders whose actions directly and indirectly influence health. Input was also sought from scientific partners and relevant professional groups, civil society and policy communities.

Engaging all stakeholders in the Health 2020 process

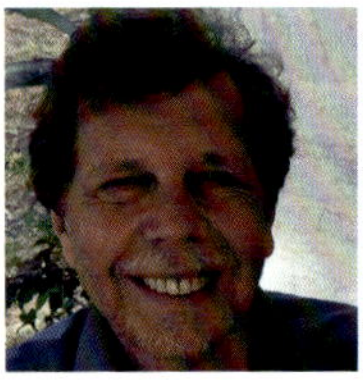

When Zsuzsanna asked me to help lead the development of this new health strategy for Europe, I was really thrilled because I knew that it was a great opportunity to launch a new era for public health in Europe that would be consistent with new developments, evidence and opportunities in the world.

I already had a deep conviction that such an instrument, such a frame, could make a huge difference in our efforts to engage and commit countries, to not just have development in the commonly understood way, but also to reach to a higher level of values and principles of modern health developments. My conviction was deeply rooted in my previous experience with Health for All.

So, our first challenge was to find a way to engrain in it all the features we knew had worked before; to make sure that it was value-based, informed by the best available evidence and would not shy away from addressing some of the most challenging issues that relate to health. We quickly understood that Health 2020 and its development process had to be an instrument for change, reform and transformation of not only health systems but also of the way countries and political systems understood and dealt with health.

We understood that this meant it was not a document to be developed by a committee, but a document that had to be developed with the backing of strong and determined leadership. This is what we had de facto with our new Regional Director.

Zsuzsanna understood well that our policy instrument not only had to be up to date with evidence, but also robust and courageous in setting a clear agenda for health development and sustainable development that was fully consistent with our times and the global calls for putting health much, much higher on the agenda of politicians and countries.

The development of WHO strategies and policies is always the result of absolute consensus, not by majority. Achieving this consensus for Health 2020 meant that it had to engage the widest possible range of internal and external stakeholders. First, it was important, in fact vital, to get the House on board, not only to support the document but also to engage and commit the House to see this as the main framework for the work of the whole office.

The Division of policy and governance for health and well-being that Zsuzsanna set up to lead the process of developing Health 2020 was cross-cutting and designed to work horizontally with all parts of the House. My first and most important task as director of this Division was to broaden in-House understanding of the strategic value of Health 2020 for the implementation of the Organization's goals. Health 2020 was to become the integrated political and strategic framework for change and innovation.

A dynamic conceptual drafting process was developed that also enabled continuous input from the evidence-gathering initiatives commissioned by the Office (social determinants of health, multi-level governance for health and economic impact). Sequential drafts went through several politically important and technical processes and rounds. So, we learned very quickly that it was important to listen carefully to all voices and process any difficulties that emerged.

One key challenge we faced, for example, was the new way we were asking people to think about health and governance. Tension arose in the beginning about some of the 'whole-of-government' and 'whole-of-society' approaches that we were putting forward. Some felt that this was beyond the remit of health ministries. Some Ministers would say they understood the concept, but this was not something that they could commit their governments to…and so on. This concern was addressed through what I call an 'osmotic process'. It was not a linear change process; rather, several factors or events combined to help reframe people's thinking.

First, within our political meetings, some articulate, vocal, highly respected, well informed countries would influence fellow Member States to be open to such visions. Testimonies from experts like Sir Michael Marmot, talking about determinants and repeatedly making a strong case about the importance and the role of other sectors was crucial in helping Ministers to understand how they could be empowered by becoming champions for health in their own government.

Secondly, we were beginning to see a new type of health leader emerging; like mayors in cities who, in most cases, did not have any direct responsibility for health services but had through their policies and programmes a very significant influence on a wide range of determinants of health, equity and well-being in their cities. Health 2020 promoted this new role.

Third, the world was changing during the period Health 2020 was being developed. The G8, for example, started talking more about health, so everybody could see that health was now becoming a key issue, high on the agenda of the top political leaders of the world.

This is why I am saying by 'osmosis'. It was a process which slowly, as we were debating and presenting those issues, allowed everybody, to come to the same denominator, and to begin to see that it would have been pointless to just stay in the 20th century or in, let's say, traditional public health approaches to those issues.

I should add here that at one point, precisely because the main frame of Health 2020 was so political and strategic, we decided to dissociate it from the technicalities of the constantly changing evidence and concluded that it was best to have a short and a long version of the document. We knew that the long version of Health 2020, when it was launched, would be state of the art, but six months later some of the aspects there would have been outdated by new evidence. So, we produced the short version which could stand the scrutiny and the passing of the time without losing its power and its relevance.

We didn't want to come to Malta without knowing we had a consensus. We had a meeting in Israel in the final stages of the process where we worked to ensure that the document was both acceptable to all Member States and, most importantly, would retain the punch, the strength, the power and the vision of what we were proposing; be value-based and deeply rooted in evidence and principles that smell and ooze and relate to the real contexts and challenges that we were all facing.

Very importantly Health 2020 was not only about health, but it also put emphasis on well-being and launched a vision that was strongly linked to sustainable development.

We had our 'red bottom lines' as it were that we didn't want to have to modify. We knew them. We knew what they were. And here again the key element is strong political leadership that understands how to frame issues in ways that engage and not only keep everyone on board but instil in everyone a pride and enthusiasm for being part of such a historical process.

We knew after the Israel meeting that we were not going to have to come to Malta with a watered-down strategy. We knew that we had a package of ideas and concepts that had depth; a framework which was strong, value-based, and evidence-informed that commits countries to take action on issues that can be difficult even to talk about let alone do something about.

Agis Tsouros, Former Director, Policy and Governance for Health and Well-being, WHO Regional Office for Europe

Our aim was to strengthen existing evidence, know-how and support for action on achieving better health for Europe. All important policy decisions were discussed and agreed at a series of meetings of a Health 2020 Steering Group which I convened. Sequential drafts were placed on our website for comment and reviewed by the Standing Committee of the Regional Committee at their regular meetings. This process aimed to engage actively our governing bodies and broader public health community in the development process and give them all a sense of ownership of what was agreed. The resultant document was presented and approved unanimously by the Regional Committee in Malta in 2012.

Health 2020 was a 'hectic' process

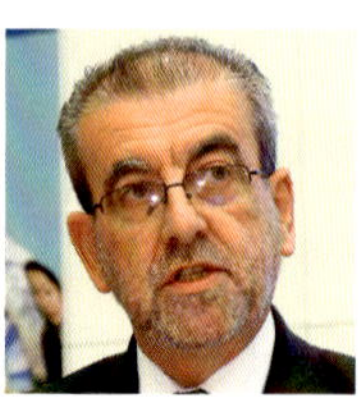

Health 2020 was 'hectic'. 'Hectic' not in a bad way but in an intense way. The Secretariat and everyone involved really worked very hard. Through a process of multiple reiterations based on feedback, comments and new evidence, it became a key document with evidence-informed guidance that all could use. It was truly a co-production of a broad range of stakeholders; including Member States, academics, practitioners and civil society.

I was involved from the very beginning. I remember when it came to the SCRC, we went through it with a 'fine toothed comb'. The document was revised and reworked through each review. There was not much disagreement on issues of substance but a lot of long discussions on what words to use to best communicate the concepts to different stakeholders across our very diverse European Region. We could all see that it was growing stronger, clearer and more useful through the process. A very good decision was made near the end to have two versions. That I believe was a real turning point for the process. A short political version was added. This was written specifically for decision-makers without detailed knowledge of the health sector. This importantly acknowledged and communicated that we were 'practising what we were preaching' about whole-of-government approaches and that we wanted to engage with all sectors, all decision-makers on all levels from presidents to mayors to community leaders and advocates. This second shorter document has proved to be very valuable.

And then in Malta we had the honour of hosting the Regional Committee meeting at which Health 2020 was formally adopted. That was a proud moment for us all.

Ray Busuttil, Former Director General, Public Health Regulation Department, Ministry for Health, the Elderly and Community Care, Malta

A common platform and common vision

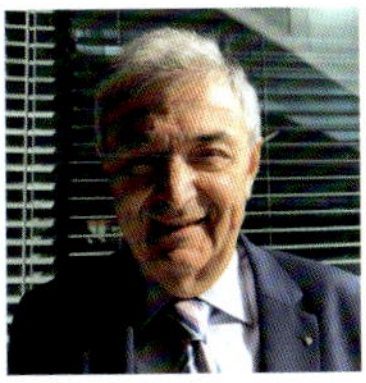

What the Member States needed was a mechanism that could put them on a common platform to elaborate a common vision. The situation had changed completely since 1998 when Health 21 was developed…and there was a need to have a new and updated 'common flag' under which all the diverse groups and countries in the Region could be united…

The WHO Office conducted a very participatory 2-year process … not for a prescriptive policy but a framework with options … a menu card…but with important priority areas that were acceptable to all.

I remember several very 'extended' talks and discussions… with sceptical countries; for example, one very liberal country said health was just the responsibility of individuals and could not see the need for a policy which calls for so many societal and environmental interventions… Slowly, slowly this country, and all others, came on board after much evidence and arguments were presented … and finally, in Malta in 2012, Health 2020 was unanimously adopted.

Mihály Kökény, Former Minister of Health, Hungary

We needed the best available impact and cost-benefit evidence. Existing evidence was systematically reviewed. When gaps were identified we supplemented our reviews with new data and recommendations made from specifically commissioned European studies on social determinants, governance and economics. In order to assure that the evidence generated to support the policy would be accessible, understandable, useful and recognized as robust and 'the best available' in all parts of the Region, I reactivated the Office's European Advisory Committee on Health Research (EACHR). The aim of the EACHR was to promote and strengthen the use of research evidence for public health decision-making and to inform policies for the development of health research in the Region. It started its work by reviewing drafts of the Health 2020 document.

Chief Scientist – Reactivating the European Advisory Committee on Health Research (EACHR)

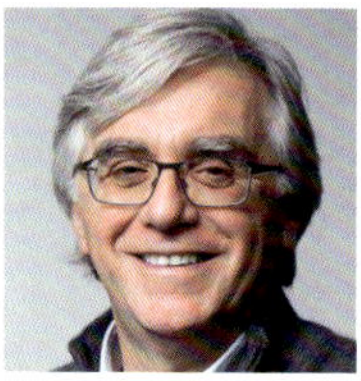

One of the first steps made after the Regional Director election, was the appointment of a Chief Scientist. This was a sort of message given to the rest of the Office saying, "OK, science is back! We want to move according to evidence. We want to give a clear message that WHO believes that knowledge is the basis of any model for change in responding to the challenges of the time."

One of my first acts as the newly appointed Chief Scientist was to reactivate the EACHR that had not been functioning for some time. This was a way of convening key public health scientists around the Region to make sure we had some sort of appropriate representation of overall European research interests and capacities. I have to say that it was not easy. It was difficult at the beginning to identify leading scientists equally from the western and eastern parts of the Region. It was difficult to shape this Committee and give it a useful and visible role for the overall work of the WHO Regional Office. Members of the Committee at first thought they were convening around the table to do some sort of priority research exercise. However, the Committee was more of a supporting body to evaluate the scientific basis of the work of the Office and to identify 'research capacity need' priorities.

One of the first tasks the EACHR carried out was a review of the scientific basis of Health 2020. This aimed to verify whether statements were actually fully based on scientific evidence.

Some primary studies were also carried out on the research capacity in the eastern part of the Region, one of which showed, for example, that one of the main challenges people faced was tailoring effective policies and 'best buys' to the actual needs and practices of different populations. What was missing was some type of applied research capacity at a country level. We documented this type of problem and this became a broader message – that there is a need for schools of public health to develop research capacity in their communities of practice which are able to verify the validity and appropriateness of different strategies in each country's context.

Roberto Bertollini, Former WHO Representative to the EU in Brussels and Former Chief Scientist of the WHO Regional Office for Europe

Helping to prioritize the public health research agenda–EACHR

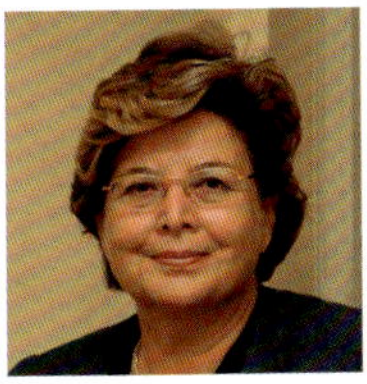

We were working in a multicultural context around the table. We started by introducing ourselves and explaining what research we were doing. Then we started to try and prioritize the topics mentioned around the table. It was not easy to distil a few major themes, but we were able to all agree a few related to equity, cultural context, gender issues and human rights.

We saw these were issues that in many places were still not mainstreamed into research agendas. We agreed that our research work around Health 2020 could help to change this.

We also moved into new ways of looking at research. As a group we knew we had this unique opportunity to view topics with many different experiences to what health and to what research is all about. Soon we were able to talk about how we could gather evidence about the issues we cared about, and we talked priorities for Europe that we thought funders should start to support with grant money. And funders started to listen to us. The EU and EC, for example, sent representatives to listen to our discussions. We became and have continued to be a unique intelligence source for research funders and funding.

I think one of the biggest achievements of this group is that we can attract the attention of the funders and help them focus on two or three major issues and meaningful solutions. I am not saying that they based their funding on what we said, but that it helped them focus. Prior to this their funding had a bit of a 'mosaic' feel. They are funding something here and there as an issue caught their attention. They would fund something in Uzbekistan, something different in Sarajevo, and then something different in Italy. It was a bit of a mishmash of issues. I think we helped them prioritize.

Tomris Turmen, Chair of the European Advisory Committee on Health Research (EACHR), Turkey

Health 2020 and the EAP-PHS aimed to make clear to everyone that the WHO Regional Office for Europe had made a strong and renewed commitment to public health, an area with long and proud traditions in many European countries. We wanted to stimulate more interest and investment into public health and placed emphasis on the need to further develop its service, training and research capacities and contribution.

To accomplish this, we identified ways to make a stronger economic and political case for the increased investment in health promotion and disease prevention needed to decrease the disease burden and the pressure on health care systems. We simultaneously advocated for action to support the training and development of adequate human resources to promote and deliver public health effectively.

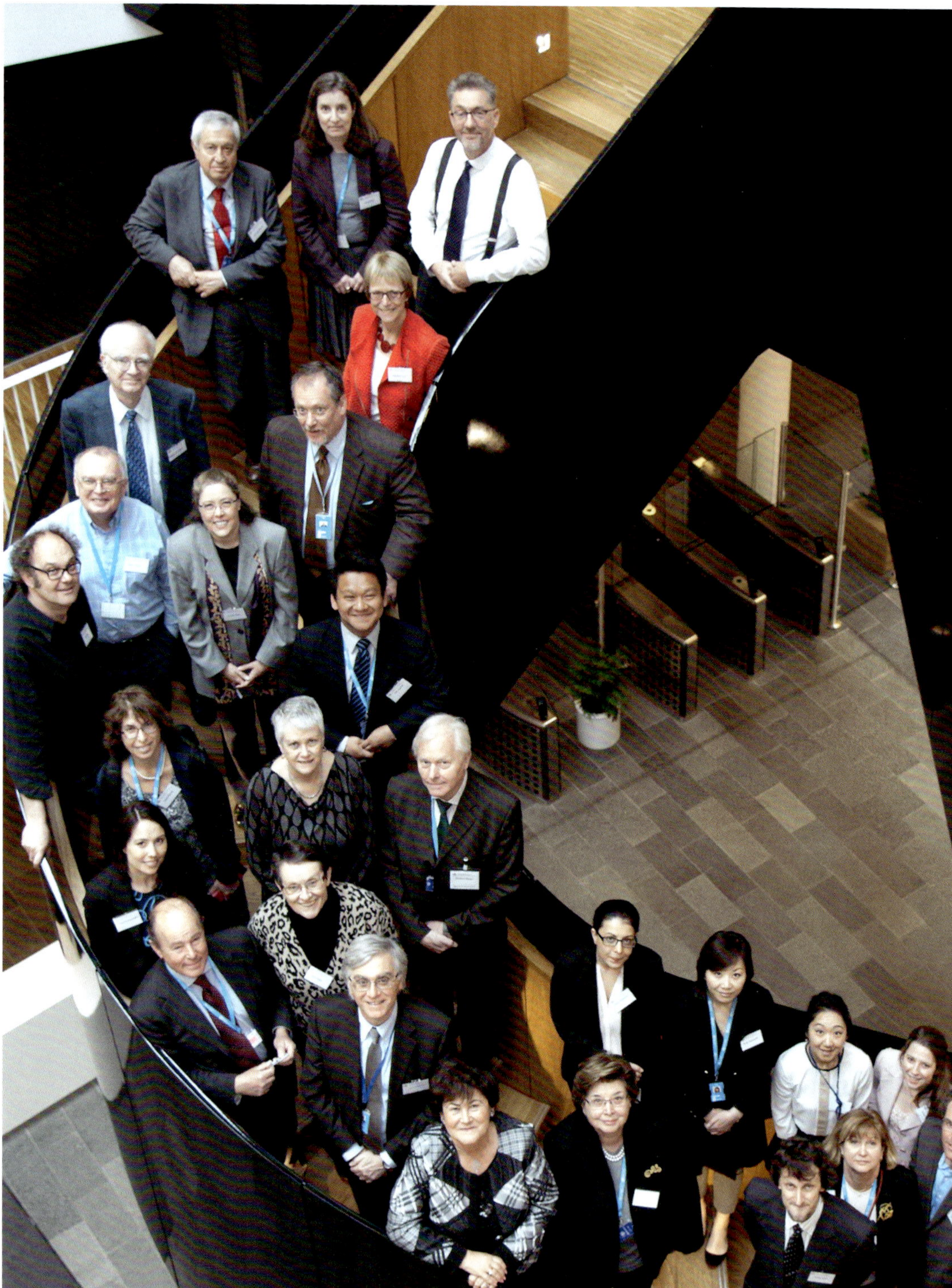

Participants from the sixth meeting of the European Advisory Committee on Health Research (EACHR), held in Copenhagen, Denmark, on 15–16 April 2015. © WHO

During the participative consultation around Health 2020 we touched many sectors and settings and engaged many people. The new policy framework demonstrated how far the territory of health had expanded and positioned health as a critical domain in development. We made linkages between public health and health systems, with an emphasis on primary health care, as foreseen in the holistic approach to health systems articulated in the Tallinn Charter. Importantly, we wanted to promote health strongly as a societal responsibility overall, and a whole-of-government responsibility advocated and led by Ministers of Health.

We encouraged and supported all Member States to use the new common Health 2020 framework to further develop, renew or update their national health policies, strategies and plans, whilst considering ways to adapt and adopt the two Health 2020 key objectives and the four priority health areas to their national circumstances and priorities (see Box 4).

Box 4. Health 2020 Objectives and Priority Health Areas

Health 2020 Objectives

1. Improving health for all and reducing the health divide

Actions on social determinants are described. They address the development of approaches that build health into all policies. The aim is that of improving the health of everyone as well as targeting interventions focused on those most affected. Strong new arguments are presented that relate to health, human rights and economics for improving health and addressing health inequities. Health for all and its values of the right to health, equity, solidarity, participation and social justice are championed.

2. Strengthen leadership and participatory governance for health

New collaborative approaches to leadership are described. They bring different partners together and mobilize broad-based political and cultural support for health development. Insights are identified into the new roles, opportunities and types of leadership needed to reach out more effectively to others within and outside government in order to identify and implement joint solutions to major health priorities. Health 2020 identifies how citizen and patient empowerment can serve as key elements for improving health outcomes, health systems' performance and satisfaction.

Health 2020 Priority health areas

Priority 1: Invest in a life-course approach and empowering people

Health 2020 shows how supporting good health and its social determinants throughout the lifespan leads to increased healthy life expectancy which can yield important economic, societal and individual benefits. Children with a good start in life learn better and have more productive lives; adults with control over their lives have greater capacity for economic and social participation and living healthier lives; and healthy older people can continue to contribute actively to society. Healthy and active ageing, which starts at birth, is a policy and major research priority.

Priority 2: Tackle Europe's major health challenges

Health 2020 focuses on a set of effective integrated strategies and interventions to address major health challenges across the Region related both to noncommunicable and communicable diseases. Both areas require determined public health action and health care system interventions. Evidence points to the need to underpin these interventions with actions on equity and social determinants of health.

Priority 3: Strengthen people-centred health systems, public health capacity and emergency preparedness, surveillance and response

Strengthening people-centred health systems has been high on the agenda of countries throughout the European Region, with new approaches and innovations for improving health and health equity. Key focus areas of Health 2020 include: improving the delivery of public health and health care services, enhancing vital health system inputs such as human resources and affordable equipment and medicines, strengthening health funding arrangements and enhancing governance.

Priority 4: Creating resilient communities and supportive environments

People's health chances are closely linked to the conditions in which they are born, grow, work and age. Resilient and empowered communities respond proactively to new or adverse situations, prepare for economic, social and environmental change and cope better with crisis and hardship. Communities that remain disadvantaged and disempowered have disproportionately poor outcomes, in terms of both health and other social determinants. Health 2020 provides a systematic assessment of the health effects of a rapidly changing environment, especially in the areas of technology, work, energy production and urbanization. Optional actions are identified to ensure positive benefits to health.

It was also important that Member States should monitor and report on their achievements using an agreed set of indicators. Member States therefore agreed a set of targets (see Box 5), 19 core and 18 additional indicators and a monitoring process for the policy framework in 2013, with 2010 set as the baseline *(28)*.

Box 5. Health 2020 Targets for the WHO European Region

1. Reduce premature mortality;
2. Increase life expectancy;
3. Reduce inequalities in health (social determinant target);
4. Enhance the well-being of the population;
5. Ensure UHC and the 'right to health'; and,
6. Set national goals and targets related to health.

I believe that the agreement to monitor targets was a crucial step in the Health 2020 implementation process. By agreeing to report on progress towards common targets and indicators, both the Regional Office and the Member States reinforced their commitment to the policy and demonstrated their willingness to be publicly accountable for the outcomes and impacts of implementation. The process of data collection also identified the need to strengthen collection mechanisms in some countries and develop some new ways of measuring outcomes.

Most of the agreed indicators are quantitative, drawing on already established data collection mechanisms. However, there are limitations with such data. Some limitations reflect poor data collection systems in some countries. Others reflect the inherent difficulties in capturing complex human experiences, for example well-being, in quantitative terms. So, the monitoring framework quite deliberately went beyond quantitative information to also include qualitative indicators for monitoring policy development and implementation.

It is my annual task, as Regional Director, to report on progress towards the Health 2020 targets. I deliver monitoring reports to the Regional Committee as part of my yearly address. Additionally, the Regional Office publishes annual Core Health Indicators reports and includes monitoring data in our European Health Reports which are organized around the Health 2020 targets (see Box 6). These reports are also now made available through the European Health Information Gateway which is the Regional Office's web portal and data warehouse, supported by a European Health Statistics mobile application *(6)*.

Box 6. European Health Reports

Our European Health Reports have been tracking progress related to the six targets set out in the Health 2020 framework (see Box 5). These reports are published every three years and document the European Region wide process to develop a more expansive approach to measurement where conventional statistical forms of data are complemented by an array of qualitative evidence from new sources.

The European health report 2012: charting the way to well-being provided an assessment of the improvements in health in the WHO European Region, emphasizing the uneven health distribution between countries. This was supported by a web-based Atlas of Health Inequalities *(219)*.

The European health report 2015. Targets and beyond – Reaching new frontiers in evidence recognized a paradigm shift in public health, in which the focus had already started to move from death and disease to health and well-being *(220)*.

European health report 2018: More than numbers – evidence for all (3) described how Member States had begun to expand the evidence base beyond numbers and statistics, taking in data from the medical humanities and social sciences and collecting real-life narratives that captured subjective experience. These new holistic approaches allow analysis of health trends that probe the social and cultural drivers of health and well-being. They also allow us for first time to go beyond descriptions of 'what' and 'how much' with explanations in terms of 'why'.

The European Health Information Initiative also conveys progress on implementation of Health 2020 through other information channels *(29)*. These include country reports of good policy and practice in the Regional Office's bilingual (English and Russian) journal *Public Health Panorama*. In addition, the Regional Office has revised the Country Profiles and Highlights on Health series to provide more detailed information on progress in Member States.

Health 2020 was focused on implementation of policies and programmes, and since its adoption in 2012 the WHO Regional Office for Europe has worked with its Member States and partners to achieve this. We have striven to build and sustain political and societal support to improve health by encouraging presidents and prime ministers to commit to health investment and outcomes as a key goal of public policy and as a marker of governmental and policy success. We have urged governments, as well as local communities and decision-makers across public and private sectors, to establish mechanisms for the implementation of whole-of-government, whole-of-society and health-in-all-policies approaches, and for monitoring and reporting on progress over time. We have helped countries analyse their public health and governance situations, as well as identify country assets and needs, and make recommendations for policy priorities and ways to implement and monitor impact through the agreed targets and indicators. We have also supported capacity development and know-how transfer about new forms of leadership, governance, engagement and communication, where needed and requested.

Evidence was to be at the core of Health 2020. During its development, the Regional Office commissioned several major studies to fill gaps in knowledge that were noted in our systematic reviews or reported to us by Member States. Commissioned studies looked at the social determinants of health, governance, economics, and environmental determinants. Beyond existing and new evidence, we wanted, across the Office, to continuously update the evidence and have it reviewed and adapted by the EACHR.

Reframing the value of evidence

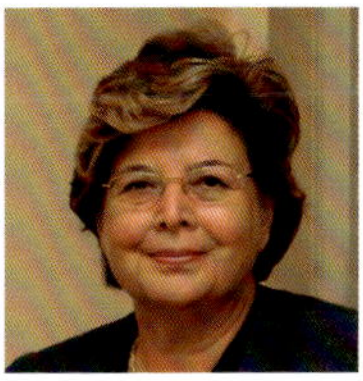

The EACHR became a cornerstone of Health 2020 policy related dialogue even though we are just a handful of people and have no budget. What we do have, though, is the ability to bring research concerns to the attention of governments. Our input is part of the evidence base justifying resolutions for action governments were being asked to take. This process has been part of the Regional Office strategy for research to be in the forefront of the public health agenda. And the evidence we are talking about here is not clinical; it is not, about the best treatment for this or that infectious diseases, it is evidence that addresses the core issues of Health 2020. It is evidence, for example, about how best to set up public health programmes that benefit everybody. It is about evidence that can inform policy-making! And the importance of research in the forefront of any debate in the governing bodies has improved apace so we are happy to see that.

We report directly to Zsuzsanna, the Regional Director. It is very rare that you report to the head of an agency from a committee. There is usually some secretariat in between, but it is not so here. Zsuzsanna has coordinated the process so that individuals in the research field, in academia and in the governments are sitting together and speaking the same language. And she always references/uses our research in her speeches and in her meetings with ministers of health, presidents and prime ministers.

In these ways the EACHR has been given the opportunity to communicate evidence much more directly to policy-makers and help make health the political choice.

Tomris Turmen, Chair of the European Advisory Committee on Health Research (EACHR), Turkey

2.2 The Review of social determinants and the health divide in the WHO European Region

The Review of social determinants and the health divide in the WHO European Region was initiated in 2010 *(7)*. It was coordinated by the University College London Institute of Health Equity and chaired by Professor Sir Michael Marmot. It brought together a cross-disciplinary consortium of leading researchers from Europe and beyond. The aim was to answer demands from policy-makers and public health advocates for practical guidance on 'policies that work' to reduce inequities in health between and within low-, middle- and high-income countries in the WHO European Region.[6]

Sending a signal

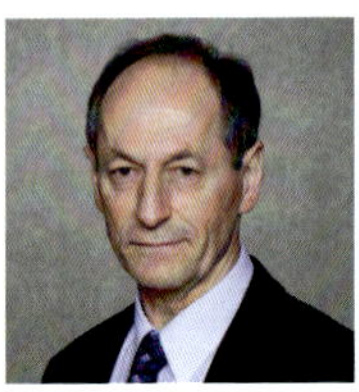

Shortly after Zsuzsanna Jakab was elected Regional Director and before she'd taken office, she asked me if I would consider doing a European review of social determinants of health. My first reaction was that, "I've done the WHO Commission on Social Determinants of Health *(30)*. That's global. I've done an English review of social determinants and health inequalities, the Marmot review in England *(31)*. That's national. Why would she want me to do one for a WHO Region?"

Zsuzsanna immediately explained to me her strategic thinking here. She told me that one of her biggest priorities was reducing the east-west health divide. She believed that a review of social determinants of health would provide crucial context specific evidence and recommendations about both what could be done internally in each country to address inequalities in health through action on social determinants, and what could be done to address the health divide across the European region. She convinced me of the importance of this work. I agreed to conduct and coordinate a multi-centre European review to gather evidence and importantly make specific recommendations for action.

I next met Zsuzsanna on her very first day as the new WHO Regional Director for Europe in February of 2010. She asked me to come to the Office that day to 'send a signal' to the whole Office of how important this Regional Review was to her strategic plans. When I got there, she welcomed me graciously and we discussed our plans for the review. She then asked if I would give a staff seminar the next day. Being asked to give a seminar with no notice was something of a surprise but nonetheless I said, "Yes, I've got my laptop here. I am sure I could put something together. But nobody will come, will they? I mean, if you tell them on a Thursday lunchtime that there is a seminar Friday morning." When three hundred people turned up, I began to understand what she meant by 'sending a signal' to the Office. She wanted to show the staff not only how important she thought inequalities in health and action on social determinants of health were, but also that she was taking immediate action to inform and engage the whole Office in this priority work area. This was her very first staff meeting and of course

6 The term "inequities in health" is used to describe unfair systematic differences in health between social groups that are avoidable by reasonable means.

everyone came. It was a terrific experience. It also sent me and my team a signal that this was indeed a number one priority for the WHO Regional Office and that we had the full support of the Regional Director.

The global financial crisis had brought conditions of great hardship to parts of the Region. There was therefore an even more pressing need for action on the social determinants of health to ensure that a commitment to health equity survived and was enhanced. Our aim was to provide both the evidence and the recommendations on effective ways to make this happen.

Sir Michael Marmot, Director,
University College London, Institute of Health Equity, United Kingdom

Thirteen task groups were set-up, each chaired by an expert in the relevant content field. The task groups gathered, analysed and synthesized evidence about what was possible and what worked in addressing the various social determinants of health and health inequities. Interim reports were made broadly available for public review and input.

The *Review* identified several key findings. Firstly, that avoidable health inequities exist within and between countries, with social, economic and environmental causes which are amenable to interventions. Secondly, that the wealth of a country is not the only factor determining its level of health and health equity. Government choices and policies can also make a positive difference, at any level of gross domestic product (GDP). The *Review* clearly identified the need and ways to accelerate the rate of improvement for those countries with the worst health. Effective approaches identified, included:

PART 1

- taking a life-course approach to health equity;
- addressing the intergenerational processes that sustain inequities;
- addressing the structural and mediating factors of exclusion; and,
- building the resilience, capabilities and strength of individuals and communities.

The study consortium advocated strongly for some key policy imperatives, including promoting a good start in the life of every child; supportive and active labour market and employment policies; and a comprehensive review of social policy measures. The *Review* produced an unprecedented "How To" policy guide on tackling health inequities and reducing the health divide across the WHO European Region. The key message was: 'Yes we can!' The *Review* presented a well-structured set of evidence-based policy recommendations to improve health and reduce inequities.

Significant progress in reducing health inequities can be made with the right choice of policies, across all countries, including those with low incomes. The *Review* recognized that countries in the European Region were at very different starting points with diverse contexts and priorities. Therefore, the *Review* identified 'best buy' priority action areas, for low-, middle- and high-income countries, and called for a 'proportionate universalistic approach' that delivered programmes with an intensity that related to social and health needs.

The *Review* recommended twelve priority action areas for policy interventions (see Table 1).

Table 1. SDH Review themes, recommendations and examples of specific action areas for policy interventions

4 Policy themes	12 recommendations-intervention action areas	Examples of specific actions
Life-course Pregnancy, early childhood, work and old age	Ensure conditions exist for good quality parenting and family building. Promote gender equity. Provide universal high-quality and affordable early years education and care. Eradicate exposure to unhealthy/unsafe work. Secure access to employment and good-quality work. Take intersectoral action to tackle inequities in older ages/prevent and manage chronic morbidity.	Provide sexual and reproductive health services. Ensure women of childbearing age/families with young children benefit. Include children most at risk in education. Protect employment rights of most vulnerable. Address youth unemployment. Address age discrimination.
Wider society Social protection, local communities, social exclusion	Improve the level and distribution of social protection. Address local determinants of health through co-creation and partnership with those affected and civil society. Focus on groups most severely affected by exclusionary processes.	Increase spending and the effectiveness of social protection. Recognize people's right to health. Ensure public engagement and community participation. Give socially excluded groups a real say in decisions that affect their lives.

4 Policy themes	12 recommendations-intervention action areas	Examples of specific actions
Macro-level Social expenditure and sustainable development and health	Promote equity through the effective use of taxes and transfers. Plan for the long term and safeguard interests of future generations – identify links between environmental, social and economic factors and their centrality to all policies and practice.	Maintain and/or improve social spending to current European average. Prioritize health and social consequences of austerity in addressing the financial crisis. Apply principles of sustainability development to all policies. Do health equity assessments.
Systems Governance, priorities for public health, ill health prevention and treatment, measurements/ targets	Improve governance for social determinants of health and health equity. Develop a comprehensive and intersectoral response to preventing and treating ill health equitably. Undertake regular reporting and public scrutiny of inequities in health and its social determinants.	Build partnerships for health and inclusive growth. Ensure UHC. Set transparent and measurable targets to improve health and reduce health inequities (Level up). Enhance UN mechanisms to improve addressing inequities in health and its social determinants.

We have been supporting the uptake of these best practices within Member States through policy dialogues, training courses and intercountry initiatives and networks. The Regional Office has produced and made available a package of evidence-based guidance and materials to support implementation of these priority actions (see Section 2.4).

Health 2020 and social determinants of health

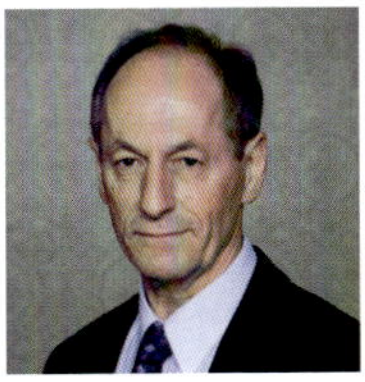

Over these last ten years we have seen that Health 2020 has provided an exceptional platform upon which countries have been able to take the new evidence on social determinants of health and consistently and strategically use it to enhance the political and social commitment to action of governments, civil society, transnational bodies and academic institutions. Actions being taken across the European Region are ultimately helping to translate the evidence into the reality of a more equitable and sustainable Europe.

Sir Michael Marmot, Director, University College London, Institute of Health Equity, United Kingdom

2.2.1 Governance for health studies

We commissioned studies aimed to help both the Regional Office and policy-makers in countries understand better and advocate for the new policy environment, as well as develop the skills and capacities needed to implement the vision of Health 2020 *(32, 83)*. Living in today's knowledge-based societies means that power and authority are no longer concentrated solely with governments. Our governance studies gathered strong evidence supporting an emerging consensus that population health can no longer be understood as an outcome produced by a single ministry, namely the Ministry of Health. It requires a synergetic set of policies involving a wide range of actors from the different ministries and beyond to deal with current and emerging public health problems. Informed citizens, conscientious businesses, independent agencies and expert bodies all increasingly have a role to play.

A political science lens on health

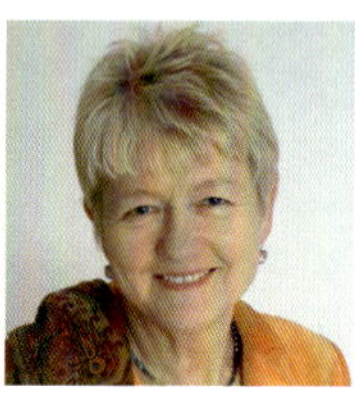

Our research work on governance for health, what is sometimes called health in all policies, highlights that a major part of health is created through other types of policies. We try to make clear that it is not just an issue about intersectorality, but that in principle, it is the way we deal with the complexities of governing in the 21st century and include all the actors. This kind of thinking was not yet happening in WHO or most Member States in 2010.

Our hope was that by looking at this through a political science lens, not something WHO had done before, we could help inform and influence the Health 2020 process; how health was approached, how it was formulated, and the kind of priorities that were set. It was, of course closely linked to the work that Sir Michael Marmot was coordinating on social determinants and inequalities. Our work focused on how you address the wide range of determinants described and documented, and how you work collaboratively with other sectors towards a healthier society.

Ilona Kickbusch, Director of the Global Health Centre, The Graduate Institute Geneva, Switzerland

Nevertheless, governments have the ultimate responsibility for ensuring the human right to health, and for meeting the international commitments contained in the SDGs. All government sectors have a vital role in managing governance for health, setting norms, providing evidence and making the healthier choice the easier choice.

Our commissioned research identified case studies of innovative governance initiatives across the Region as ways to increase understanding of and competence in providing new 'smart' forms of leadership for health in the changing governance contexts of the 21st century *(83)*. These studies presented practical examples of how policy-makers and public health advocates are bringing together diverse actors, coalitions and networks, including community, government and business representatives, within the whole-of-government, whole-of-society and health-in-all-policies approaches.

Key messages included:

- There is no one-size-fits-all approach. Certain constitutional, political, institutional and cultural characteristics shape governance approaches at all levels within societies. Hence whole-of-government and whole-of-society approaches must be adapted to each country's unique context and background. Implementing whole-of-government approaches has been found to be more feasible and effective where a common ethos and strong unified sense of values exist, helping build trust across sectors. This said, no policy fits perfectly in all contexts, and learning from others what works, and why, is vital. This is especially true for common challenges such as the noncommunicable disease epidemic and demographic shifts.
- Joined up (net)working is possible. A culture that is supportive of thinking and acting across agency borders can be attained through incentives and rewards that encourage organizational flexibility, and people's adaptability and openness to creative and innovative policy-making. Adding value through partnerships, mutual gain or co-benefit strategies has become a common theme in governance for health.
- New roles for new times. Health sector policy-makers and advocates have new roles to play; for example, they can act as: brokers, diplomats, catalysts, animators, educators and partners, in much more participatory, non-hierarchical processes. Health 2020 supports and encourages health ministries to bring together key stakeholders from different sectors in a shared effort to promote health and protect people and populations.

2.2.2 Economic studies

We also commissioned economic studies to help policy-makers, practitioners and advocates better understand and promote the economic case for investing in health promotion and noncommunicable disease prevention *(33)*. These studies, produced in partnership with the European Observatory on Health Systems and Policies (see Section 5.6) and Organisation for Economic Co-operation and Development (OECD) (see Section 5.2), went beyond looking at just the economic benefits of actions within health care systems and analysed the added benefits for investing 'upstream' across the whole economy prior to the onset of illness and before health care services are required.

These studies identified a wide variety of areas where appropriate policies can generate health benefits at an affordable cost, reduce health expenditure in the short term and help address health inequalities at the same time (see Box 7) *(34)*. These studies reinforced the value of making solid economic cases for investment in health. They showed that investing in public health policies and interventions can be cost saving and provide high returns for health and sustainable development across the Region.

Getting the numbers down

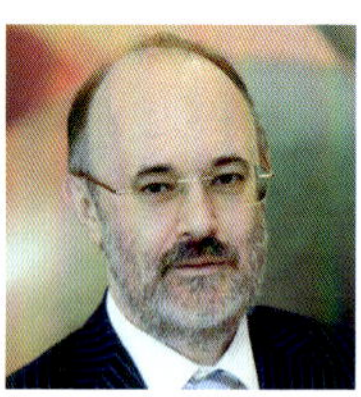

Ten to fifteen years ago, we didn't have our numbers down. At that time, we didn't have a holistic view of the cost and spending structure of our complex fragmented health care systems. When I started my job in 2003, one of my bigger challenges was the tax redistribution framework with our regions. This is a national exercise we do every four years, how to redistribute the tax allocation etc.

In that first year, we had a single chart of numbers in front of us and when we presented them to the regional ministers, they were able to tear them apart within the first 15 minutes because they were wrong. We didn't have an adequate level of accurate information.

Since then we have gotten very serious about health systems research and making our economic arguments. We have made tremendous progress over these last 10 years and now do monitoring reports on health costs and analyse optional policies twice a year. Regional economic studies from WHO and others have been most helpful in this process.

Clemens Martin Auer, Special Envoy for Health, Austria

Box 7. The economic evidence for investment in health: some examples

1. The current WHO 'best buy' interventions (the most cost-effective interventions) for NCDs show several 'upstream' interventions that are highly cost-effective, including tobacco and alcohol legislation; reducing salt and trans-fats; and increasing physical activity *(35)*.
2. The most cost-effective tobacco control policy, for example, is raising taxes *(36)*. A 10% price increase could result in 0.6 million to 1.8 million fewer premature deaths in eastern European and central Asian countries, at a cost of only US$ 3 to US$ 78 per disability-adjusted life year (DALY) in the short run.
3. Overall it is estimated that every US$ 1 invested in the WHO 'best buys' for NCDs will yield a return of at least US$ 7 by 2030, and that implementing the WHO 'best buys' can generate US$ 350 billion in economic growth between now and 2030 *(37)*.
4. Similar findings are available at the country level, for example indicating that avoidable economic losses from NCDs are equivalent to 3.9% of gross domestic product in Kyrgyzstan and 5.4% in Belarus *(38, 39)*.
5. In the United Kingdom, a highly cost-effective intervention is the screening programme for older women at high risk of hip fractures, as it suggests a cost per quality-adjusted life year (QALY) gained of US$ 4,11 *(40)*.
6. As a cost-saving initiative, in Italy, a return on investment analysis suggests that the universal hepatitis B vaccination will return US$ 2,78 for every US$ 1 invested from the health system, with the programme breaking even within 20 years *(51)*.
7. Health promotion and disease prevention can bring results: a 10% reduction in cardiovascular diseases could save €20 billion per year in lower- and middle-income countries. Investing in early childhood development is estimated to produce a 17-fold return for each euro invested. Preventive approaches could contribute between 50–75% to the reduction of cardiovascular mortality in high-income countries and 78% globally *(33)*. Meanwhile, in 2016 the cost of physical inactivity globally was estimated at US$ 67.5 billion in health care expenditure and lost productivity *(41)*.

These examples clearly show that cost-effective preventive approaches can contribute to improvements in health outcomes, whilst achieving lower and more sustainable costs. The level of savings achieved can be huge and could, for example, potentially be used to support the implementation of UHC.

Tackling inequalities could also bring huge savings to the health system itself. In England (United Kingdom), for example, socioeconomic inequalities – which in turn drive health inequalities (the social gradient) – were estimated to cost the National Health System £4.8 billion in 2011–2012 as a result of excess hospital admissions *(42)*. There are also significant macroeconomic effects. Studies show that reducing health inequality by 1% per year in low and middle income countries would increase a country's annual rate of GDP growth by 0.15% *(43)*. In 2011, it was estimated that, in the European Union, inequality-related losses to health reduce labour productivity and take 1.4% off GDP each year. Moreover, health inequality related welfare losses were estimated to be €980 billion per year, or 9.4% of GDP *(44)*.

These economic studies strengthen and reinforce our arguments. Our challenge has been and continues to be finding effective ways to use these new data to convince politicians at all levels, including most particularly those involved in economic and fiscal matters, of these facts and the economic savings and benefits that could flow from greater investments in public health and well-being.

Complementary reports and the moral case

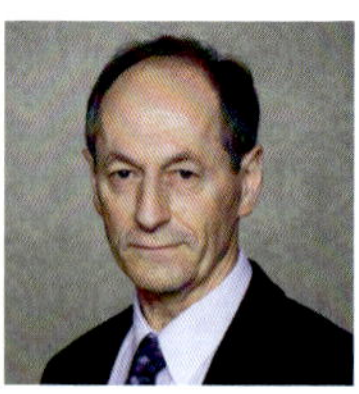

I think it was very good to have these complementary governance and economic reports. The fact that Ilona Kickbusch was doing her report on governance meant we could do less on that in our commissioned review. I was very pleased that Ilona saw social determinants of health as vital to what she was doing. And I was pleased that she was talking about how you do it, how you develop whole-of-government approaches to address social determinants.

The economic case evidence was also very helpful. But that's not the case we were making. We were making a moral case, that you should reduce health inequalities because it is the right thing to do.

Avoidable health inequalities are unjust, and that's why you need to take action. Not for economic reasons. If the economic case helps, great. But that was not our rationale.

Sir Michael Marmot, Director, University College London, Institute of Health Equity, United Kingdom

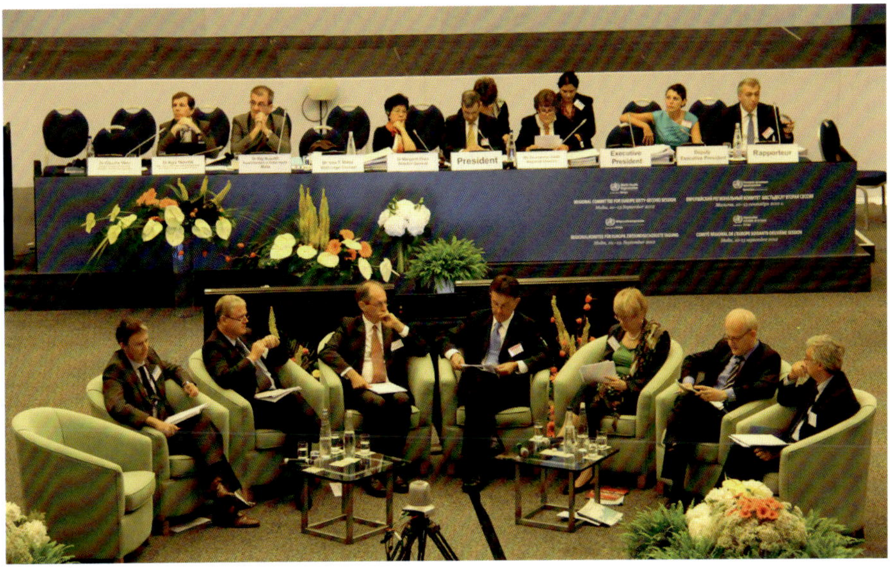

Panel discussing Health 2020 and its evidence base at the 62nd session of the Regional Committee for Europe in Malta, 10–13 September 2012. © Brian Cassar

2.2.3 Environmental determinants

WHO Headquarters and the Regional Office have also commissioned studies on environmental health determinants and risk factors, for example in relation to water and sanitation, air quality, chemical safety and climate change *(45–48)*. The stronger, broader evidence base that resulted supports better policy responses. It also helps political negotiations, typically involving different sectors, where health remains firmly in the debate if not centre stage. Here our key priority has been to raise and maintain awareness, and protect population health, from present and future environmental threats, e.g., climate change *(47)*.

A highly effective and constructive cooperation

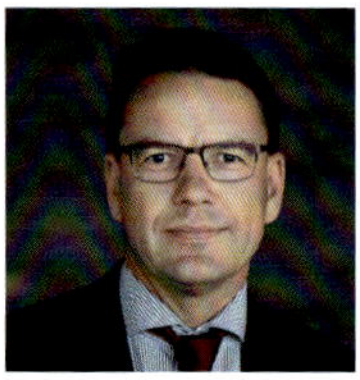

During my years as Executive Secretary of UNECE, I found the WHO Regional Office for Europe to be a very constructive and innovative partner. WHO is at the forefront of understanding the very complex linkages between environment and health, and engaging very constructively as a UN partner in a non-dogmatic and very forward-looking manner.

We have, for example, a very important and extremely effective cooperation under the convention on the trans-boundary effects of air pollution. The convention and its implementation have greatly benefitted from the scientific work done by the WHO European Centre for Environment and Health (ECEH) in Bonn. Work done under that convention over some decades has shown significant results in terms of lowering the number of pollutants by 40–70%!

Air pollution is the biggest challenge in Europe when it comes to loss of life expectancy and environmental-related diseases.

Christian Friis Bach, Former Executive Secretary, United Nations Economic Commission for Europe (UNECE)

Health 2020 also focused on the effects of living circumstances within communities on health experience. Our environmental research looked at the lived environment within the places and communities in which people spend their lives with the aim of helping the creation of health enabling and resilient communities *(49)*.[7]

As I indicated earlier these Health 2020 concepts such as community resilience and the life-course approach are strongly influenced by cultural contexts, and require new types of evidence and measurement, often qualitative rather than quantitative in nature. The WHO Regional Office for Europe therefore established an expert advisory group on the cultural contexts of health and well-being to recommend innovative ways in which this communication might be done *(50)*.

[7] Resilience is related to processes and skills that influence good individual and community health outcomes despite negative events, serious threats and hazards.

2.3 The European Action Plan for Strengthening Public Health Capacities and Services

We understood that Health 2020 could not be implemented without a strong public function within our societies supported by capable public health services. We therefore consulted widely on how to proceed to achieve this public health strengthening. Subsequently the EAP-PHS was adopted by the European Regional Committee alongside Health 2020 in 2012, as a key pillar of Health 2020 implementation. In 2018, we enhanced that commitment when the Regional Committee endorsed a new vision paper: *Advancing public health for sustainable development in the WHO European Region (51)*.

Throughout the last decade Member States and the Regional Office have been working together with partners to make public health stronger by reinforcing relevant laws, institutions, practices and human resources. In support, the organization and delivery of 10 Essential Public Health Operations (EPHOs) *(52)* were developed as a key component of the EAP-PHS (see Box 8), most importantly including the training and capacities of the public health workforce. To further support Member States, a self-assessment tool was developed to assist review of the performance of current public health capacities and services against the expectations of the EPHOs, as well as the identification of needed improvements.

PART 1

Box 8. The 10 Essential Public Health Operations

1. Surveillance and assessment of the population's health and well-being;
2. Identification of health problems and health hazards in the community;
3. Health protection services (environment, occupation, food safety);
4. Preparedness for and planning of public health emergencies;
5. Disease prevention;
6. Health promotion;
7. Assurance of a competent public health and personal health care workforce;
8. Governance, financing and evaluation of quality and effectiveness of public health services;
9. Communication for public health; and,
10. Health-related research.

Taking action to implement the EAP-PHS

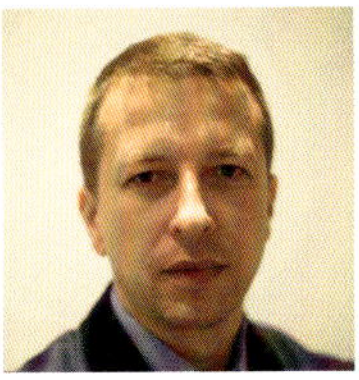

We, along with many other public health agencies and practitioners, were involved in the consultation process for Health 2020. When our members and partners gathered together in 2012 at the 5th European Public Health Conference in Malta, it was a little more than a month after Health 2020 and the EAP-PHS were unanimously adopted by all 53 Member States of the European Region, we felt a sense of 'co-production' and 'co-ownership' and were all ready to jump into implementation! United under the call: "Public Health is back!"

Follow-up on the EAP-PHS evolved over time. First, working groups for each of the 10 EPHOs (see Box 8) were set up for the initial analysis of the situation, followed by a more concerted approach to design joint initiatives focusing on the previously neglected enabler functions (EPHOs 6–9 in particular: governance, workforce, funding and communication).

ASPHER led from the start on the efforts focusing on EPHO 7 – the development of the public health workforce. We were very pleased to be able to bring the need for public health professionalization to the agenda – addressing not only the regulated professions (e.g., medical doctors, nurses and pharmacists) but also a wider workforce context.

This has led to and opened up some great opportunities for relevant development within countries which we are now observing. We already have our first success stories showing strengthened professionalization of the wider public health community and their improved abilities to address the challenging agendas in Health 2020's cross-sector, cross-discipline, cross-professional, inclusive manner.

Robert Otok, Director, Association of Schools of Public Health in the European Region (ASPHER), Belgium

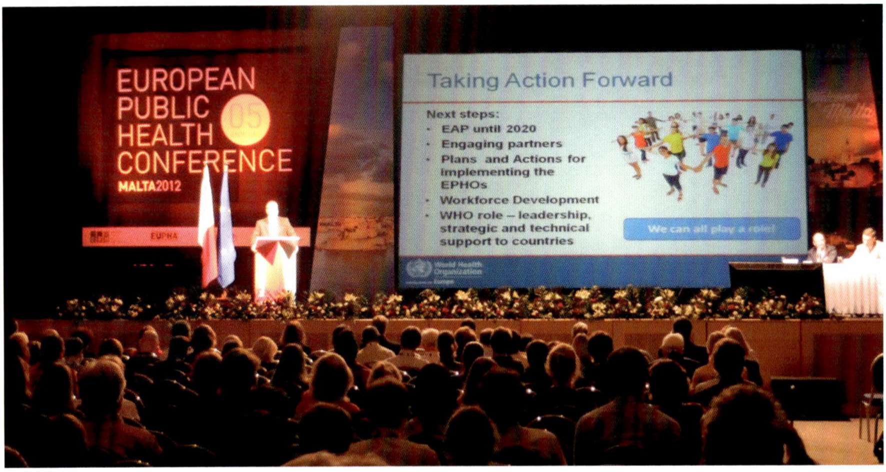

The WHO European Action Plan for Strengthening Public Health Capacities and Services is discussed at the 5th European Public Health Association (EUPHA) conference in Malta, November 2012. © Helen Corvus

Building public health competencies

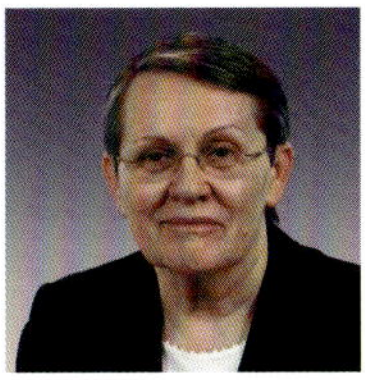

In common with other countries in the Central Eastern European bloc, from the Second World War until 1990, Hungary had a public health history based on the Semashko model. Within this model public health was primarily focused on controlling infectious diseases, so the main skills and capacities of public health practitioners related to hygiene and vaccination immunization against different infectious diseases.

While this led Hungary and other eastern European countries to maintain high levels of immunization in line with or better than the rest of Europe unfortunately it didn't prepare us well enough for the 'epidemiologic transition'. NCDs became overwhelmingly dominant as causes of morbidity and mortality among the populations of our countries.

Our key challenges today remain controlling NCDs; addressing lifestyle and environmental factors; appreciating the very strong influence of socioeconomic determinants and the needs of our most vulnerable groups e.g. Roma; and applying and understanding whole-of-government and whole-of-society approaches. These public health interventions were missing, not only in my country, but in practically all the countries of the former Soviet bloc in the European region.

We have welcomed the activities of WHO to help strengthen public health capacities and services. The activities of WHO, ASPHER and many other bilateral or international funding agencies have helped in establishing and reorganizing schools of public health. The new approaches are becoming more understood and accepted among educational authorities responsible for national accreditation in these countries *(53)*.

Róza Ádány, Professor of Public Health, University of Debrecen, Hungary

Since the adoption of the EAP-PHS the Regional Office has continued to advocate for strengthening public health institutions, for example, through the development of the Coalition of Partners (see Section 9.3.4.9) and continued joint work and publications with the Organisation for Economic Co-operation and Development (OECD) *(55)* and the European Observatory on Health Systems and Policies on the economic case for health promotion and disease prevention *(33)*. To strengthen the evidence base for reforming public health institutions, for example, the WHO Regional Office for Europe and the European Observatory on Health Systems and Policies produced a comparative study on organizing and financing public health services in the European Region *(56)*.

First, we need a sustainable, high-quality workforce

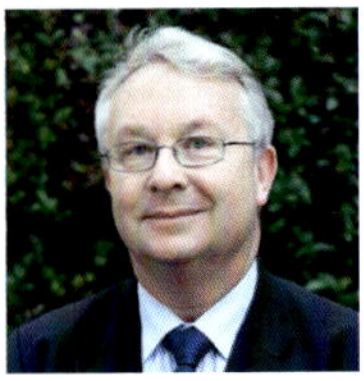

To understand the challenge in terms of competencies we really need to step back and look at the overall public health work force because there is no point in trying to promote competencies if there is nobody there to do the work.

The difficulty is that in public health, expertise in Europe is very highly concentrated. There are a number of countries that have well-established career pathways, and highly motivated, highly skilled individuals. Looked at objectively, in terms of high impact of research outputs some countries, like the United Kingdom, Sweden, the Netherlands, Italy, and Spain, have high levels of expertise. Such outputs and contributions are lacking in other parts of the Region. I think that's partly because we've been unable to develop the career pathways, funding streams and incentives for health professionals to stay in public health who might otherwise go into areas like clinical medicine. So, the first thing is to have a sustainable high-quality work force, and the next step is to make sure they have the appropriate competencies.

I think most of that work has to take place within individual countries because the amount of money that's involved is way beyond the resources WHO or any other international organization would have.

The WHO Regional Office for Europe has been providing some major intellectual contributions in support of people advocating for that, as well as making the case somewhat indirectly. Regional Committees, for example, now have very good scientific and technical presentations, and a lot of expertise.

When I first was working with WHO in 1995, I was told we do not do research, we promote values. That has now changed. It is a much more technical Organization, and over the last ten years, especially, has created a culture of knowledge-sharing, with much more data and evaluative research being presented at Regional Committee meetings, as well as high quality publications.

I think Member States' Governments have realized they have to keep up with all of this; they need the capacity to do the things that need to be done. Coupled with that also there has been the recognition that public health has changed. Now the degree of sophistication of epidemiology, certain monitoring surveillance systems, the data explosion with the internet, etc. have completely transformed what public health professionals need to do.

We need highly skilled people, and the challenge is that we are now competing for such people skilled in information technology with very highly paid jobs in the financial services and pharmaceutical industries. I think there is a long way to go to ensure that we can provide competitive rewards.

Martin McKee, Professor of European Public Health, London School of Hygiene and Tropical Medicine (LSHTM), United Kingdom

2.4 New tools and approaches to support Member States

Our Regional Office staff worked hard to make Health 2020 accessible and practical for all Member States – to make Health 2020 the 'easy' choice.

2.4.1 Implementation package

Immediately after Health 2020 was adopted by the Regional Committee in 2012, we started working on the creation of a 'package' of implementation methodologies and tools which could provide guidance to Member States. We also developed, a self-assessment tool for national health policies, strategies and plans and examples of best Health 2020 practices and applications. This implementation package and other tools are now on-line and are regularly updated *(26, 57)*. Practical materials for use and adaptation at national and local levels are included in the package – for example, communication materials to introduce Health 2020.

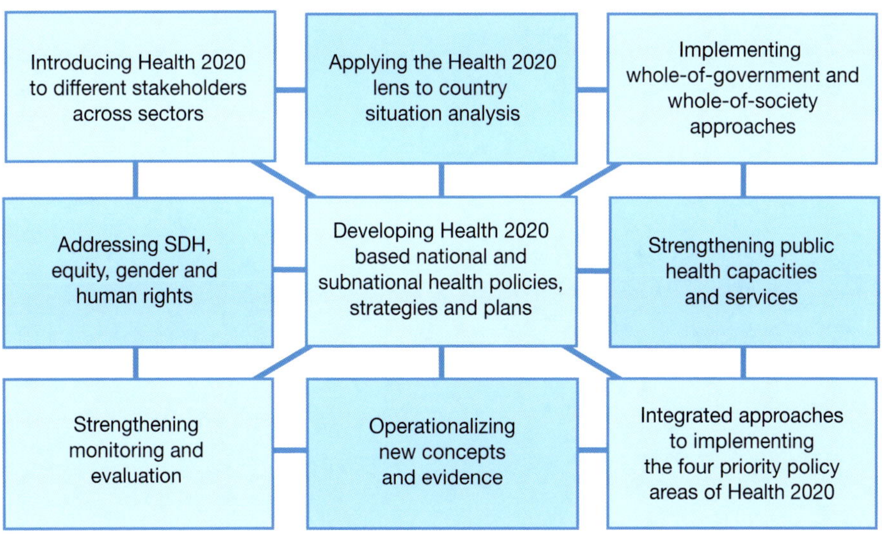

Fig. 7. The WHO Regional Office for Europe Health 2020 implementation package.
Source: Health 2020 implementation package *(218)*.

'National glasses'

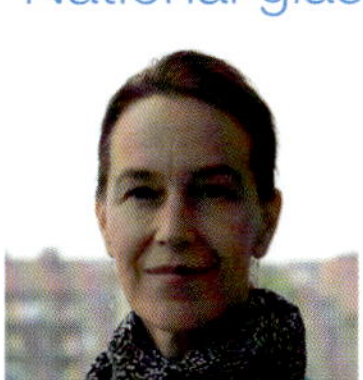

A key success factor for adaptation of Health 2020 to national level, is to read the framework using your own 'national glasses' – and see the challenges and solutions from your own country context.

Director General, National Board for Health and Welfare, Sweden

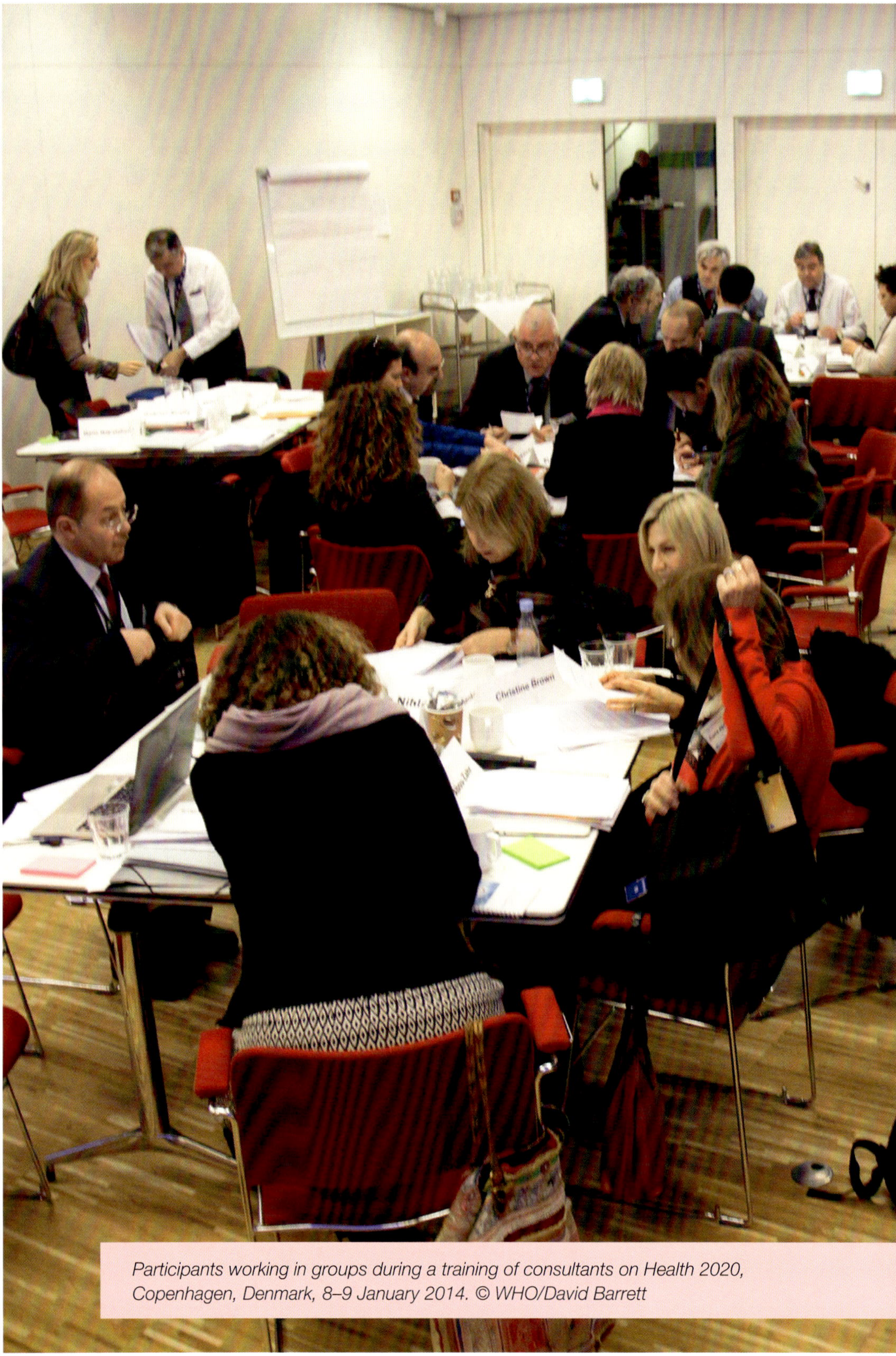

Participants working in groups during a training of consultants on Health 2020, Copenhagen, Denmark, 8–9 January 2014. © WHO/David Barrett

2.4.2 Building intersectoral support

Intersectoral action supporting Health 2020 has been highly visible in several intercountry dialogues. Examples include the sub-regional high-level event on Health 2020 implementation in Tashkent, Uzbekistan, in November 2014; technical meetings in Paris, France, and Berlin, Germany, in April 2015; the International Health Forum to Commemorate the 20th Anniversary of the National Health Programme of Turkmenistan in Ashgabat in July 2015; the South-eastern Europe Health Network ministerial meeting in Belgrade, Serbia, in June 2015; and the Second High-level Meeting of the WHO Small Countries Initiative in Andorra in July 2015.

The high-level conference 'Promoting intersectoral and interagency action for health and well-being in the WHO European Region' held in Paris on 7–8 December 2016 was of great importance. It focused on strengthening intersectoral cooperation between the health, education and social sectors in the WHO European Region, to achieve better, more equal health and social outcomes for children and adolescents, and their families. The discussions helped to increase understanding and build stronger policy synergies across sectors, benefiting health and health equity. It was the first time a WHO high-level meeting had brought together representatives from the respective ministries for the three sectors to discuss how to implement intersectoral and cross-governmental policies to ensure that no child is left behind – a cornerstone of both Health 2020 and the United Nations 2030 Agenda for Sustainable Development.

PART 1

The conference culminated in the adoption of the Paris Declaration 'Partnerships for the health and well-being of our young and future generations, and a 'Proposal for the establishment of an Ad Hoc Regional Platform for Working Together for Better Health and Well-being for All'. In the Declaration, Member States committed to work together across the three sectors to increase understanding and build stronger policy synergies to benefit health and health equity. WHO, and other international organizations and agencies, committed to continue on this path, both through the Regional platform, and other future initiatives.

One direct success of the platform was the establishment of the UNESCO Chair and WHO Collaborating Centre for Research in Education and Health a joint WHO–UNESCO initiative to build on the achievements of the Paris conference and ensure continued collaboration between the health and education sectors. A further successful outcome has been the commitment of all 1400 WHO Healthy Cities in the European Region to ensuring that every school within their city is a WHO health promoting school.

There have also been several collaborations between the WHO Regional Office for Europe and other organizations and institutions on strengthening intersectoral action. Some examples included:

1. supporting the development of intersectoral environment and health action plans in countries *(58)*;

2. assisting countries to improve the overall quality of their laboratory services, through the Better Labs for Better Health initiative *(59)*;
3. facilitating joint action by the transport, interior, health, finance and urban development sectors in policy areas from legislation and enforcement of laws to rapid access to emergency trauma care, as well as promotion of social marketing campaigns to modify risk behaviours *(60)*;
4. playing a catalytic role with other sectors in achieving a 50% reduction in road traffic injury mortality in Europe *(61)*; and,
5. signing a Protocol on Water and Health in 1999 providing a holistic policy framework for the WHO European Region in achieving improvements in safe water, sanitation and hygiene (WaSH) at Regional and country levels *(62)*.The WHO Regional Office for Europe, together with the United Nations Economic Commission for Europe (UNECE), continue to provide secretariat services to the Protocol and support Member States in setting and implementing national targets.

UNECE and WHO – good and historic colleagues

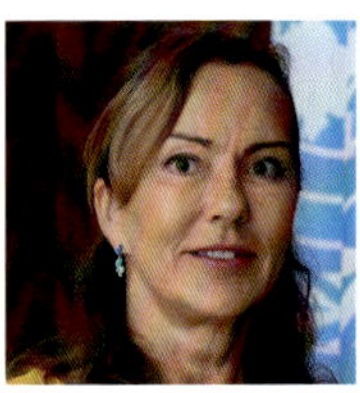

UNECE and WHO are very good and historic colleagues with a long tradition of cooperation. We have been doing work together since the 1990s and now with Agenda 2030 our work together is improving, strengthening and deepening.

We work on many programmes together. For example, we jointly created the Pan-European Programme on Transport, Health and Environment (THE PEP) in 2002. The forward-looking programme is driven by our Member States in the European Region and promotes the inclusion of environment and health issues into transport policies. THE PEP brings together a wide range of multisectoral stakeholders which has helped to identify green jobs in the transport sector, promote cycling and walking and has developed a variety of unique and powerful tools for measuring the impact of transport, environment and health policy-making.

The Protocol on Water and Health is another example. This Protocol is under our UNECE Convention on the Protection and Use of Transboundary Watercourses and International Lakes. Under this protocol, together with WHO, we are able to provide strong support to our Member States in the Region in achieving clean water, safe sanitation and hygiene for all.

We have good cooperative activities in many other areas, as well. These include a joint task force on health aspects of air pollution, an interagency coordination group for industrial and chemical accidents and road safety. We benefit from WHO's expertise on health impact assessment under our protocol on strategic environmental assessment.

WHO Europe is also involved in UNECE environmental performance reviews. Our cooperation is very rich and has been really strengthening over time.

Olga Algayerova, Executive Secretary, United Nations Economic Commission for Europe (UNECE)

2.5 Aligning national policies, strategies and implementation plans with Health 2020

One of the great privileges I have had as Regional Director has been the opportunity to visit so many countries and to participate in national launches and debates on Health 2020, as well as in national health policy development. I have met with presidents and prime ministers to discuss how health can be improved equitably using whole-of-government, whole-of-society and health-in-all-policies approaches.

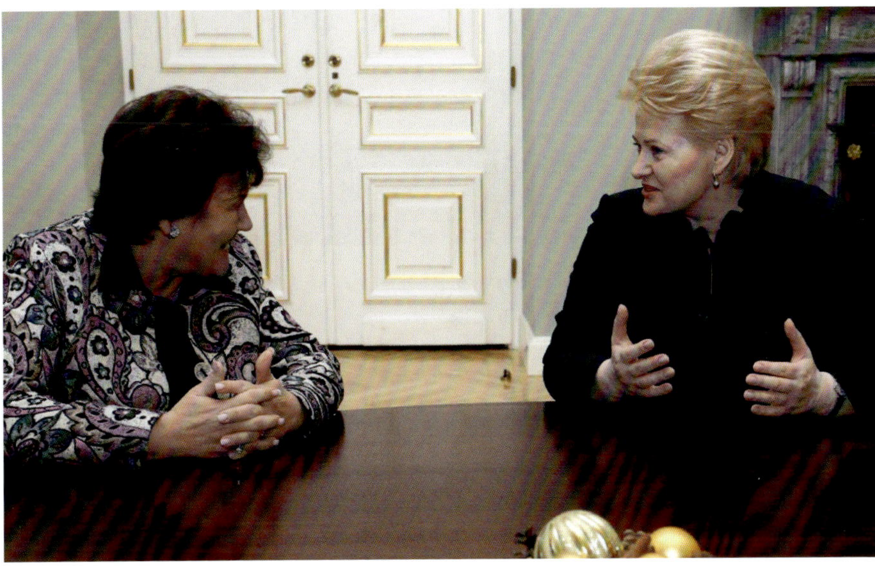

Zsuzsanna Jakab, WHO Regional Director for Europe, meeting with Dalia Grybauskaite, President of Lithuania, during her visit to Lithuania, 28–29 November 2012. © WHO

PART 1

Progress has been rapid in aligning national policies, strategies and implementation plans with Health 2020. By 2016, 93% of 42 responding countries indicated that they had a national health policy aligned with Health 2020; 35% more than in 2010. In addition to having aligned policies, 86% of countries reported having implementation plans, and 98% of the responding countries reported having a policy or strategy to reduce health inequities, an increase of 10% since 2010. By 2016, 88% of responding countries reported that they had defined targets or indicators for Health 2020, which was 15% higher than in 2010 *(54)*.

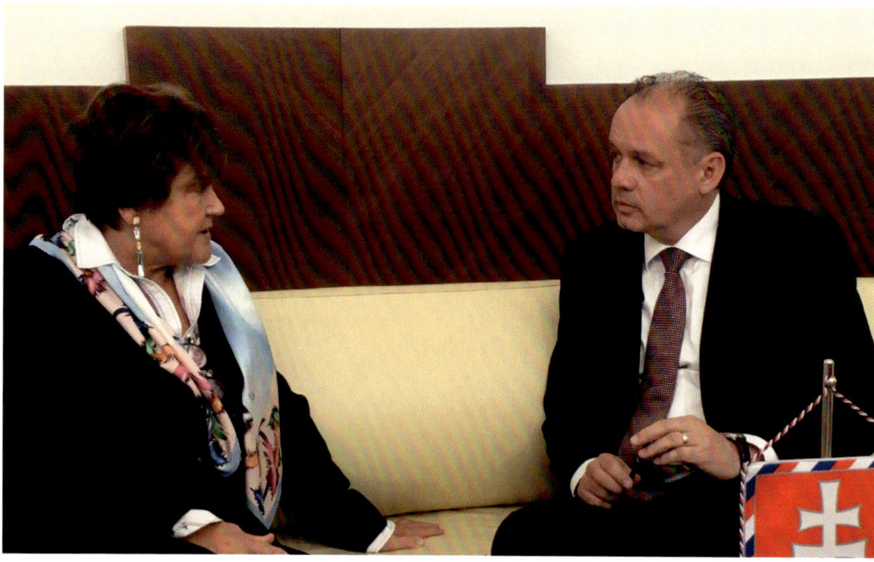

Zsuzsanna Jakab, WHO Regional Director for Europe, meeting with Andrej Kiska, President of the Slovak Republic in 2016. © WHO

Since 2012, countries have also introduced a variety of new Health 2020 related and inspired policies with broadened scope of application. Increasingly, these policies reflect Health 2020 values, key objectives and action priorities. They emphasize, for example, addressing social determinants of health such as poverty, the importance of resolving health inequities, helping disadvantaged groups, creating the conditions for a healthy start in life, expanding UHC, and improving the environment. They do this with a solid political commitment to the idea of 'Health as a Political Choice', and to the underlying values of health as a human right, and to solidarity, equity and the gender perspective (see Box 9).

Box 9. Examples of national plans aligned with Health 2020

1. Portugal – The National Health Plan is a value-based and action orientated instrument, designed to be adopted at national, regional and local levels. The Plan covers most of Health 2020 policy framework elements. The Plan has the values and principles of transparency and accountability that allow the confidence and appreciation of the stakeholders. These principles include involvement and participation of all stakeholders in the health creative processes; reduction of health inequalities as a basis for the promotion of equity and social justice; integration and continuity of care provided to citizens; a health system that responds quickly to needs, making

the best use of available resources to avoid waste, and; sustainability, in order to preserve these values for the future *(63)*.

A number of health goals are set out under this Plan: reducing premature mortality at or under 70 years to below 20%; increasing healthy life expectancy at 65 by 30%; reducing the prevalence of smoking in the adult population and eliminating exposure to environmental tobacco smoke; and controlling the incidence and prevalence of overweight and obesity in children and schoolchildren.

2. Ireland – The Healthy Ireland Framework 2013–2025 calls for all sectors of society and the whole of government to be proactively involved in improving the health and well-being of the population, as it is based on an understanding of the wider determinants of health, e.g. economic status, education, housing, the physical environment, as well as policy decisions taken by Government, the individual choices people make, and the participation of people in their communities. The Framework explicitly recognizes the importance of working across the whole of government and the whole of society *(64)*.

   To ensure the former, a cross-sectoral group comprising high-level representatives from government departments and key state agencies has been established to support the implementation of Healthy Ireland. The group monitors and evaluates implementation and provides clear communications channels across Government. The membership includes health, social, environmental and economic sectors. For example, the Environmental Protection Agency (EPA) in its draft strategic plan commits to 'the development of stronger and more robust approaches and promoting the essential role that protecting the environment plays in improving the health of the population'.

   The Healthy Ireland Council was established. This is a multi-stakeholder national forum that provides a platform to connect and mobilize communities, families and individuals into a national movement with one aim: supporting everyone to enjoy the best possible health and well-being. The Council comprises 35 members from a wide range of sectors including health, academia, older people, sport, nongovernmental organizations, media, youth and diversity. They are recognized leaders and influencers in their respective fields who have a genuine passion for health and well-being.

Health 2020 policy and strategy documents have been translated by the Office into all official languages and by some Member States into other national languages. These have been disseminated widely in support of awareness-raising campaigns and other work by WHO country offices. Health 2020 has also been presented and debated in public health journals and media across the Region.

Health 2020 – involving county councils and municipalities in Sweden

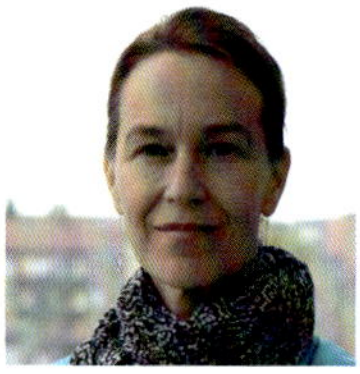

Government agencies in Sweden, such as my own agency and our Public Health Agency, have been very much involved in Health 2020. It meant active participation in consultations, delivering input and discussing issues of relevance for us, and we are glad to have taken part in this work.

We took the opportunity to use the finished product by translating the summary into Swedish so we could send it to all county councils and municipalities and get them involved in the work.

We were also proud to host the Nordic-Baltic High-Level Meeting on Health 2020 in October 2016.

Olivia Wigzell, Director General, National Board for Health and Welfare, Sweden

Health 2020 in Tajikistan

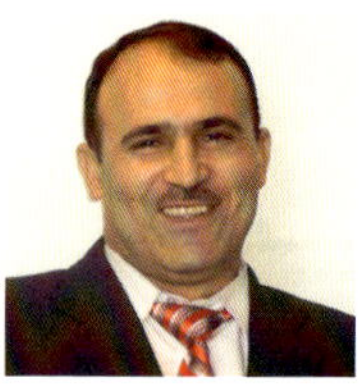

Health 2020 became a good source of inspiration and guidance for Tajikistan in further developing of our National Health Strategy for 2010–2020.

As a Member State of the WHO European Region, Tajikistan is involved in a variety of different regional Health 2020 informed programmes, including: IHR, immunization, NCDs, AMR, tobacco control programmes, reduction of traffic accidents, oncological diseases and diabetes.

Disunity of actions, inefficient health care systems, especially at primary health care (PHC) level and the high-cost of health programme implementation forced us to seek new problem-solving approaches to address our difficulties. Challenges included introducing new health financing mechanisms, managing PHC facilities, recruiting doctors and nurses, providing affordable medicines, etc.

Starting from 2010, we initiated an Annual Health Summit, where all national and foreign partners discussed questions of health strategy development and solutions, as well as helped us prioritize our next year's implementation plans.

Improved organization and strengthening of national and regional agencies were achieved with the support of Ministries and Departments involved in healthy lifestyle formation, integration of relevant structures with primary health care facilities, training of medical staff and development of family medicine. They all contributed to the improvement of health indicators at national level, for example, in children and maternal mortality; the reduction of infectious diseases, and improvement of indicators on human resources for health.

The Health 2020 framework encouraged us to expand the participation of other Ministries (Ministry of Finance, Ministry of Economic Development and Trade), regional, city and district khukumats (administrations) in finding solutions to existing health system problems.

The annual message of the President of the Republic of Tajikistan further promoted participation of other relevant Ministries and Agencies (Internal Affairs, Justice, Finance, Education and Science, Women's Affairs and Sports Committee) to allow Tajikistan to address specific challenges related to HIV/AIDS, tuberculosis, tobacco control and improvement of population physical activity.

Another important development has been the establishment of the National Health Council under the Government of the Republic of Tajikistan, where all health sector problems are discussed and settled on a cross-sectoral basis.

Salomudin Jabbor Yusufi, Head of the Department of Medical and Pharmaceutical Education, Health Personnel Policy and Science Ministry of Health and Social Protection, Republic of Tajikistan

Health 2020 in action – Georgia

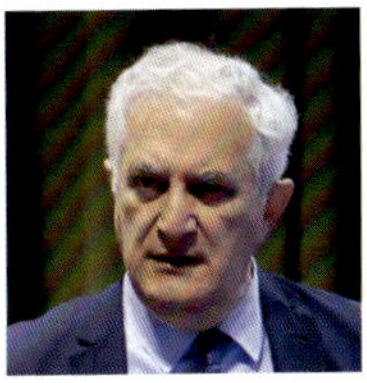

I am happy that Georgia has introduced actions recommended in the Health 2020 policy framework for developing universality in health policies and interventions to improve population health, affordability and accessibility to health care services, and reduce the effect of negative social determinants.

WHO's role was significant in integrating Health 2020 approaches and principles in Georgia. The WHO Regional Office for Europe, the WHO Barcelona Office for Health Systems Strengthening and WHO representatives played a very important role in advising and helping to advance universal health coverage, thus expanding access to the health care services for all, and promoting financial protection.

The most enabling factor in the country for implementing Health 2020 principles was a supportive political situation in 2012 and strong political commitment, unlike the different political vision of the previous Government, which was more oriented on targeted health care, thus hindering implementation of Health 2020 principles.

Amiran Gamkrelidze, Director General of the National Center for Disease Control and Public Health, Georgia

Health 2020 Development – Finland

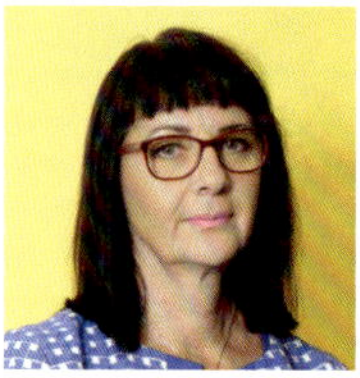

We have a long tradition of developing and implementing broad health policies in Finland. Already in the 80s we were one of the pilot countries for primary health care and the WHO European Health for All programme. And we have continued playing such a Regional 'pioneering' role with our health-in-all-policies work during our EU presidency in 2006. Health 2020 is in line with what we are and have been doing in Finland with its broad health policy perspective, intersectionality, Health for All policies, equity, etc.

Because of that, we have been very actively involved. We are very pleased with how it has developed over these ten years. Health 2020 is a valuable action framework on which we can now all more easily build our sustainable development implementation work.

Taru Koivisto, Director of the Department for Wellbeing and Services, Ministry of Social Affairs and Health, Finland

2.6 Aligning Regional strategies with Health 2020

Since its adoption, all WHO European Regional strategies, action plans, ministerial conferences and other high-level meetings have been based on the principles and content of Health 2020. This integrated approach has increasingly improved coherence within the work of the Office. The Health 2020 policy framework provides a strategic overview for health improvement and helps solve operational issues in both health and health services.

One example of a transformational ministerial conference that used the Health 2020 approach to expand both strategic and operational understanding of health improvement was the ground-breaking WHO European Ministerial Conference on the Life-course Approach in the Context of Health 2020, held in Minsk, Belarus, in October 2015. Here, we discussed the evidence and policy implications of new research findings on the genetic, social, economic, commercial, and behavioural determinants of health, and the interactions between these factors in the living environment of human beings across their life-course.

Standing up to commercial interests

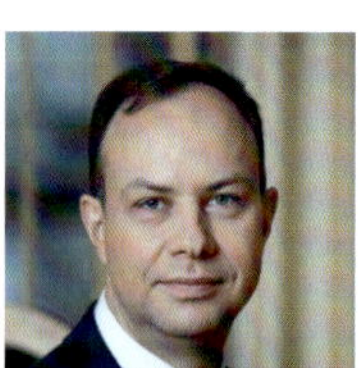

We had a very tough case on vaccine procurement. We asked the company for a preliminary price and planned our budget accordingly. After the decision to purchase, the company came with a much higher price, 25% higher. So, we asked the WHO Regional Office for help. First, for their opinion about the specific vaccine being offered. Second, about the particular vaccination scheme we were interested in because countries use different schemes and different formulations. These have big implications for price.

We asked WHO to make a cost-benefit evaluation for us. They came back to us with the price of a vaccine they thought would be pharma-economically effective. It was a fantastic price and one which we knew we could afford. So even though we knew that no one would get the vaccine for that price, we used that for the negotiation with this company. They were very unhappy and told us that this price was crazy. So, I asked them, can I tell the WHO that your official opinion about their experts' estimate is that it is ridiculous and crazy? This 'somehow' got to the media… and the company lowered their price to the initial price they gave.

At the beginning they were scaring us that they could not provide us the vaccine at this price, and so on. But WHO expertise helped us a lot with the negotiations and now we can protect our children with this vaccine.

Aurelijus Veryga, Minister of Health, Lithuania

The Minsk Declaration summarized actions to consider and commitments agreed to at the Conference, which reflected the objectives and priority action areas of Health 2020 (see Box 10) *(65)*.

Box 10. Minsk Declaration – Actions to consider

1. Strengthen or develop healthy and health-promoting conditions, structures and processes in settings where people work, learn or live that take into consideration the life-course approach: from kindergartens to schools, workplaces, districts or cities, and homes for the elderly.
2. Create environments free of tobacco, alcohol, recreational drug use and violence, where access to affordable healthy diets is facilitated, physical activity is promoted; and settings where public engagement and active leisure pursuits are encouraged.
3. Create safe, decent and family-friendly work environments with as much job security as possible, aiding individuals in their search for employment as well as stimulating businesses in the creation of secure jobs and providing working conditions that minimize occupational exposures to psychological and environmental risks and injuries.
4. Protect parents and children from stresses that may affect the next generation, including protection from adverse environmental exposures, the effects of which are likely to be irreversible and may also become heritable.
5. Strengthen the capacity of health professionals and health systems to act in a person-centred fashion with respect for all, coordinating the needs of individuals and groups, fostering interdisciplinary approaches, and empowering dignity and autonomy, self-help and self-care.
6. Take multisectoral actions to promote health partnerships, policies, programmes and coordinating mechanisms.
7. Raise awareness that the irrational use of natural resources by our present generation is threatening the well-being and even survival of our children and succeeding generations.

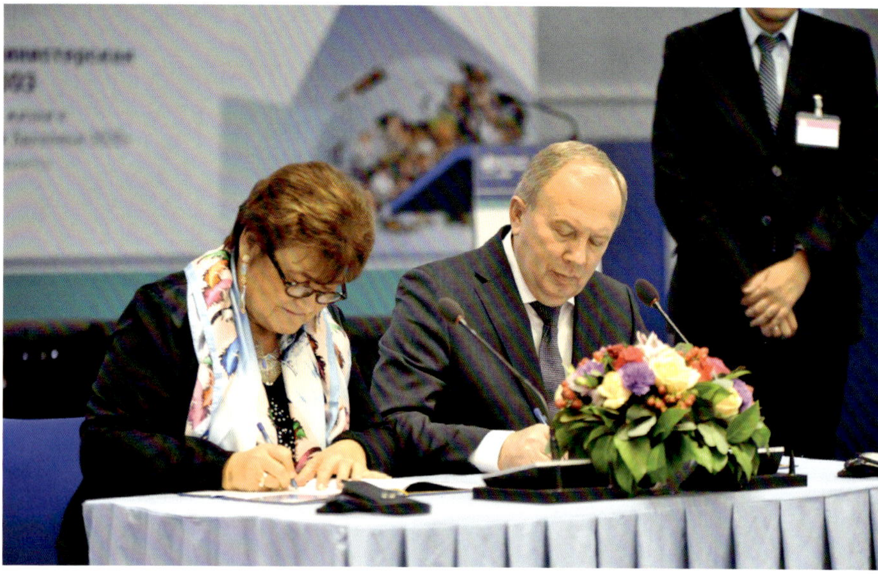

Zsuzsanna Jakab with Vasily Zharko, Minister of Health of Belarus, signing the Minsk Declaration, Minsk, Belarus, 12 February, 2015. © WHO/Evgenyi Krech

Another example of transformative Regional policy action, built on the Health 2020 framework, focused on the development of strategies for women's and men's health and well-being across the life-course, and a new commitment to gender-responsive health policy.

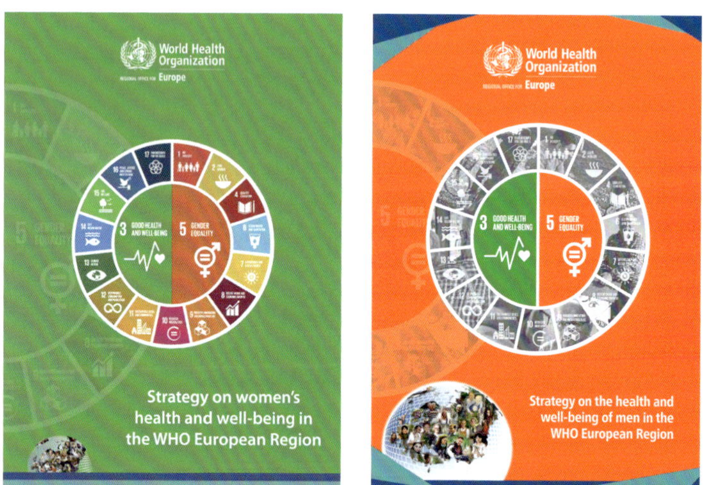

Fig. 8. The WHO Regional Committee for Europe adopted strategies on women's (2016) and men's (2018) health and well-being in the WHO European Region.
Source: Strategy on women's health and well-being *(66)* and Strategy on the health and well-being of men *(67)*.

Gender relations include how power and access to, and control over resources, are distributed between the sexes. Since gender relations are a social construct, they can be transformed over time to become more equitable. When individuals do not fit established gender norms, they often face discrimination or social exclusion – which adversely affects health.

In all countries, health indicators present differences among men and women across socioeconomic groups and across the life-course in health outcomes, exposure to main risks, adoption of healthy behaviours, access to and use of services, response from providers, and use of formal and informal care. Biological factors in men and women are important in shaping these differences, but they cannot be explained by biology alone. Gender is a social construct that interacts with, but is different from, biological sex. It refers to the socially constructed roles, behaviours and attributes that a given society considers appropriate for women and men.

Acknowledging, understanding and acting upon the impact of these norms is using a gender approach to health and well-being. This approach strengthens the interconnections between SDG 5 goal on gender equality and empowering of women with the health-related targets under SDG 3.

Enhancing gender and rights action

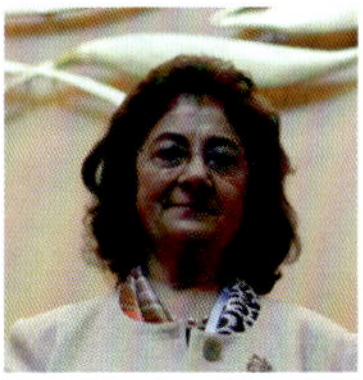

Gender and rights issues usually do not get their deserved attention in many countries, even in the WHO European Region.

I remember when I was a member of the Standing Committee of the Regional Committee (SCRC) in 1999 we sent a questionnaire to the Member States asking about the most important health related issues in their respected countries. Very few countries even mentioned gender issues and none as a priority.

I noticed that after Dr Jakab became Regional Director, programmes on gender and rights issues were strengthened at the Regional Office. She was able to recruit professionals who were qualified in gender and rights topics.

For the first time our University was able to work with staff in the WHO Regional Office and carry out studies on gender and rights analyses of national legislations. The Regional Office has also started to have more collaboration with the WHO headquarters where there is an established Gender and Rights Advisory Panel (GAP.)

Ayse Akin, Professor Public Health, Maternal and Child and Reproductive Health, Baskent University, Ankara, Turkey

In the WHO European Region, the *Strategy for women's health and well-being (2016)* and the *Strategy for the health and well-being of men (2018)* provide a comprehensive working framework for improving health and well-being in Europe through gender-responsive approaches *(66, 67)*. Both strategies highlight the importance such an approach for improving health and well-being among men and women and for decreasing inequities across the Region and within countries. They are also consistent with SDGs which highlight the importance of gender and human rights-based approaches in accelerating transformative and sustainable progress *(68)*.

The recommendations of the strategies illustrate how factors affecting notions of masculinity and femininity and the way gender roles are defined in societies have a massive effect not only on exposure to risk factors, but also on the responses given by health systems. Moreover, they highlight the many interlinkages between gender equality and health policy and explain how better policy coherence between the two would accelerate health progress for both women and men.

The adoption of the two strategies represented a landmark achievement as the WHO European Region became the first region with a comprehensive framework for how to address gender in health policy and practice.

Moreover, the Strategy on the health and well-being of men is the first-ever WHO strategy addressing men's health issues from a gender perspective. This comprehensive strategic framework aims to support Member States to develop policies and programmes that are rights-based and gender responsive in order to improve health service delivery and reduce health inequities.

Key lessons learned for the effective integration of gender approaches in Member States, based on the recent experiences in the WHO European Region, include the necessity to have a strong evidence-based technical programme on gender and gender equality; the usefulness of governing body processes to bring different parts of the organization together with a common aim; and the need for strong support by senior management for the approach and process.

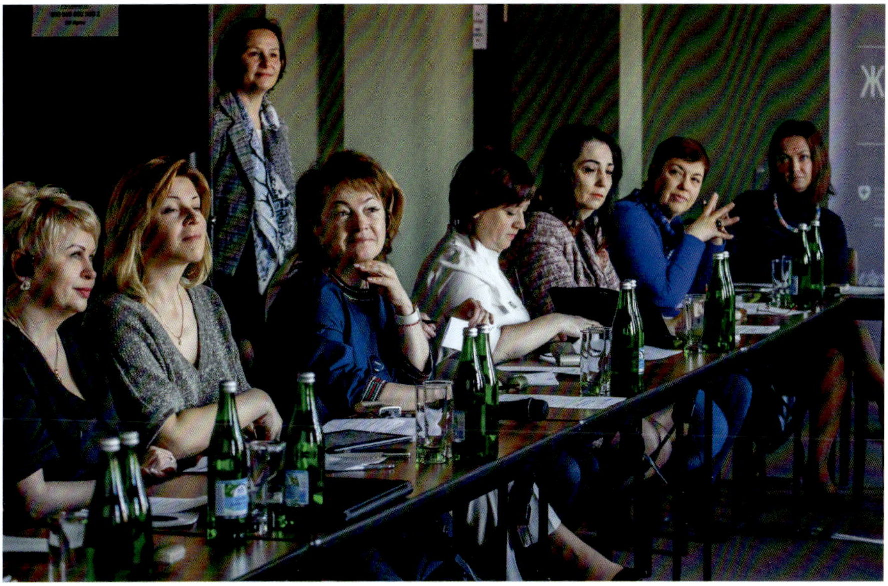

In order to empower and support the development of female leaders who drive and will drive public health reforms, the Ministry of Health of Ukraine, with technical support from WHO and contributions from ASPHER and Maastricht University, organized a seminar on "Women Leadership in Public Health" held in Kyiv, Ukraine, 16–18 May 2017. © WHO

The commitments made in these strategies are reflected in Member States' statements from high-level meetings and other forums, one example being the outcome statement from the High-level Regional Meeting: Health Systems Respond to NCDs held in Sitges, Spain, in April 2018. Another example was the *Action Plan for implementation of the European Strategy for the Prevention and Control of Noncommunicable Diseases 2012–2016*, together with a set of related policy mandates adopted in Ashgabat and Vienna. These included declarations on alcohol, tobacco, food and nutrition, and physical activity *(12, 69, 70)*.

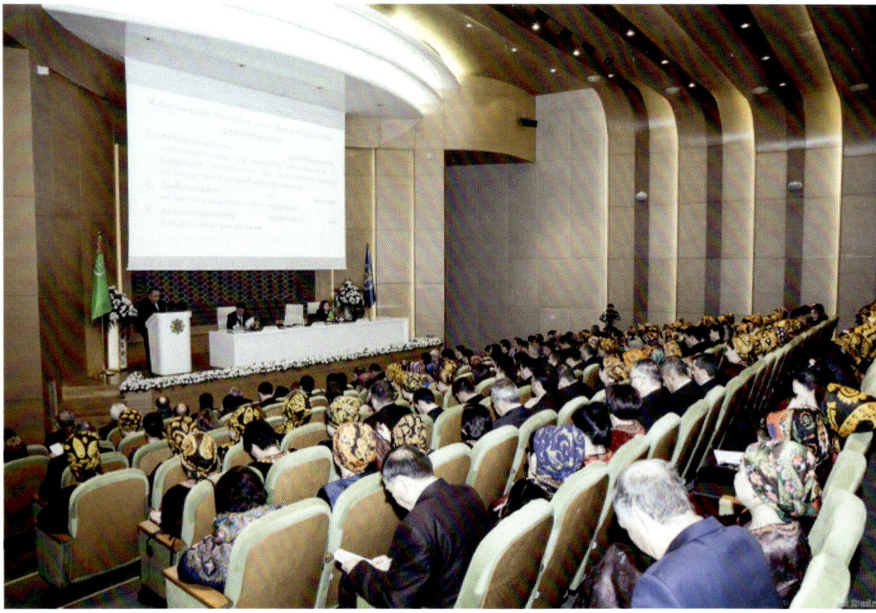

On 4 December 2017, Turkmenistan marked the 4th anniversary of the implementation of the Ashgabat Declaration on the Prevention and Control of NCDs in the Context of Health 2020 by hosting a conference dedicated to reviewing achievements in this area and setting objectives for the future. © WHO

The Action Plan adopted core elements of the prevention of NCDs as a contribution to reducing health inequities in the European Region.

Amongst the NCDs, the largest group of causes of premature mortality in the Region are cardiovascular diseases and their risk factors. These contribute greatly to the differences we see in life expectancy between the eastern and western parts of the Region. On a positive note, the European Region has seen a narrowing of that gap over the past decade, and the achieving of greater equity among countries. Most of this progress is due to improvements in countries with the highest premature mortality. However, the absolute differences between countries remain large. Sadly, examples of inequities abound, including the inadequate detection and management of cervical cancer in women, and premature deaths from heart attack or stroke in men.

The European environment and health process (see Box 11 and Section 9.3.5.1) is another good practice example in the development of national health polices, strategies and plans based upon all determinants of health, and constructed around the principles and institutional requirements of multisectoral action.

The foundations were laid through large changes in institutional processes and the power of environmental Ministries and were supported through a series of conferences: Frankfurt (1989), Helsinki (1994), London (1999), Budapest (2004), Parma (2010) and Ostrava (2017), which together drove this process.

Box 11. The European Environment and Health Process (EHP)

The recognition in Health 2020 of the importance of environmental determinants of health has given emphasis to the European Environment and Health Process (EHP), which was initiated in the 1980s by the Member States of the European Region to help eliminate the most significant environmental threats to human health. Progress towards this goal is driven by a series of ministerial conferences held every five years organized by WHO in collaboration with the United Nations Economic Commission for Europe (UNECE). WHO European Member States have nominated representatives from the health and the environment sectors to the European Environment and Health Task Force.

The EHP thus represents a pioneering experience of the intersectoral collaboration which is advocated in Health 2020. Under the programme additional partnerships have been developed, such as the THE PEP – a joint WHO and UNECE policy platform.

The EHP was reviewed in 2015 in the light of implementation of the commitments made at the Fifth Ministerial Conference on Environment and Health in 2010. This discussion was framed and inspired by Health 2020, and produced consensus on a roadmap, which includes 'traditional' risk factors – such as air pollution, access to safe water, and chemical safety – as well as broad areas – such as climate change, energy, waste, and cities – that reflect the emphasis placed by Health 2020 on the determinants of health.

The political commitment to address environmental determinants was strongly renewed at our Sixth Ministerial Conference on Environment and Health, held in Ostrava, Czechia in June 2107 (see Section 9.3.5.1). It was another excellent example of strategic partnerships. In the Declaration, Member States committed to enhance implementation through the development of national portfolios of actions on environment and health by the end of 2018.

All Regional and global strategies and action plans reviewed and/or adopted by the WHO European Regional Committee in the years just prior to and since Health 2020 have been (re)considered and implemented in alignment with Health 2020. Examples (see further discussions in Part II) include:

- *Strategy and action plan for healthy ageing in Europe, 2012–2020 (71).*
- *Investing in children: the European child and adolescent health strategy 2015–2020 (72).*
- *Investing in children: the European child maltreatment prevention action plan 2015–2020 (73).*
- *Action Plan for Sexual and Reproductive Health: towards achieving the 2030 Agenda for Sustainable Development in the WHO European Region – leaving no one behind (74).*
- *European Vaccine Action Plan 2015–2020* as a regional interpretation of the *Global Vaccine Action Plan 2011–2020 (75).*
- *European strategic action plan on antibiotic resistance (76).*
- *Advancing food safety initiatives: strategic plan for food safety including foodborne zoonoses 2013–2022 (77).*
- *European strategic directions for strengthening nursing and midwifery towards Health 2020 goals (78).*
- *Action plans for the prevention and control of HIV/AIDS and of viral hepatitis in the WHO European Region 2016–2021 (79, 80).*
- *Framework for control and prevention of soil-transmitted helminthiases in the WHO European Region 2016–2020 (81).*

2.7 SDGs and Health 2020

Member States of the European Region had a head start in tackling the health-related SDGs as Health 2020 anticipated the global processes that led to SDG development and the United Nations 2030 Agenda for Sustainable Development. The goals of both the SDGs and Health 2020 are universal, integrated, interdependent and indivisible. Indeed the catchphrase of the SDGs –'leaving no one behind' – applies equally well to Health 2020.

Improved health and well-being depend substantially on political commitment. Both the SDGs and Health 2020 advocate for high-level leadership for health and well-being, and strong intersectoral mechanisms to address the many risk factors and determinants of health. Both also focus on whole-of-government, whole-of-society and health-in-all-policies approaches.

As shown in Fig. 9 below, of the 17 SDGs, SDG 3 is the key health goal. It commits countries to 'ensure healthy lives and promote well-being for all at all ages'. Each of the SDGs has one or more targets directly and/or indirectly related to health, reflecting the complex pattern of health determinants. Within SDG 3, target 3.8 commits to 'achieve universal health coverage, including financial risk protection, access to quality essential health-care services and access to safe, effective, quality and affordable essential medicines and vaccines for all'.

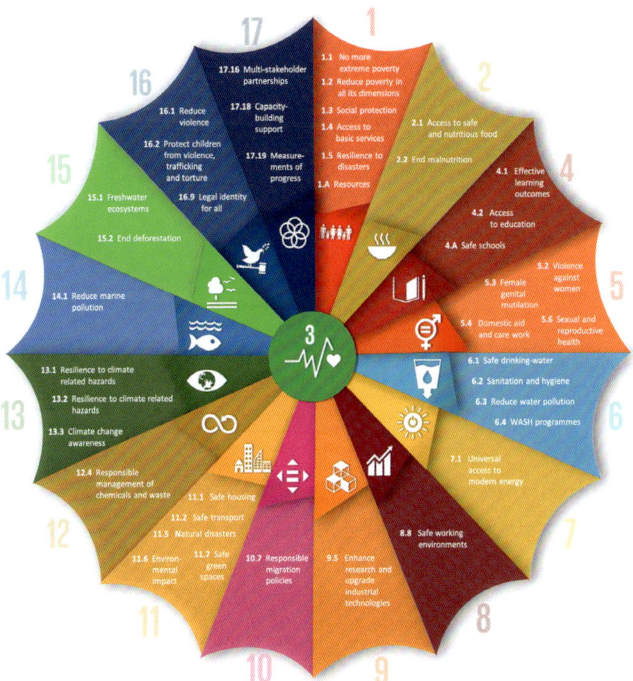
17
17.16 Multi-stakeholder partnerships
17.18 Capacity-building support
17.19 Measurements of progress
1
1.1 No more extreme poverty
1.2 Reduce poverty in all its dimensions
1.3 Social protection
1.4 Access to basic services
1.5 Resilience to disasters
1.A Resources
2
2.1 Access to safe and nutritious food
2.2 End malnutrition
4
4.1 Effective learning outcomes
4.2 Access to education
4.A Safe schools
5
5.2 Violence against women
5.3 Female genital mutilation
5.4 Domestic aid and care work
5.6 Sexual and reproductive health
6
6.1 Safe drinking-water
6.2 Sanitation and hygiene
6.3 Reduce water pollution
6.4 WASH programmes
7
7.1 Universal access to modern energy
8
8.8 Safe working environments
9
9.5 Enhance research and upgrade industrial technologies
10
10.7 Responsible migration policies
11
11.1 Safe housing
11.2 Safe transport
11.5 Natural disasters
11.6 Environmental impact
11.7 Safe green spaces
12
12.4 Responsible management of chemicals and waste
13
13.1 Resilience to climate related hazards
13.2 Resilience to climate related hazards
13.3 Climate change awareness
14
14.1 Reduce marine pollution
15
15.1 Freshwater ecosystems
15.2 End deforestation
16
16.1 Reduce violence
16.2 Protect children from violence, trafficking and torture
16.9 Legal identity for all
3

Fig. 9. The Sustainable Development Goal health-related targets.
Source: Compiled by C. Wippel and B. Menne and used with permission *(221)*

The Health 2020 development and implementation process successfully generated and promoted country commitments to SDG targets, helped develop enabling partnerships, and identified practical ways to link strategic and policy processes to financing.

SDGs and Health 2020 – platforms for intersectoral action

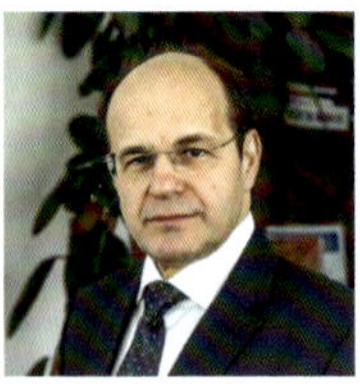

Here in Bosnia and Herzegovina, we use the SDGs and indicators as our goals and targets that initiate activities and intersectoral cooperation in the fields of air pollution; hazardous chemicals, water and soil pollution and contamination; mortality rates attributed to household and ambient air pollution; and the burden of disease attributable to unsafe water, unsafe sanitation and lack of hygiene.

Addressing these issues is in line with the Health 2020 policy and reducing health inequality because they relate to both developing cities and underdeveloped areas.

Considering that Bosnia and Herzegovina does not have a health strategy, the SDGs serve as our specific strategic course in the field of health. This means that our health sector is involved in solving the above problems together with environment, industry and other sectors. Thus, the health sector will not be alone in dealing with the consequences of air and water pollution and soil contamination, but actively engaged with their sectors in resolving the causes of these problems. In the past period relevant authorities in Bosnia and Herzegovina implemented several intersectoral initiatives which have targeted vulnerable population, especially children, as the highest priority. From 2009–2014, in collaboration with UNICEF, entity health, education and social welfare authorities together with the Ministry of Civil Affairs of Bosnia and Herzegovina, implemented the SPIS Project (Strengthening Social Protection and Inclusion Systems). This was an intersectoral model of integrated municipality social protection promoting a comprehensive approach to social protection and inclusion of children. This programme resulted in adoption of several policies and documents that are a part of the today's policy foundations and proved the success of collaboration of interconnected sectors, working with the same vision and aspirations.

Adil Osmanovic, Minister of Civil Affairs, Bosnia and Herzegovina

In order to achieve the SDGs and Health 2020 goals, governments, the United Nations system, the private sector, civil society and many other stakeholders are challenged to work together in a transformative way. All the WHO Regional Office work on Health 2020 has supported and helped Member States to transform their governance and policy development and implementation arrangements to work in this way.

Paving the way to SDGs and GPW13

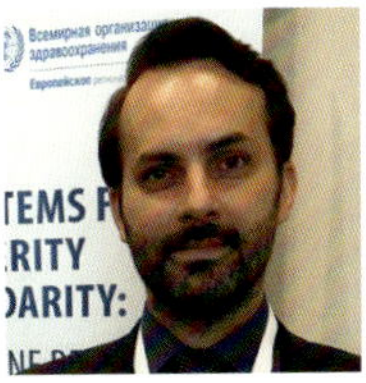

Health 2020 paved the way for prioritization at national level of our preparations and involvement in SDG's, and successful participation in the GPW13 consultation process.

Slovakia welcomes the inclusiveness and openness of the SDG and GPW13 processes. Our country, for example, presented during GPW13 draft negotiations, several priorities, including: aligning the programme with SDGs, UHC, responding to demographic change and intersectoralism; links to social affairs, family, education and environmental sectors; fighting tuberculosis; focusing on marginalized groups; the impact of the Internet and digital marketing; extremism; addiction among children and youth; engaging communities, patients and their families, particularly the vulnerable.

Jozef Suvada, Head of Projects, Standard preventive, diagnostic, therapeutic procedures, Ministry of Health, Slovakia

Health 2020 and SDGs as communication platforms

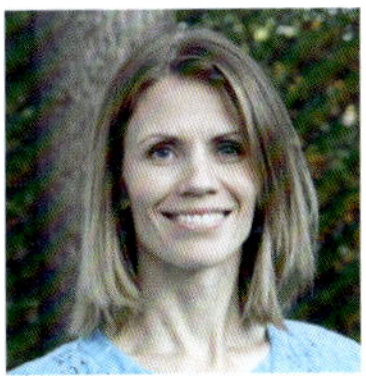

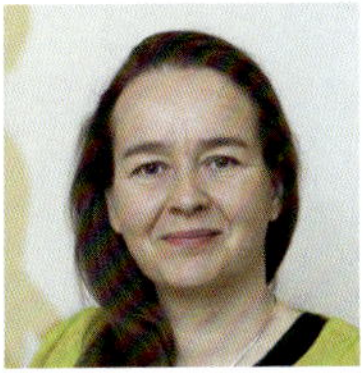

Finland is indeed committed to take actions to achieve the goals of Health 2020 and the SDGs. We have taken relevant content and included it to national and city level plans.

In Finland we have had a well developed cross-sectoral approach for several years, e.g. most of the municipalities have a cross-sectoral well-being working group. Health 2020 and SDGs provide platforms that make it easier to communicate on these common goals. This makes it easier for us to continue our work and try to find new areas in which to collaborate with different people on all levels. We are, for example, trying to stress the importance of all sectors in cities to participate in the preparation of the city health and well-being reports.

The Finnish Healthy Cities network works in collaboration with the Ministry of Social Affairs and Health, providing good opportunities to exchange information. The network has been active in developing and piloting the structures of the health and well-being promotion of municipalities that are now in the legislation – health and well-being report, prospective health impact assessment, and health and well-being coordinators in municipalities.

We cooperate because our ultimate goals are the same, namely healthy people. Our roles are different, but they support each other, which is why it works so well.

Sanna Ahonen, Healthy Cities National Network Coordinator, Finland and Heli Hätönen, Ministerial Adviser at Ministry of Social Affairs and Health, Finland

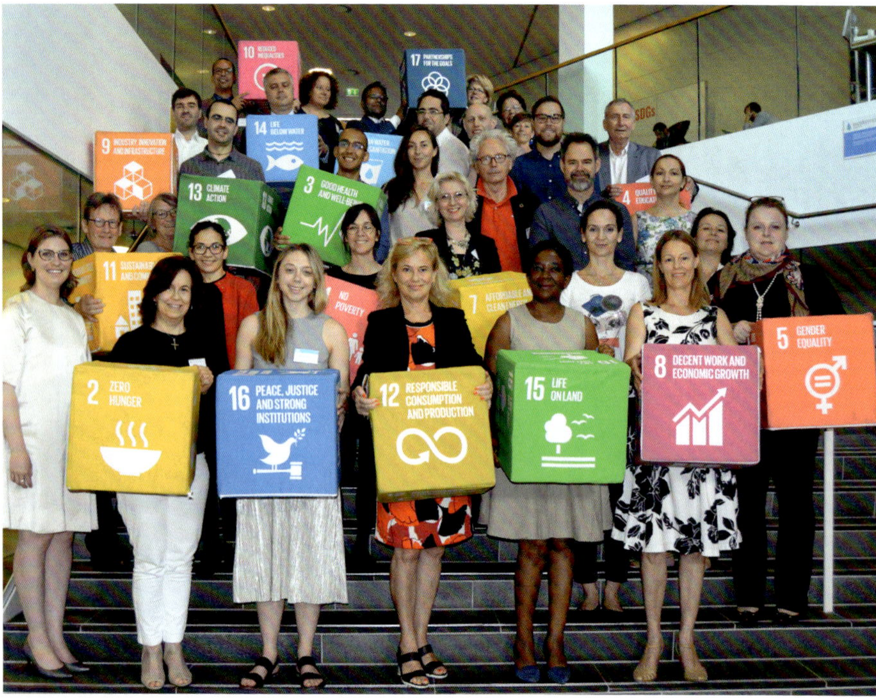

A Health and Sustainable Development Goals Advisory Meeting was held at the WHO Regional Office for Europe in Copenhagen, Denmark on 18-19 June 2019. The purpose of the meeting was to discuss and revise a draft SDG Guide and its associated technical resources. © WHO/Ramy Srour

In September 2017 the WHO Regional Committee for Europe endorsed the *Roadmap to implement the 2030 Agenda for Sustainable Development, building on Health 2020, the European policy for health and well-being* (hereafter called the SDG roadmap) *(82)*. This SDG roadmap was developed to assist Member States in the implementation of the 2030 Agenda for Sustainable Development and the SDGs, to strengthen the capacities of Member States to achieve better, more equitable and sustainable health and well-being for all, at all ages. The roadmap has five strategic directions and four enablers (see Fig. 10), which build on Health 2020, and go beyond.

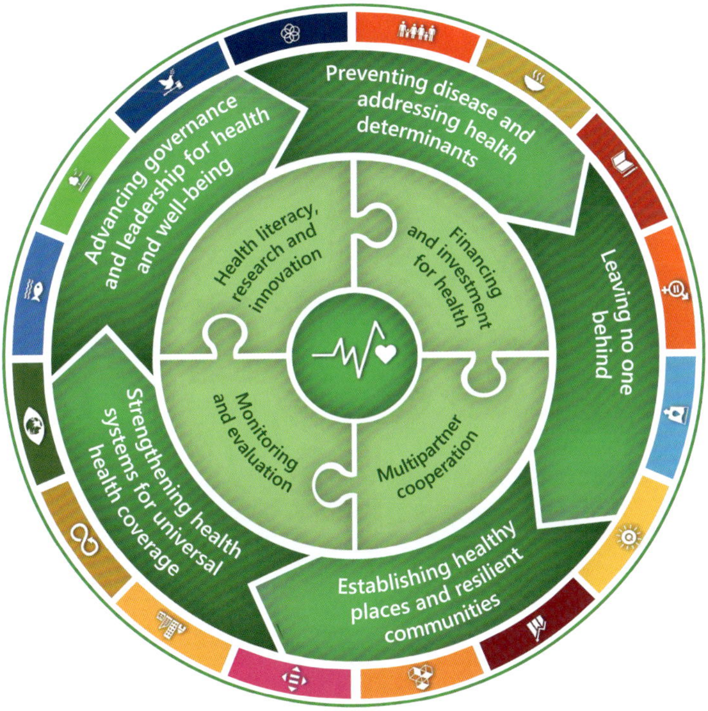

Fig. 10. The strategic directions and enablers of the WHO SDG roadmap.
Source: WHO Regional Office for Europe *(222)*

Several prime ministers, deputy prime ministers and ministers of health have promoted the SDG roadmap and its implementation. Many countries have reported progress using the roadmap as a means of implementing the SDGs (see Section 6.3).

PART 1

Implement SDGs to leave more answers for future generations

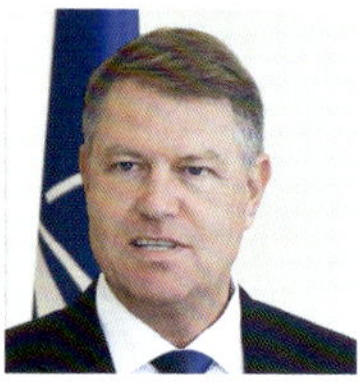

On the occasion of the policy dialogue, addressing the environment and health challenges and priorities in Romania, the institutional arrangements and instruments for intersectoral collaboration in this field with the aim of supporting the implementation of the Sustainable Development Goals, I want to emphasize my strong conviction that if we want a population with a good health status, more safety in the field of public health or a prosperous society, there is one answer: health in all policies.

I believe that it is time to act now, through such an integrated approach, to address future challenges, including those related to demographic change. I believe that we are connected by this common approach and the desire to find integrated solutions.

The closer we bring this approach to the people and talk about it with determination and courage, the more chances there are to make it a reality and to leave for the future generations more answers and not so many problems to solve.

Klaus Iohannis, President, Romania

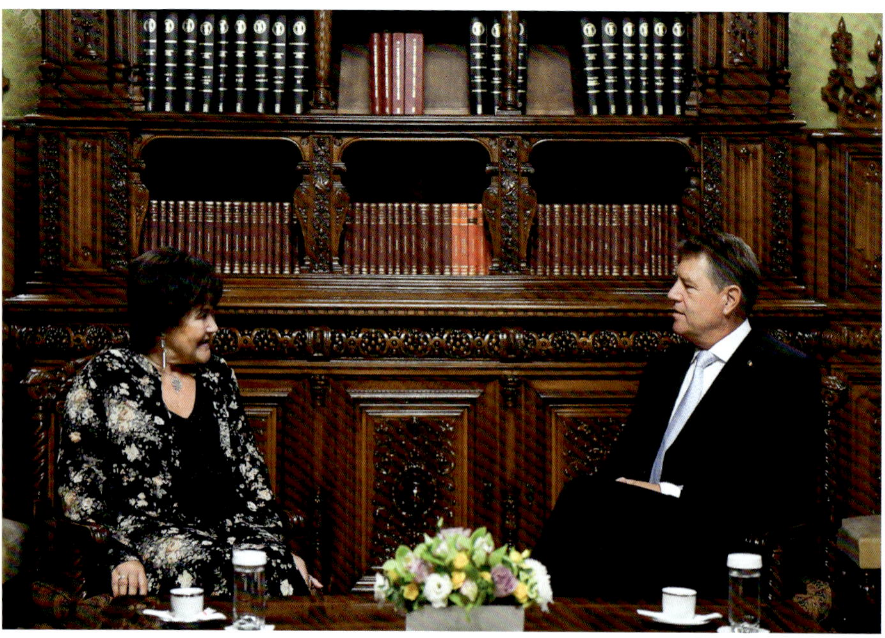

Zsuzsanna Jakab, WHO Regional Director for Europe made an official visit to Romania on 30–31 May 2018, at the invitation of His Excellency Klaus Iohannis, President of Romania. © Presidential Administration of Romania

R O M Â N I A

PREŞEDINTELE ROMÂNIEI

Dr. Zsuzsanna Jakab
WHO Regional Director for Europe

Bucharest, March 2019

Dr Jakab,

As your second term as WHO Regional Director for Europe comes to a close, I would like to take this opportunity to thank you for your contribution to a better health for Europe: more equitable and sustainable.

Over the past four years, we have had a strong cooperation, mainly oriented towards the Sustainable Development Goals implementation in Romania, to which your participation in the policy dialogues organized at Cotroceni Palace, your visits in our country and our discussions on health topics of major importance had a great contribution.

Let me take this opportunity to express my appreciation for your constant support and the international expertise offered through the WHO Country Office, aspects that are essential for Romania in the area of public health.

It is a great pleasure, on behalf of the Romanian people and myself, to wish you continued success in your future endeavors.

I reiterate my commitment taken at the UN Summit in September 2015 to contribute to the implementation of the 2030 Agenda on Sustainable Development and I look forward to our further cooperation.

Please accept, Dr Jakab, the assurances of my highest consideration.

Klaus Werner Iohannis
President of Romania

Fig. 11. Letter to Zsuzsanna Jakab from His Excellency Klaus Iohannis, President of Romania.
Source: Reproduced with the permission of the Office of the President of Romania

2.8 The Thirteenth General Programme of Work (GPW13)

The Thirteenth General Programme of Work 2019–2023 is the latest in a series of exercises to guide the Organization in terms of its strategic priorities and provide the operational management and budgeting of WHO *(132)*.

The GPW13 is strongly informed by the United Nations 2030 Agenda for Sustainable Development and the SDGs, and particularly SDG 3 on good health and well-being. GPW13 states that WHO will promote public health impact in every country and lead a transformative agenda that supports countries in reaching all health-related SDG targets. These objectives are fully consistent with our Health 2020 processes and identify clear and strong organization-wide outcome and impact-oriented targets.

In order to accelerate progress towards SDG targets, GPW13 focuses on three interconnected areas:

1. achieving UHC;
2. addressing health emergencies; and,
3. promoting healthier populations.

The GPW13 commits WHO to 'triple billion' targets related to each area. WHO aims to help ensure that by 2023 one billion more people benefit from UHC; one billion more people have better protection from health emergencies; and one billion more people enjoy better health and well-being.

Our Director-General, Dr Tedros, is absolutely committed to these goals, and I am strongly supportive. I believe these goals are achievable and that our Regional Office will continue to take a leadership role in identifying effective ways to achieve these targets.

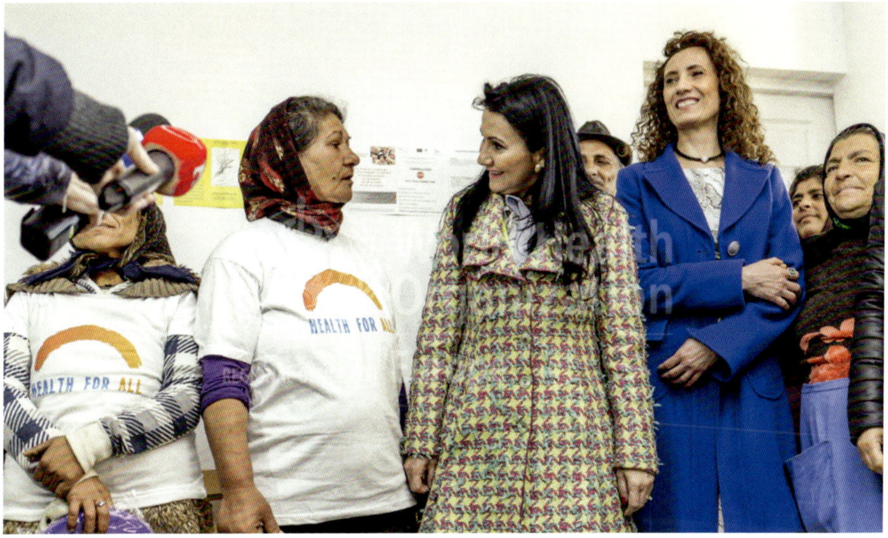

Marking World Health Day (WHD) 2018 in a rural community in Giurgiu county, Romania. That year's WHD marked the start of a 2-year campaign to raise awareness and advocate for action towards UHC. © WHO/Costin Simion

PART 1

Summary reflection

Health 2020 – developing the policy and its evidence base

Message 1: Never underestimate the power of a common vision

Health 2020, as a value-driven evidence-informed European health policy framework and as a coherent vision for equitable improvement in health and well-being, created new scientific information on the social determinants of health, governance for health, and the economics of health intervention. It provided a strategic approach to health and well-being dealing with all determinants through national health policies and, most particularly, the social and political determinants. It saw investment in health as a major contributor to development, using economic alongside health arguments to promote investment in public health, the benefits of health promotion and disease prevention, and the value of reducing co-payment percentages for the provision of health services.

Health 2020 was developed through a broad co-production exercise to engage the widest possible range of internal and external stakeholders concerned with public health in Europe and beyond. We quickly learned the process was not just about making sure that we put the right words in the document but that we truly engaged people in both policy development and implementation.

We needed not only to get those involved in public health on board, to express their views and provide their inputs but also, and more importantly, all diverse stakeholders in the community. The main goal was to create a sense of unity among the different sectors of society, a feeling of a common cause and ownership shared by all. To accomplish this, we knew we needed to put these principles into practice ourselves. We needed all our staff to reframe our work around Health 2020 values and approaches; and to look at our own governance approaches, intersectoral working patterns, partnerships, life-course approaches, etc. We needed to model the behaviours and approaches we were proposing; to act not just in words, but to really, truly, embrace and practice what we were advocating.

This catalysed a major change process in all our offices. There were evidence gaps around, for example, the social determinants of health, governance and economics, and new research and evidence gathering was needed. So, we used our collective experiences to inform our research agendas. We learned also how our behaviours could reinforce and strengthen the reception and application of our technical norms and standards.

Health 2020 has had significant impact. Within the Regional Office all work has been reframed and aligned with Health 2020 objectives and priorities. Most positively, our Health 2020 approaches were consistent with, and to some extent anticipated, global developments, most notably the United Nations 2030 Agenda for Sustainable Development and the SDGs, and helped prepare us to take leadership roles in this area.

An important added value has been that Health 2020 provided an entry window into the SDGs with political decision-makers on all levels and from different sectors. We have had many opportunities to visit prime ministers, presidents and parliamentarians, as well as ministers of health, to remind them that their countries have adopted this approach. We have persuaded and helped them to frame any health challenges they are concerned about within the consistent Health 2020 values of equity, participation and solidarity over, for example, tobacco taxation, migration, co-payments, etc. In doing so we have been able to help cement the commitment of the country on issues that have previously been difficult to even talk about, let alone do something about.

3. Improved governance in the WHO European Region and in the Regional Office

When I took office, I made a commitment to strengthen the governance structures in the Regional Office, under the guidance of the Regional Committee and Standing Committee of the Regional Committee (SCRC). The role of the Regional Committee has been strengthened and all important decisions on policy, strategy, regional action plans, partnerships, budget and oversight are now taken by the Regional Committee. What is more, all governance reforms in the WHO Regional Office for Europe have been both based upon, and contributed to, the processes of global WHO reform.

Over the years, the Secretariat has continued to earn trust and respect from the Member States and the conduct of business in the Regional Committees has become smoother with the spirit of consensus prevailing on all items, including difficult ones. It is encouraging to see that this determined approach and the investment has paid off and now every part of the Region is equally active in the discussions.

Throughout the main principles to be achieved have been public health excellence, together with transparency, efficiency, accountability, and inclusiveness. The SCRC with an improved oversight function and increased representation has played a crucial role in ensuring these principles have been put into practice as well as in achieving consensus among Member States.

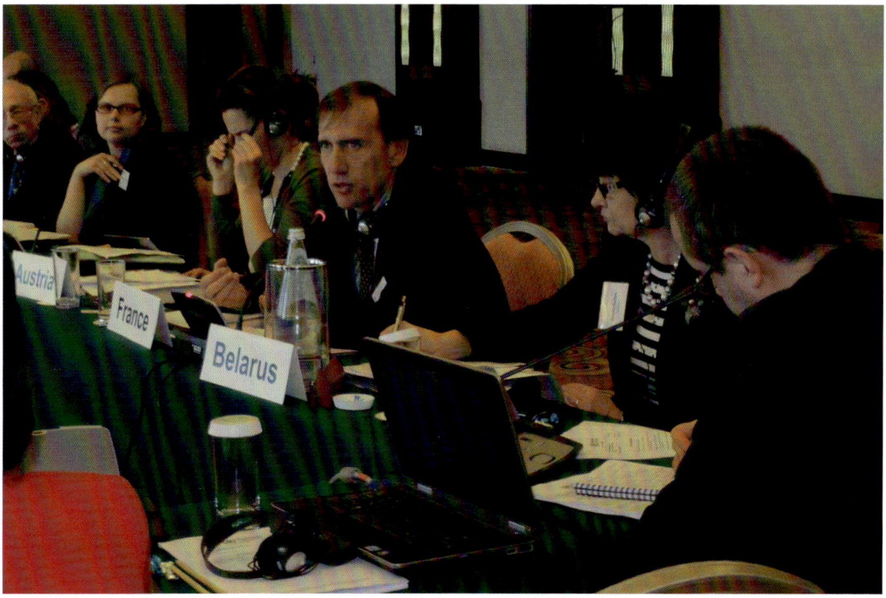

Members of the WHO European Standing Committee of the Regional Committee (SCRC) at a meeting, Malta, 16–17 December 2013. © WHO

The SCRC now plays a more significant role in the Region and it enjoys a higher level of trust with the Regional Committee. This governance reform in the European Region has been inspirational for some of the global developments.

Innovative Regional governance benchmarks

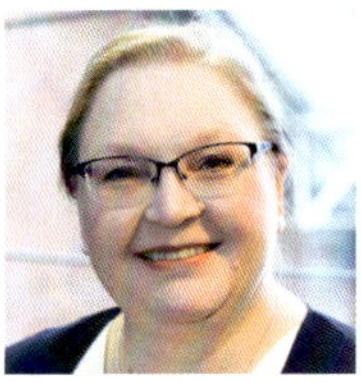

Over the last ten years, the European Region has taken many steps to improve how our governance structures work. We've implemented changes and made innovations that are now benchmarks for the whole Organization.

One such example is the sunsetting of resolutions. We have passed many resolutions, over the decades, resulting in reporting requirements that are overlapping, and which become obsolete. We created principles on how to review resolutions and the Secretariat did a mapping exercise of what resolutions we have, and what are the reporting requirements. Based on the recommendation of the SCRC, the Regional Committee decided to cease the reporting requirements of old obsolete resolutions. Now when we propose a new resolution, it states which ones it replaces and what the time limit for the reporting is … so, you do not have conflicts about what is in place.

Another governance reform relates to the election process for the Regional Director. We revised the set of rules governing the process and introduced a code on how the candidates should act. One of the issues we wanted to avoid was for every candidate having to travel to every country to make their case. Instead we would ask them to come to Regional meetings, where they could all be present and have the same access to countries. So, it would not be a question of how much money you had in your budget or if you were able to reach out to countries.

We also looked at how we shortlist candidates, how we interview them and what issues they need to include in their applications so that they are relevant to the decision-making process in countries. To increase access, we introduced a web forum, where countries can put questions to the candidates. The most important change was to arrange an interview of all candidates at the May SCRC meeting, so that everyone has a chance to hear them.

We've made some changes in how we evaluate all the candidates that countries put up for positions on the WHO Executive Board and SCRC. We now look at both the individual candidate's national and international qualifications; their experience in the governing bodies, their other international collaborations and experience. We also now ask for country statements about how they intend to use their governing body and SCRC memberships, and what their priorities are.

We have put in place timelines for processes like setting the agenda, and for proposing resolutions and amendments, in an effort to have earlier notice. We can see already that documentation has improved tremendously in both quality and timing of delivery.

> We've also changed the rules in the Regional Committee about how we engage with NGOs ... I think that the overall approach to non-State actors in the European Region has been very proactive and positive.
>
> I think Member States are very proud about the reforms we've taken, and with the support of Regional Director Zsuzsanna Jakab, we've presented many of them as good practices to be taken forward at the global level.
>
> **Outi Kuivasniemi, Chair of the Regional Evaluation Group 2014, Finland**

Within the Regional Office we have identified five strategic approaches to SMART governance that we have tried to build into our own practise and to promote with Member States *(83)*. These included:

1. the value of collaboration to facilitate communication, trust, commitment and understanding;
2. the importance of engaging citizens to encourage participation, transparency and accountability;
3. the use of a mix of regulation and persuasion to support health and engage actors;
4. the provision of evidence through independent expert bodies such as federal agencies, commissions, regulators and auditors; and,
5. the importance of adapting quickly and anticipating future needs through improved forecasting and promoting multiple small-scale interventions at local and community levels.

Programme budgeting can be a powerful tool of governance, and the European Regional components of the WHO global Programme Budgets have been developed and used as a 'strategic tool of accountability'. We employed a commonly agreed 'results chain', using a bottom-up planning based on the BCAs and defined outcomes as a 'contract' between the Regional Office and Member States. These concepts used in the European Regional Programme Budget have also provided a major contribution to the global planning process. We have also aligned our resource mobilization procedures with those of Headquarters.

We have also organized governing bodies (Executive Board and SCRC) members visits to country offices to review programmes, and to make the role of the country offices and the backup from the Regional Office better understood. The aim of these visits has been to elicit input widely and enhance the knowledge and awareness of governing bodies members about needs, assets and the impacts of country activities. This is important because such visits provide Member States the opportunity to:

- understand more about how WHO operates in the countries. In the past there was less engagement of the governing bodies with this level of WHO activity. As the vision of Dr Tedros and GPW13 is now based on an increased and improved country focus and impact, Member States want to understand better how we operate at this level before they approve investment in more funding. The WHO Regional Office for Europe, for example, has a specific business model: we have modest technical capacity in the countries and a large part of our technical support and cooperation with Member States comes from the Regional Office. This is the only model the Office can afford financially, based on our limited budget and the high number of WHO Member States in our Region. In order to increase our impact, we also provide some of our technical assistance through interactions with multiple countries. These country visits give governing bodies' members insights into these different ways the Regional Office supports countries;

- witness how decisions made by the governing bodies are realized in countries; and,
- see how we interact with other United Nations organizations and partners within the framework of the United Nations reform processes.

SCRC country visits – seeing how decisions are translated into action

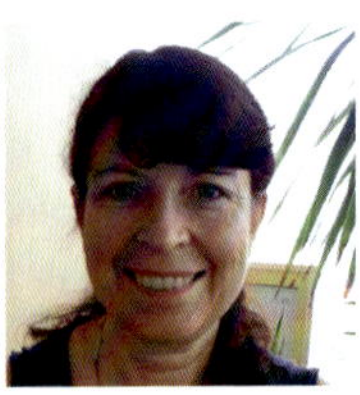

As a member of the SCRC I had the opportunity to visit countries and get a better understanding of our country work. Our group visited offices in Georgia, Russian Federation and Turkey. I was privileged to also organize a visit for SCRC and EB members in my own country, Slovenia. We could see how well the WHO offices perform in each of the countries and with partner agencies. We could see how we are working to get things right with the UN, research community and civil society. Most important, it was great to get a chance to witness first-hand the impact of the work of WHO and its partners, and to see how decisions taken during sessions of the Regional Committee are then translated into concrete action plans and implemented at the country level.

Vesna-Kerstin Petrič, Head, Division for Health Promotion and Prevention of Noncommunicable Diseases, Ministry of Health, Slovenia

Summary reflection

Improved governance in the WHO European Region and in the Regional Office

Message 2: Complex problems need congruent 'joined up' solutions

We learned a lot about governance for health in the WHO European Region and in the Regional Office, through supporting and publishing research on governance, making the concept of governance mainstream, and retraining frontline staff in country offices and others in health diplomacy.

In addition, transparency and involvement in the internal governance of the WHO European Region has improved through staff training and the strengthening of SCRC and Regional Committee processes. Our new approach is helping to transform health and health service dominated approaches to governance to health-in-all-policies, whole-of-government, whole-of-society approaches.

Importantly, it has also changed the way our staff think, work, plan and address the health challenges we confront. We have also learned a lot about the new skill mix and capabilities that today's public health leaders need to meet their current health challenges and achieve change; including:

- initiating and informing policy debates;
- advocating for polices for health;
- assessing health needs and capacity for health gain;
- creating innovative networks for change;
- stimulating change in complex and sometimes 'wicked systems' where change often comes from relationship-building, advocacy and negotiation, rather than direct control; and,
- acknowledging the newly important role of health diplomacy.

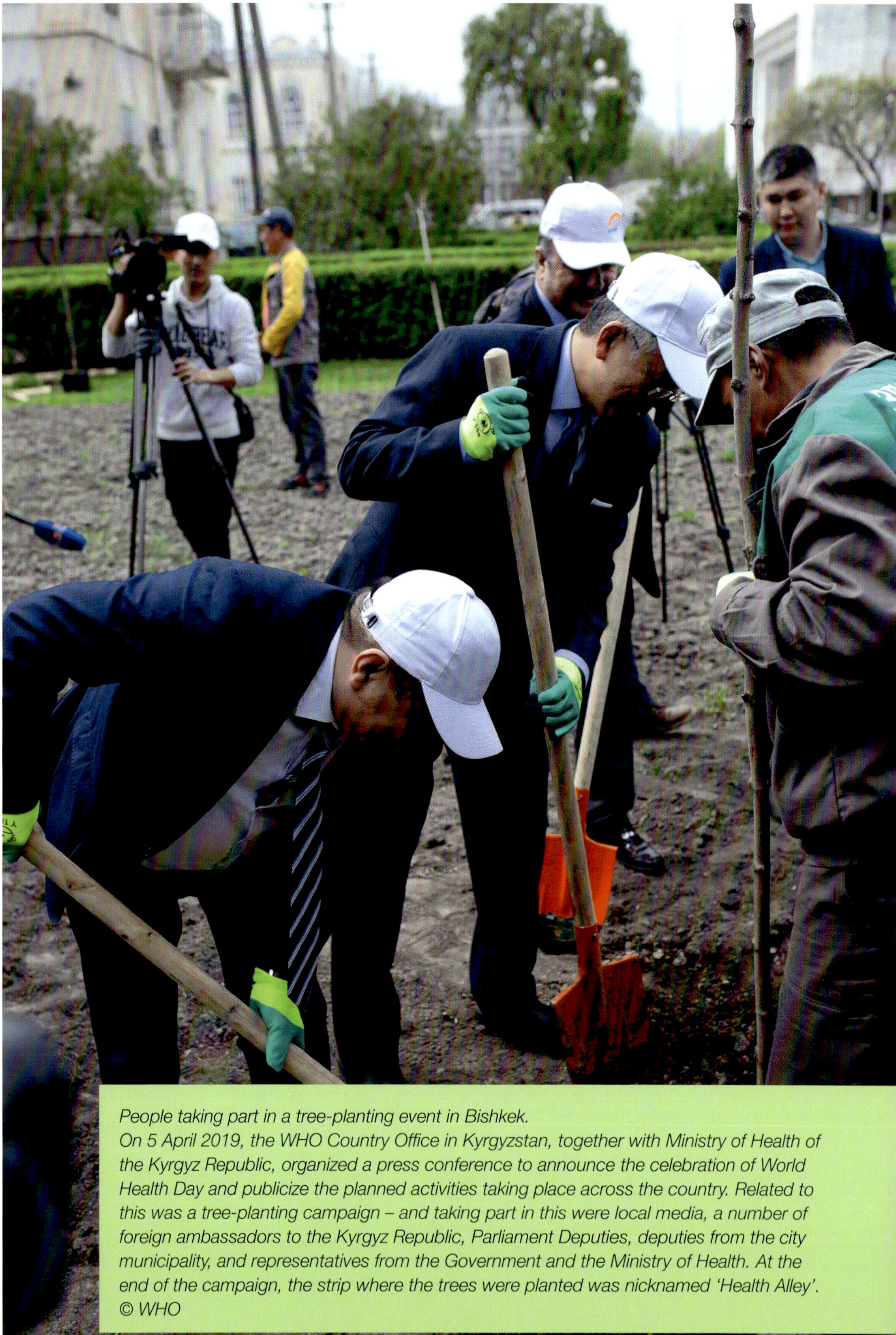

People taking part in a tree-planting event in Bishkek.
On 5 April 2019, the WHO Country Office in Kyrgyzstan, together with Ministry of Health of the Kyrgyz Republic, organized a press conference to announce the celebration of World Health Day and publicize the planned activities taking place across the country. Related to this was a tree-planting campaign – and taking part in this were local media, a number of foreign ambassadors to the Kyrgyz Republic, Parliament Deputies, deputies from the city municipality, and representatives from the Government and the Ministry of Health. At the end of the campaign, the strip where the trees were planted was nicknamed 'Health Alley'.

4. Strengthening collaboration with Member States

A main priority for our Office over these last 10 years has been to improve the way we work with, in and for countries. At the start of my mandate in 2010, I emphasized to Member States that I wanted to further strengthen collaboration with Member States.

Here the development of Health 2020 was vitally important. For implementation I wanted to combine our Office resources, with the resources in Member States and across the Region. Many Member States had developed institutions, skills and knowledge, and there were already many highly competent academic, research and public health institutions in Europe. There was therefore an enlarged pool of expertise with which we could work.

I also wanted to improve the way we worked with countries. In September 2012, I presented an interim country strategy to the Regional Committee outlining the Regional Office's plan for strengthening its country-specific focus. New ways of working were identified and adopted, including changing ways the Regional Office was being represented in countries, strengthening network and institutional partnerships, and reorganizing how country work is managed and supported within the Office.

A decision was taken for the WHO Regional Office for Europe to be better represented in all Member States. We initiated changes to the Region's country offices from liaison offices led by nationals of the country concerned to internationally led offices (see Section 4.1). In countries without offices, we worked to expand our networks of national counterparts. Thematic focal points were also appointed for each of the major areas of work of Health 2020 and for 12 key disease and programmatic areas.

The Regional Office has also helped to strengthen existing political and technical networks, including, among others, the South-eastern Europe Health Network (SEEHN), a newly established Small Countries Initiative (SCI), the Visegrad for Health Initiative as well as networks representing healthy settings such as the Regions for Health Network (RHN) and the WHO European Healthy Cities Network.

A Strategic Relations with Countries (SRC) unit was established to replace the country 'helpdesk' in the Regional Director's Office and ensure a closer coordination between technical divisions in the Regional Office and countries. The SRC collates country information, helps ensure timely support by technical programmes in response to requests from countries, provides regular information to countries when required (through country offices and national counterparts), and prepares guidance and standard operating procedures applicable at the Regional Office and country levels. The team has also been responsible for bottom-up planning and development of

BCAs, assisting the roll-out of the later developed country cooperation strategies (CCSs) to the countries that requested them and has taken responsibility for liaising with all 53 countries in the development of country support plans (see Section 4.1).

Also as part of improving our links with Member States, our country assessment capacities and training programmes have expanded, helping the Office develop new areas of technical assistance. Assessments have helped countries to review different aspects of their national polices and identify actions to strengthen them. New Regional training programmes for high-level decision-makers in countries, as well as technical experts, have proven to be popular and in demand. These have focused on commitments in international health and global and regional policy issues; noncommunicable disease interventions; impacts of financial crisis; UHC, health financing and financial protection; health diplomacy; and migration and health. Assessments have helped countries to review different aspects of their national polices and identify actions to strengthen them.

WHO collaborating centres are also an important point of contact with Member States. These are leading national academic, research and public health institutions which carry out activities in support of WHO's programmes at all levels and ensure the scientific validity of its work.

The centres themselves benefit from being part of this global network by obtaining greater visibility and recognition from national authorities, and by attracting more public attention to the health issues that they address. They also have increased opportunities to exchange information and develop technical cooperation with other institutions such as public health schools and institutes, and universities.

The WHO collaborating centres were reviewed in terms of their activities and contributions to WHO's work, and to ensure that those relevant to the European programmes continued to supplement research, knowledge-sharing and training provided by these programmes, in fields of particular interest in Europe.

The WHO Regional Office for Europe's added value – Denmark

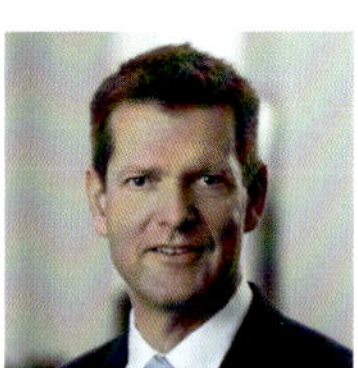

We really have appreciated the help of the Regional Office with the challenges we have faced over our child immunization programme. We have always had a very strong childhood immunization programme, but we were hit with some problems in 2014 and 2015, specifically regarding HPV vaccines for 12-year-old girls. There was a sudden post-factual erosion of confidence among parents about the safety of the vaccine, fuelled by social media. And we were struggling with that, trying to help parents regain confidence. We were very thankful for the help we received from the Regional Office. They brought us together with Member States, like Ireland, that faced similar challenges. Now Italy is facing them. It shows why collaboration with the WHO is important, because many public health challenges are not just a single-country issue. The Regional Office brought us knowledge – technical know-how that we really appreciated. We also used WHO independent health authority positioning in our local campaigns; letting people know that we are backed by the WHO.

Søren Brostrøm, Director General, Danish Health Authority, Denmark

The WHO Regional Office for Europe's added value – Slovakia

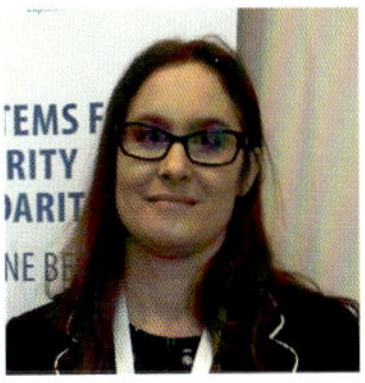

Slovakia developed many projects inspired by WHO. WHO helped us, for example, in the prioritization of Slovak health policy development. Specific priority topics included: TB control activities, medicine policy, standards, child and adolescent health, ethical issues, data and e-health and health system effectiveness measurement. We also believe that WHO sponsored Global and Regional activities, for example Immunization Week and World Health Days are important to help all countries give coordinated and coherent messages on key health challenges and topics.

Zuzana Foldesova Motajova, Director, Department of health insurance and macroeconomics, Ministry of Health, Slovakia

WHO relevance – Finland: a proactive partner

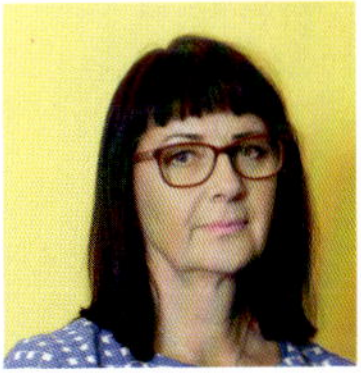

Our connections with WHO have always been very important for us. We are a small country and for us it's important to have advice from WHO but also to be involved and supported, and to provide the experience which we have. WHO is important to us in many ways – in terms of technical input and as a convenor and provider of exchange platforms where we can talk about what we do and get feedback and perhaps influence others. By being in such Region and Global discussions and having an opportunity to network with others we can share and learn. WHO gives us a very good forum for that. This said, its important to be proactive with WHO. I and other Finish colleagues have always taken active roles in governing bodies. These experiences have been especially important. It's really valuable to hear the discussions and have an opportunity to be involved and participate and be a part of a decision making resource which is important for all countries, not just us but all of us.

Taru Koivisto, Director of the Department for Wellbeing and Services. Ministry of Social Affairs and Health, Finland

To further strengthen country collaboration, I have visited many Member States, meeting presidents, prime ministers, ministers of health and other sectoral ministers, as well as a wide range of other partners for health. I have always tried to use these visits to advocate for putting health and well-being higher on the governments' political and policy agendas, for Health 2020, for our jointly agreed country priorities, and for the promotion of intersectoral work and mechanisms.

High-level political advocacy

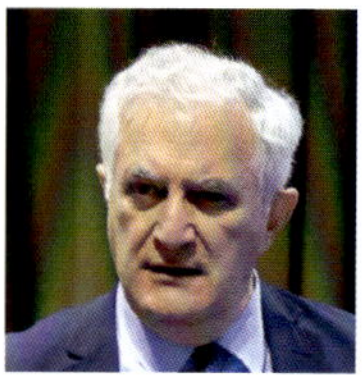

One of the major challenges of public health over the last 10 years, to my mind, has been the need for more advocating on a high political level. We very much appreciate that despite her very busy schedule, Dr Zsuzsanna Jakab conducted several visits to Georgia, where she held high-level meetings with our Prime Minister and other Government officials. These visits were very important in advocating universal health coverage, hepatitis C, tobacco control, health system financing, NCDs, communicable disease control, immunization etc. It should also be mentioned that during her tenure, she helped Georgia advocate for more active representation in WHO governance structures. For the first time, we became a member of the WHO Executive Board and served as Chair country of the SCRC as well as European Environment and Health Ministerial Board.

Amiran Gamkrelidze, Director General of the National Center for Disease Control and Public Health, Georgia

WHO support is additional political power

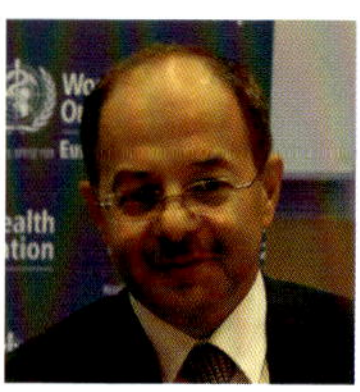

I always recommend that the directors of WHO should work in the field much more, especially with high-powered politicians whenever possible; visiting prime ministers and presidents. They are very helpful. Zsuzsanna Jakab has done that well and I believe that she did her homework very well too and has been effective. She was always very close to us when we needed to launch something in our country or get quick expert advice.

Particularly in humanitarian issues, the WHO should take control much more eagerly. Whenever it needs to, the WHO should speak loudly. Without the strong support of the WHO, in most of the countries, politicians will not do the necessary things in health care. In this way the WHO can increase their worth. When you get the support of the WHO for this kind of effort you gain additional power.

Recep Akdag, Former Deputy Prime Minister, Former Minister of Health, Turkey

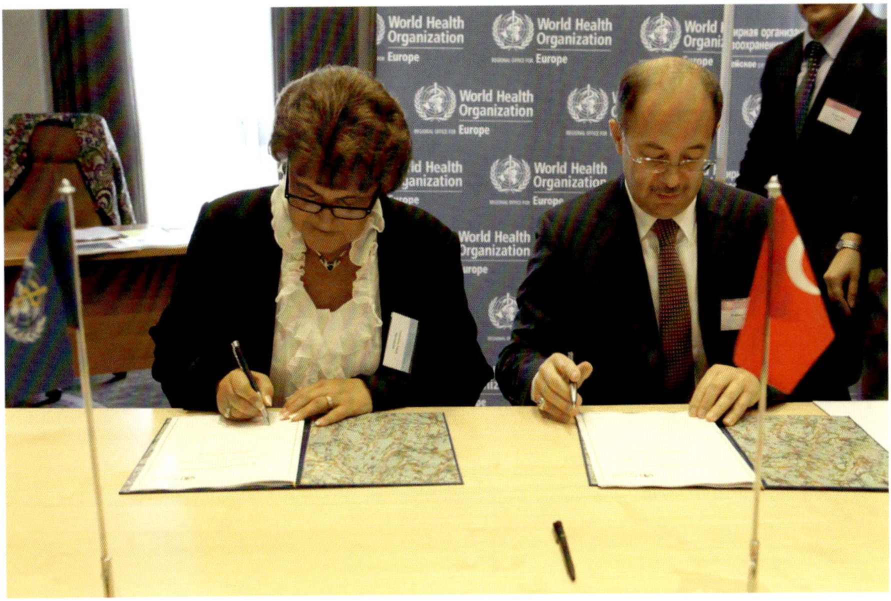

Zsuzsanna Jakab and Recep Akdag, Minister of Health of Turkey, signing the BCA between WHO Regional Office for Europe and Turkey at the 62nd session of the Regional Committee in Malta, 10–13 September 2012. © WHO/Brian Cassar

The Regional Office has also made a big effort to 'be there' for countries when and where they needed us; not only in health emergencies but also for critical parliamentary health debates and other urgent national health developments. When there was an opportunity provided by a change in the political scene, we made every effort to 'jump on the train' and identify the necessary expertise even at a short notice.

Plain packaging – Parliamentary debates in Slovenia

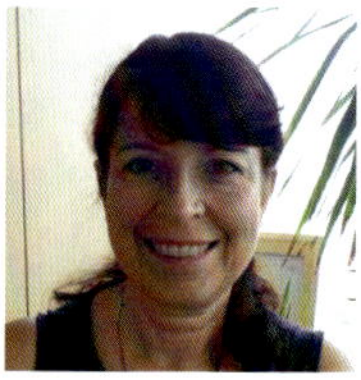

Slovenia adopted the Framework Convention on Tobacco Control with no problem. In 2007 we changed our legislation and included a total ban on smoking in all closed public places. In 2014 when the new EU directive was adopted, we thought it was time to strengthen our legislation. We asked ourselves what was there to adopt and decided "Okay let's put everything that is left from FCTC – like a total ban on advertising, even at the place of sale; and plain packaging – on our agenda". Immediately there was response from the industry. An expert who was very skilled in intellectual property rights in Slovenia was brought in to prove that plain packaging was something that we shouldn't do because we would be violating intellectual property rights and we would end up going to court, and paying enormous fines, and so on. It was a huge pressure, just as we were approaching decision-making time in Parliament.

I remember I was at home on the Friday and I thought "Oh my God, this will be a really difficult thing because there is more and more pressure on the Commission from the industry". One after another the parliamentarians expressed their doubts about adopting the plain packaging proposal. I didn't know what to do, so I called Gauden Galea, the NCD Director from WHO. I asked him if, even at such short notice, he could talk to Zsuzsanna and come and speak for us in Parliament to show that WHO is really interested and is also carefully monitoring how countries are implementing the FCTC. I said that if he was there, people would understand that it is something really serious. That is exactly what happened. He got permission immediately. Zsuzsanna did not waste time. She understands so well political processes and knew it was important and urgent.

I informed all the parliamentarians that the WHO would be attending, and that they are looking closely at all the countries and trying to understand where lobbying is so strong that things will not work, and so on. Gauden came and presented the views of the Organization, but then he also carefully wrote down everything that was discussed in the Parliamentarian commission which made a big impression. The parliamentarians now better informed and more confident that they are making the right decision, decided that Slovenia would also implement the plain packaging!

Vesna-Kerstin Petrič, Head, Division for Health Promotion and Prevention of Noncommunicable Diseases, Ministry of Health, Slovenia

I decided to continue Dr Asvall's practice of inviting newly appointed Ministers of health to visit the Regional Office in Copenhagen to learn about WHO's work. These ministerial visits to the Regional Office have been a means to ensure a more focused approach to country specific assistance. These visits have provided Ministers with the opportunity to spend a day in the Regional Office, to meet with me, but also to discuss with technical staff their country's health issues and ensure a clear plan of action directly with the relevant technical programmes. These visits also provided an unique opportunity for the Ministers to get to know the Office and for us to get to know them.

Making health the political choice

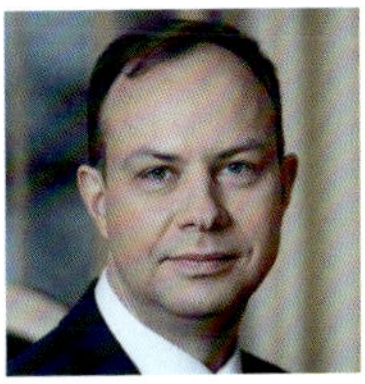

I was a very traditional medical student, I didn't even believe in public health, I was dreaming about neurology or something like that. One of my colleagues asked me, would I be interested in going into PhD studies, and I asked what this would be about. He told me this would be about tobacco control, addiction. I thought – "Wow, it is so boring. It is about printing leaflets or something, I do not want to spend my time there."

I was too serious studying medicine, which takes so much time, so I said: "I will not waste my time with tobacco control." But they were patient, and they finally took me to a WHO Regional Office for Europe conference for tobacco control – if I remember correctly in Warsaw, in Poland. And then to training in Geneva, for NGOs working in NCDs. They finally got me! And it is like an infection. When you get this one, you cannot really be treated. So, it works well.

I became a PhD and started to lead our Institute – which was a WHO collaborating centre for NCD prevention and surveillance. I worked on tobacco and alcohol prevention and control, and my research was associated with epidemiology of tobacco and alcohol, and that's how I came finally to the real politics, to the country politics.

I wrote first for one party in their election programme, a piece on alcohol prevention policy. But they didn't implement it. They used it for election purposes, but they didn't implement it. That was one of the arguments for me to go to politics. I loved my job as a researcher and teacher and medical doctor, but that was the motivation for me to go into politics – to try to implement the principles I had been working on for all of my career, at the research institute, as a teacher and a university professor.

WHO had an impact on me. I was always associated with WHO somehow – in trainings, in different activities. On entering politics, I wrote the programme for my party, very much associated with public health and NCDs prevention. Targeting all major pieces – physical activity, nutrition, tobacco, and alcohol... That's how it worked.

Aurelijus Veryga, Minister of Health, Lithuania

4.1 Collaborative agreements with countries and country offices

The Office has created new types of collaborative agreements with countries. While BCAs continue to provide the main framework for health development work in low and middle-income countries, new CCSs have been agreed with several high-income countries. Both BCAs and CCSs provide the focus for intensive strategic work in key technical areas.

New relationships and approaches – WHO and the Russian Federation

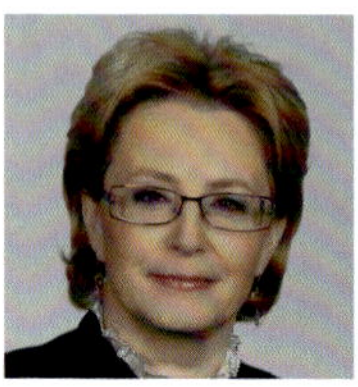

Over the last 10 years, the Russian Federation has greatly strengthened its partnership activities with the WHO Regional Office for Europe. New types of collaborations and approaches have been agreed under our current CCS with WHO. We now provide significant voluntary financial donations and technical support that enhances both Regional and Global work on prevention and NCDs and communicable diseases. Our work, for example, includes interventions to help national, Regional and Global partners to increase preparedness for health emergencies, and capacities to respond to them in accordance with the International Health Regulations (IHR); provide support for safe pregnancy programmes; strengthen maternal and child health services; and increase the use of the Russian language in WHO and the availability of publications in the Russian language.

Russian experts and institutions have been very active in various WHO programmes, inside and outside of the Russian Federation. The Russian Federation currently has 21 WHO Collaborating Centres and several new institutions are in the process of designation. These centres have an important role in both enhancing the scientific work of WHO and also in making it more accessible to countries.

The Moscow based GDO on NCDs established in 2014, has strengthened technical and scientific resources at regional and sub-regional levels and has accelerated implementation of planned measures on all levels.

The new active leadership of the Russian Federation has also resulted in a number of high level ministerial conferences: including, the first International Ministerial Conference on Road Safety (2009), the first Global Ministerial Conference on Healthy Lifestyle and NCD Control (2011) and the first Global Ministerial Conference on Ending Tuberculosis in the SDG era (2018).

These events and their outcome documents have laid the basis for high level meetings of the General Assembly of the United Nations: on NCDs (2011, 2014 and 2018) and TB (2018). These meetings were instrumental is assuring political commitments of heads of states and accelerated work towards achieving health targets of the SDGs.

Veronika Skvortsova, Minister of Health, Russian Federation

WHO representation in countries has also been strengthened. Since the start of the EUROHEALTH programme in countries of the former Soviet Union and central and eastern Europe, country offices were staffed by national professional officers (NPOs). Our strategy was for these offices to be led by international staff members (WHO representatives or WRs), who could be more independent of national interests and provide more objective advice and professional and technical contributions. These WRs, we thought, could also play a stronger interagency coordination role with the United Nations System, establish other international partnerships, and coordinate the work of the country offices more widely. By the end of my mandate, all 31 country offices will be led by international staff.

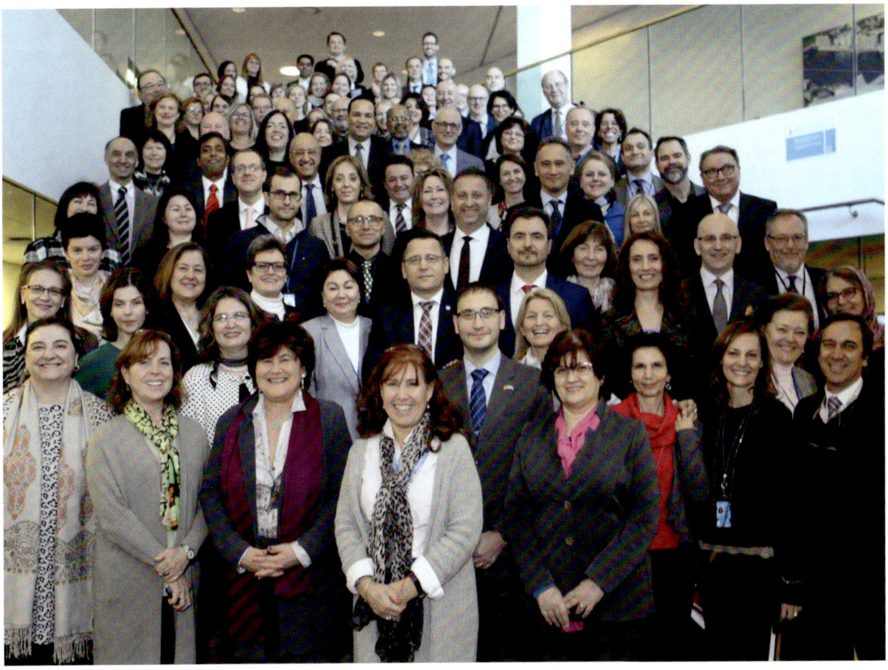

WHO Representatives (WRs) in European Member States gathered with WHO staff in Copenhagen in 2018. © WHO/Lasse Badsberg-Hansen

For example, working with the Government of Turkmenistan we were able to expand our country office there. Initially it was a very small office, with only three people. It is now a big office led by a WR, with ten staff implementing four major projects. Hence, we have become real partners, not only to the country but also to the United Nations System and other development organizations. Turkmenistan has become a donor for WHO Europe on NCDs and sponsored the WHO European Ministerial Conference on the Prevention and Control of Noncommunicable Diseases in the Context of Health 2020 in 2013 and a high-level conference on meeting NCDs targets to achieve SDGs in 2019 *(69)*. We also started a very big project funded by the Government on combating tobacco and on how to become a tobacco-free country.

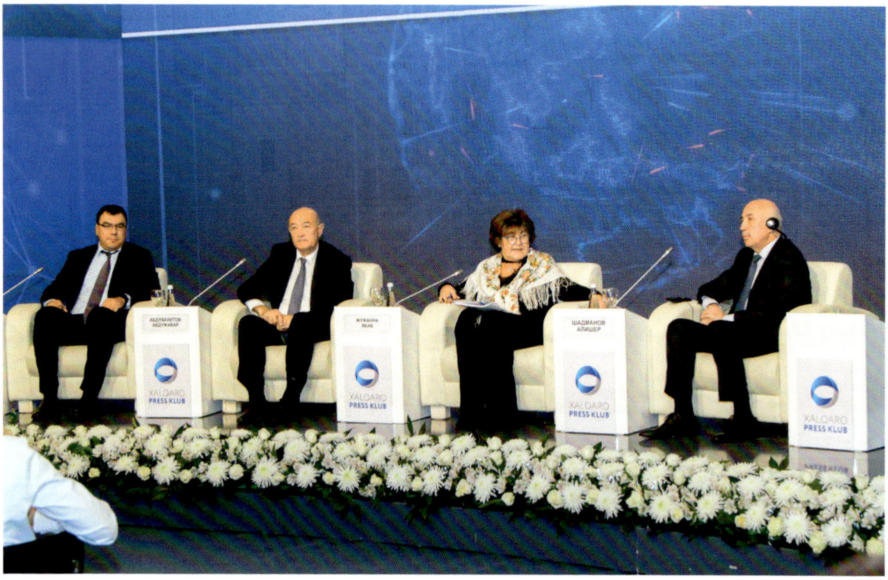

Press conference for "Uzbekistan health reform in the Sustainable Development Goals era" during official visit of Zsuzsanna Jakab to Uzbekistan on 18–21 November 2018. From the left: Aziz Abdukhakimov, Deputy Prime Minister of Uzbekistan; Abdujabar Abduvakhitov, Adviser to the President on Youth, Science, Education, Health and Sports; Zsuzsanna Jakab, WHO Regional Director for Europe; and Alisher Shadmanov, Minister of Health of Uzbekistan. © *WHO*

Similar changes have taken place in Uzbekistan, where we now have a WR and staff of 13 working in the Country Office in Tashkent. There our collaborative work has focused on tobacco control, TB diagnostics and treatment, IHR (2005) compliance and health system strengthening. I made an official visit to Uzbekistan on 18–21 November 2018. A new 'Concept of Health Sector Development' was launched during my visit at a national high-level intersectoral conference 'Uzbekistan health reform in the Sustainable Development Goals era'. It is a dynamic long-term strategic plan, seeking to advance comprehensive national health reforms and meet the health-related Sustainable Development Goals by 2030. The conference brought together high-level representatives of different sectors, such as health, education, finance, civil society, the United Nations and international agencies, to map out implementation of the reform, focusing on primary health care development, health financing and strengthening governance for health and well-being at the intersectoral level.

We have also seen the development of a new pattern of country offices. For example, the Regional Office has started work in Greece at the request of the Government, with a new country office to support the immense health reform work underway there at country level and to build stronger linkages with their refugee and migrant health programmes.

Leaving no one behind in Greece

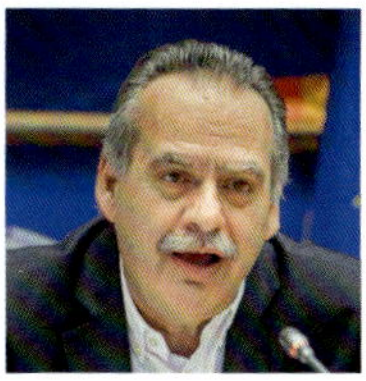

We have worked closely with the WHO European Office now through two very different governments in Greece. Amazingly, we have been able to maintain our collaborative work on transforming our health system and providing care to the many migrants and refugees who have arrived in our country.

The health system reform priorities that we have worked on together are universal health coverage, strengthening primary health care, and stopping the impoverishment of people needing health services. With WHO we constructed a 100-point document on how to deal with all these priorities. This document helped our Government and Ministry to adopt legislations and take ministerial decisions on actions to help move things forward.

Our work with refugees focused on the 1.5 million people who have arrived in Greece since 2015. WHO's guidance developed at the 2016 Rome High Level Meeting on Migration and Health helped us get started. Now we have a lot of experience to share. We worked to improve living conditions in refugee camps. We offered people access to primary health care and created an epidemiological surveillance system to inhibit the spread of any epidemic. We were guided by what WHO has been saying 'no one must be left behind'.

We understand that in public health politics, this is very important. If even a small amount of people are outside the health system, you cannot have public health security. We think that the best way is universal health coverage and access for everybody to national health services – but it is not easy to achieve.

I am pleased to say that to date we have not had epidemics in our refugee camps. We had a big campaign that provided more than 90% of refugee children with basic vaccinations. And even though we had a measles epidemic in Greece in 2018, no refugee and migrant children were infected!

Given the impact of the work we have done with WHO, we have decided to extend our collaboration and open a country office. Our plan is to build on existing programmes of health transformation and refugee work and also do work in neighbouring countries. There is trust and good will between us and we have things to do.

Ioannis Baskozos, Secretary General of Public Health, Ministry of Health, Greece

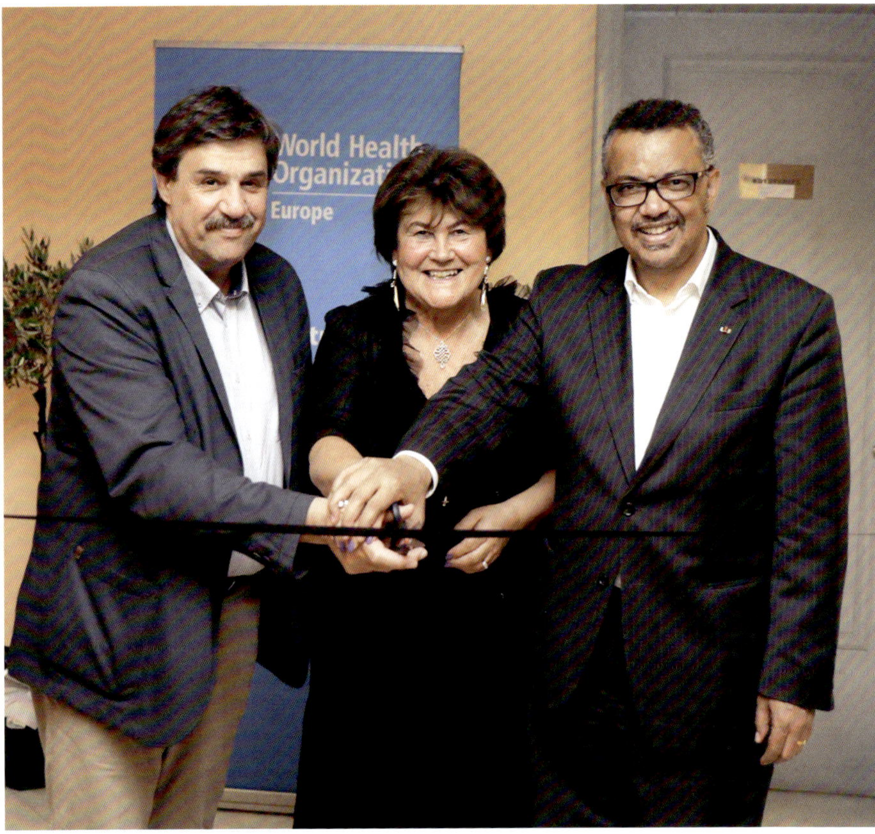

Andreas Xanthos, Minister of Health of Greece, Tedros Adhanom Ghebreyesus, WHO Director-General, and Zsuzsanna Jakab, WHO Regional Director for Europe inaugurated the new WHO Country Office in Greece on 20 June 2018. © WHO

Since country-level work is highly dependent on the capacity and knowledge of staff in the Regional Office, supported by WHO headquarters when required, the training and capacity building of staff were vital components of strengthening our work with countries. Importantly, this included our leaders at the country level, i.e. the heads of country offices and WRs, who were trained on strategic matters such as global health diplomacy, negotiating skills and leadership in the UN, but also on technical areas such as NCDs, Health 2020, and new research-based programmes such as the Evidence-informed Policy Network (EVIPNet) (see Section 7.1). Other key areas of training included communication and web-based training, writing skills, and EU project writing.

Trainings also covered ways of working better with United Nations partners within the framework of the UN reform programme, which allowed them to participate in Common Country Assessments (CCAs) contributing to the United Nations Development Assistance Frameworks (UNDAFs), in the countries where they existed.

Health diplomacy training

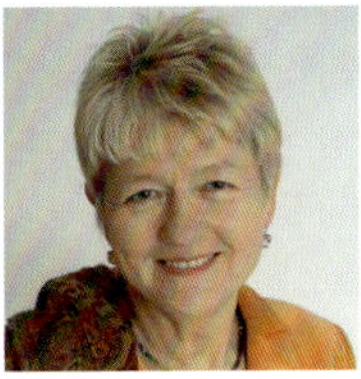

WHO staff, especially country based WRs for example, need these skills to be bridge builders and relationship developers with the forces of power within their countries, with donors and other agencies (including within the UN system). To address this need, we developed with the Regional Office a whole series of global health diplomacy training initiatives for country office staff that brought people together in a variety of ways with country representatives.

As a good technical person, you do not necessarily learn negotiation skills. You learn how to be a content expert but not necessarily how to just explain to a minister in ways they can understand and be persuaded by, for example, why a sugar tax might be important. We helped staff better understand how they can be a more active part of a political process, for example, that leads to a sugar tax. And how that requires diplomacy skills. This is different from the advocacy civil society might be doing to push a government etc. Diplomacy is always about processes of power and how you deal with them, how you play with them, negotiate with them and how you manage to influence them.

Ilona Kickbusch, Director of the Global Health Centre,
The Graduate Institute Geneva, Switzerland

Diplomacy training – enhancing the WR's skill mix

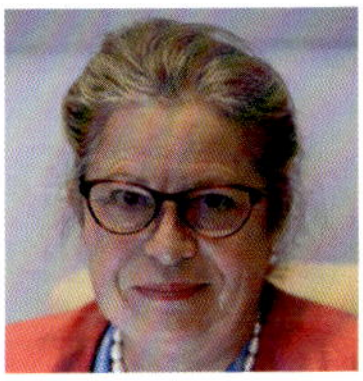

We realized that the WRs – who are the frontline leadership at country level – needed a new education. And this is where health diplomacy, the more broad-based political analyst role came in. We could no longer send epidemiologists to be the spokesperson for WHO in different countries, so the whole WR recruitment, and whole training and vetting and education was changed.

If we were going to achieve anything in countries, we could not anymore just deal with Ministers of Health. Ministers of Health are often in a weak position, despite health being on the political agenda in every single country whenever there is an election. They tend not to be the ones that are final decision-makers. And why can I say that? The Minister of Finance can, for example, overrule a Minister of Health because he believes that the taxes he is getting on tobacco is an income, and therefore he will stop legislation to stop tobacco, even though stopping tobacco is good business.

Getting the Minister of Health to understand that we should stop smoking is key but getting the Ministers of Finance to understand that this will actually protect both health and wealth, and that the Treasury will still be filled if s/he raises tobacco taxes, is most important.

Anne Marie Worning, Former Chief of Cabinet
WHO headquarters in Geneva

The main tool of cooperation in the Regional Office for Europe has been the BCAs and these have continued to be developed and implemented, with some amendments to the procedures in order to ensure a more proactive country-based approach. The SRC, as discussed above, also assists with the roll-out of CCSs to the countries that requested them and helps develop country support plans that are aligned with GPW13. I am happy to note that we have CCSs with high income countries without country offices, such as Belgium, Cyprus, Italy, Malta, Portugal, Russian Federation, Switzerland, and are currently being drafted with Israel, Kazakhstan and Turkey.

Specifically, to support the implementation of the IHR (2005) the Region has also developed new arrangements for countries to report. This can be conducted at the request of the Member States and includes the state of their preparedness and surveillance and response capacities in the context of IHR (2005), through voluntary Joint External Evaluation (JEE) with a focus on core capacities, as well as CCSs.

The Joint External Evaluation in Belgium

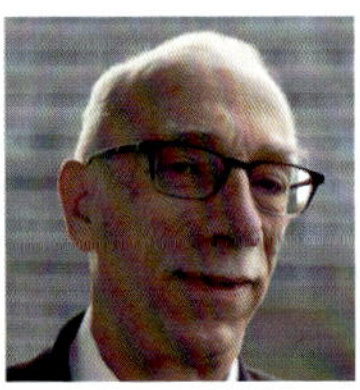

The Joint External Evaluation (JEE) provided us with a unique occasion to perform a wide and detailed assessment of the implementation of IHR core capacities in Belgium. It gave us the opportunity to gather a large panel of Belgian experts involved in the fight against public health emergencies of all origins. They came from fields like human and animal health, food safety, home affairs, disaster management, and nuclear, radiological or chemical sectors, etc.

The assessment of our strengths and weaknesses, by international and high-level experts, was most fruitful. We appreciated the positive comments as well as the areas that needed improvement, as identified by these experts. Their recommendations helped us to identify and prioritize actions, as well as providing us with a formal and necessary lever to ask for action and implement certain policies to strengthen our IHR capacities.

Before and after this exercise, Belgium sent experts to JEEs in Latvia, Switzerland, Burundi and North Macedonia. To be on 'the other side of the process' helps you even better to understand what it takes to implement the IHR, and why this is so important.

Daniel Reynders, Chair ECDC Management Board, Head of International Relations Unit, Belgian Federal Public Service (FPS) of Health, Food Chain Safety and Environment, Belgium

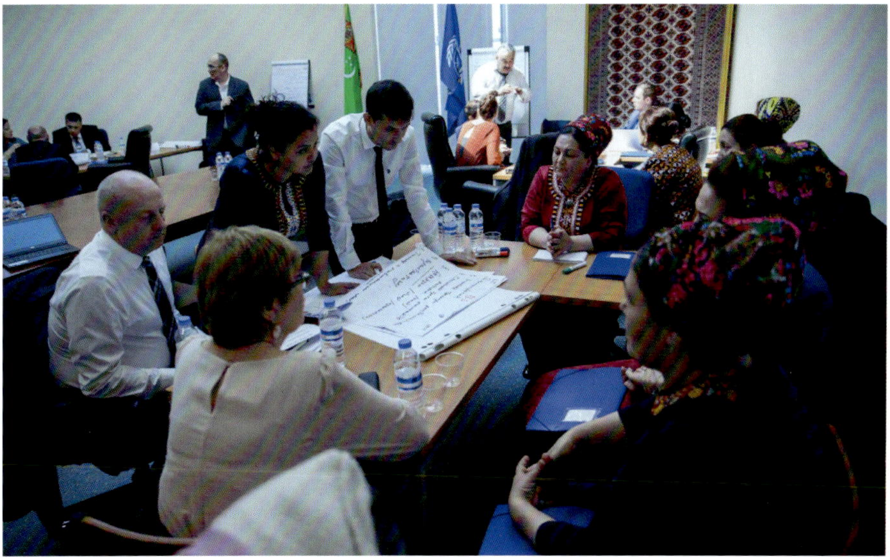

Voluntary Joint External Evaluation (JEE) of National emergency preparedness and response capabilities in Turkmenistan, 2016, in preparation for the 5th Asian Indoor and Martial Arts Games (AIMAG), which took place in Ashgabat, Turkmenistan, in September 2017. © WHO

On the administrative side, we have worked to ensure that resource mobilization (see Box 12) for country programmes and activities is in line with the approved Programme Budget, to strengthen contributor agreements, to allow more flexible funding, and to put more focus on the implementation and reporting.

We also have initiated external evaluations of programmes including peer reviews to identify barriers and means to improve efficiency and to strengthen the culture of evaluation. We have further strengthened internal management by establishing a compliance unit, for example, to increase financial discipline. This has now been replicated across the whole of WHO.

Box 12. Resource Mobilization

The Regional Office has been developing coordinated and integrated resource mobilization approaches which are aligned with global WHO guidance *(85)*. This is in line with the WHO reform and uses a four-step approach: initiate, validate, approve and report. For example, a country office (or technical unit) may come up with an idea or has a donor contact and would like to engage in a fundraising effort. In this case they may contact the Coordinated Resource Mobilization team (part of the Partnership (PAR) team in the Regional Director's Office) with information about the donor and about the area of work they want to fund raise for.

The PAR team checks the request and provides advice about the donor, e.g., whether there is a framework agreement in place with that donor, or whether there are templates for proposals. In some cases, we know that a donor is totally not acceptable for WHO and/or that there may be a conflict of interest. Based on this advice the Country Office (or the technical unit) decides whether they want to proceed with developing their proposal.

Once the proposal is finalized, the PAR team arranges for technical, budget and legal reviews of the proposal in the Office, before final review by the Divisional Director and approval and signature by myself. This is the procedure for doing all proposals and all agreements. I am glad to say that for urgent proposals we are able to do all this in a couple of days and for really urgent proposals in one day!

4.2 Geographically dispersed offices (GDOs)

The geographically dispersed offices (GDOs) were developed to create additional technical capacity and budget resources for the Regional Office through the creation of centres of excellence in different technical areas, in close collaboration with the hosting Member States. The GDOs collect and coordinate information exchanges and provide evidence-informed technical and analytical support for policy and programme development and implementation. This combined capacity has brought very good results (see Box 13).

Box 13. Geographically dispersed offices

GDOs are specialized offices established through ad hoc agreements between the WHO Regional Office for Europe and host national and/or local competent authorities. The GDOs are an integral part of the WHO Regional Office for Europe and their staff members are WHO employees and therefore part of the Secretariat. They serve all Member States of the WHO European Region in their specific technical areas of competence. They make use of financial resources and in-kind contributions by the host countries and the Regional Office for the entire duration of the respective agreement. These resources are supplemented by other donors in relation to specific programmes and projects.

The experience in the European Region during the last 10 years has been extremely positive in terms of: increased technical and financial resources for the WHO Regional Office for Europe programmes; the high quality and quantity of the outputs; and the facilitation of the implementation by the WHO European Region Member States of resolutions and other policy documents of the WHO European Region governing bodies. A number of high-quality scientific products of intercountry and global interest have been made available, which are of use both in the European Region and in other WHO Regions. A considerable proportion of the effort has been dedicated to support countries more in need and their institutions.

The GDOs have also offered to the WHO Regional Office for Europe many less visible but equally important benefits including:

1. the opportunity to work more effectively with international and intergovernmental organizations established in the host country, e.g. FAO in Rome and various UN Bodies, the European Food Safety Authority (EFSA) in Parma and the Secretariat of the United Nations Framework Convention on Climate Change (UNFCCC) in Bonn;
2. the development of many effective technical cooperation activities with the host country; and
3. an opportunity for a better and deeper understanding of the health situation in the host country.

An additional benefit of the GDOs is more flexible and efficient raising of voluntary donations. The experience acquired by GDOs through their activities has been distilled and provided as policy advice to the WHO European Region governing bodies for their wider consideration and possible use *(86)*.

When I started my term office in 2010, I wanted to look again at the role of the GDOs. That same year we conducted a review and achieved consensus with Member States at the Regional Committee on the way forward. Member States were strongly supportive of the work of the offices, so we worked to make the GDOs more visible and integrated and clarify their role under the supervision of the Regional Office.

We agreed that all core functions would remain at the Regional Office, whilst the GDOs would play their role to generate and provide evidence to the work and support the implementation in the countries. We also agreed to more clearly acknowledge the contributions of Member States that were supporting these entities. I have always felt it was important for the GDOs to serve the international community but at the same time to give special attention to the host (and funding) country. As such, the GDO would be able to promote WHO relevant themes (in collaboration with national counterparts) and be a spokesperson for WHO in the hosting country.

Our GDO in Barcelona is focused on health systems; Bonn is focused on environment and health; and Venice is focused on the social determinants of health. All have been strengthened. In addition, and with the generous assistance of the Governments concerned, new GDOs have been established, considerably strengthening our capacities to support Member States in the delivery of health services founded on the principles of primary health care (Almaty, Kazakhstan) and the prevention and control of noncommunicable disease (Moscow, Russian Federation).

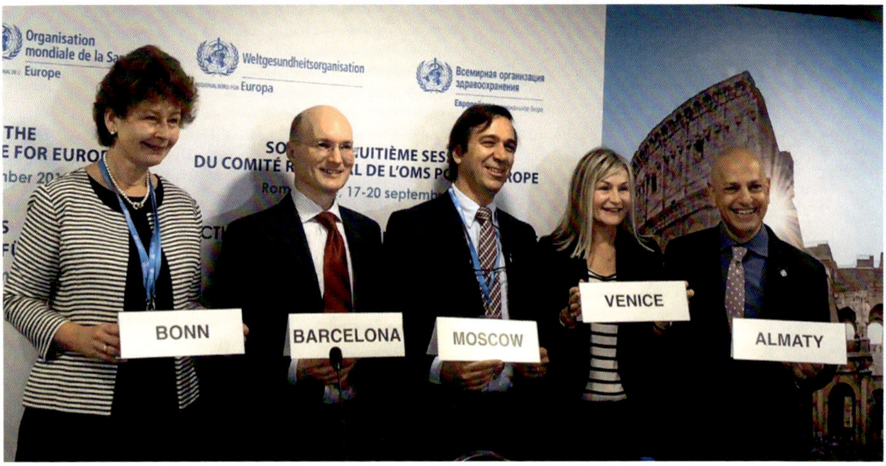

Breakfast briefing with the heads of the GDOs of the WHO European Region at the 68th session of the WHO Regional Committee for Europe, Rome, Italy, 17–20 September 2018.
© WHO

While the work of the GDOs is focused on specific technical areas, it is also aligned more broadly with Health 2020 approaches and is very much intersectoral. No office works in isolation. Connections have been created between all technical areas. To foster these connections regular videoconferencing and a yearly face-to-face retreat takes place, during which we discuss priority areas and countries.

The benefits of this GDO way of working has been recognized globally. Our GDO in Bonn helps with the development of guidelines in environment and health, for example on air quality. Our GDO in Moscow is focused on NCDs and has developed standards at the European and the global level, because of their capacity to analyse and implement at the same time. Our team at the Barcelona GDO supports work on UHC and financial protection, including reviews of out-of-pocket payments (OOPs), organizes regular flagship courses on health financing both for European health leaders, and also convenes other global courses, for example, on how health systems can be strengthened to support the management of NCDs (see Section 9.3.4.7).

The GDOs have created a unique space where they are well positioned to test and adjust analysis and insights, as well as set more useful standards based on their practical implementation activities (see Developmental reflection 1). Other WHO Regions have also followed suit, such as the Western Pacific Region which recently established a GDO on environmental health, learning from the Bonn Office.

GDO as models for other Regions

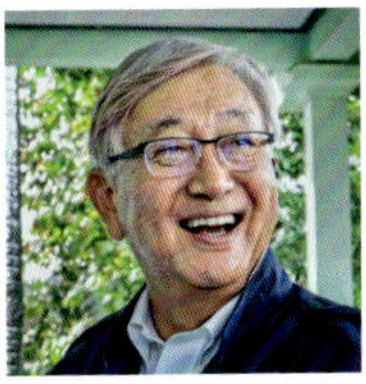

The WHO Regional Office for the Western Pacific has learned a lot from the WHO European Region. We have even adapted programmes and initiatives they have started; for example, the GDOs. They have at least five now. Essentially, they serve two functions. Firstly, they have helped raise money for the Office, and secondly, they enhance human resources for special programmes. For historical reasons, the WHO Regional Office for Europe receives less than they should from the overall WHO budget allocations which were agreed before 1990 and all the changes in the Region. These changes meant they suddenly had 20 more very challenging countries in the Region. They needed extra resources, and they came up with this idea to have Member States host some of their departments; e.g. Environment and Occupational Health in Bonn, Germany; Health Systems in Barcelona, Spain; etc. All these offices, supported by the host country, are engaged in some special activities for the whole Region. It has worked very well, and countries seem to be enjoying the status.

We're from a Region of several advanced countries, and we followed this example and now we've just started to have several GDOs. This is a very recent movement.

Young-soo Shin, Regional Director, WHO Regional Office for the Western Pacific, 2009–2019

Developmental reflection 1

Setting up the GDO on Primary Health Care – Kazakhstan

This GDO on primary health care was an idea that was launched about ten years ago. The idea was to have a centre that could implement our Alma-Ata Declaration on Primary Health Care. Early on Kazakhstan came forward to express their interest in supporting such a centre. Kazakhstan, of course has a long history of leadership in primary health care dated back to even before the 1978 Alma-Ata Declaration. As you can imagine, moving from interest to reality required a lot of political commitment and funds from the country. There was a tender offer made to all member states and Kazakhstan was the only country that proposed to support the establishment of a PHC GDO. That was in 2012. From that moment on the negotiations started. A business case was developed to show how the centre could work, what the technical areas of work could be, what was the benefit for Kazakhstan – which was of course very important, particularly for the internal and skilfully-managed negotiations of Salidat Kairbekova, the then Minister of Health. Finally, we came to an agreement.

The discussion was then about where it was to be established, and it was decided that it would be hosted by the Kazak National Medical University in Almaty. We assigned our programme manager of health services delivery to serve as acting head of the Office and he started to commute between Copenhagen and Almaty. Initially it was a small team that started to work in the area of primary health care. One year later we made the decision to merge our whole programme of health service delivery and the GDO. As a consequence, the Office expanded and started consolidating lines of activity and the team.

Country work

Our focus in the GDO was on country work for two reasons.

First, before the centre was started, in Copenhagen, we had already developed a policy for integrated service delivery that had primary health care at the centre. So, we didn't need to work on policies or strategies at this regional level. We already had a framework. Our plan was to focus on implementation in countries because that would bring more understanding, if the framework was working or not.

Second, because we had a new team, none of whom had worked in WHO before. So, it was a way to create a sort of new generation of professionals, that could focus on implementation and learn how to move an agenda at country level. None of them had much country experience – only one or two countries and sometimes just short missions. None of them had been residents abroad long enough to move an agenda. Focusing on 'moving an agenda in countries' gives you a different perspective. It requires different capacities, like learning to be simple in the messaging, being patient on how to implement, what to do, how to address country needs, etc. The GDO is working with many countries in the Region.

In the Republic of Moldova, for example, we have allocated staff to work with the Ministry to help them organize and implement their reform of primary health care. Helping them not only in the contents of their new strategies, but rather thinking through with them how we could bring sustainability to the reform itself. For example, for many years we have been working to create a model that could improve quality of care in practice. With our support they implemented this on a pilot basis and documented the experience. Based on the positive results there is now a Government Decree calling for the roll-out of this model across the whole country. So, we will now help them to do a roll-out that is targeting certain regions, etc.

In Norway, they were very interested to our surveys because they do not have enough data about the workload and satisfaction of the health workers. We have a few model survey tools dedicated to that. Norway, of course has a lot of capacity, so in this case we give them the tools and some training and then let them do the work. They give us feedback on what they have done with our materials. And in Kazakhstan, of course, we work very closely to roll-out some new ideas. It has become quite a primary care development laboratory. We have been working especially in isolated and poor regions.

Relevancy

In all our work we try to tailor our activities to be relevant for all countries. We make sure that we create tools, for example questionnaires that aim at collecting data that many countries want to compare. We also try to bring countries together and to connect them. We find that too often countries do not document their experiences, especially in western countries where many experiences are decentralized. The ones that are providing primary care services, for example, are at the local and regional levels. Therefore, we have tried to network with the regions in order to gather their intelligence and to bring it back to the national level.

This dynamic exchange also exposes the regions to international experiences. We have found that such exposure gives the regions the confidence to continue if they are going in the right direction, or to change if they see the need to modify anything.

Finally, language is important. Many concepts evolve and over time get more refined, precise and useful. For example, many will start with patient satisfaction measurement and overtime evolve to more detailed evaluation of patient experience. While there will always be cultural and contextual issues to deal with, if people or countries can see how these concepts evolve, they can either follow or jump to the next step, saving themselves years of work that has already been done by other countries. Facilitating such 'leap frogging' is one of the great benefits of GDOs' work in countries.

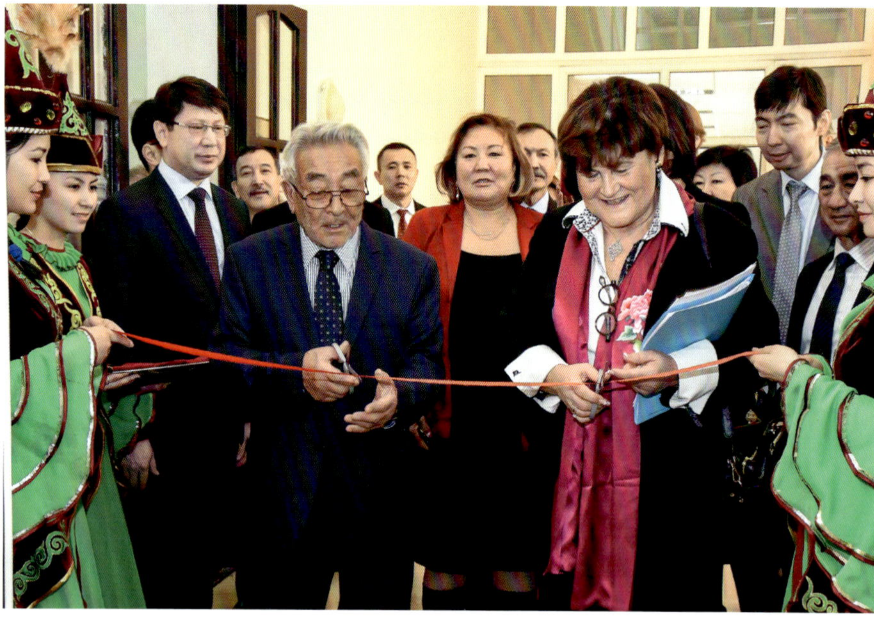

Zsuzsanna Jakab, WHO Regional Director for Europe, and Torgeldy Sharmanov, President of the Kazakh Academy of Nutrition, Former Minister of Health, Kazakh Soviet Socialist Republic, USSR, 1978, inaugurating the new centre of excellence in Almaty, Kazakhstan, 2015. © Sergey Gurzhin

Summary reflection

Strengthening collaboration with Member States

Message 3: Relevance and leadership are earned qualities

We learned that we were able to engage with all our Member States by strengthening our technical skills in areas where they had expressed a need, e.g. economic impact data concerning out-of-pocket payments, anticipating health needs, migration and health, men's health, etc. and by enhancing our resources through partnerships, networks and new GDOs.

We have been able to demonstrate our relevance and leadership in many new and established areas not only for our Region, but globally as well. Areas worth highlighting here include:

- developing a more evidence-informed focus on equity;
- re-emphasizing and reinvigorating public health through delivery of the European Action Plan for the Strengthening of Public Health Capacities and Services and a new vision for advancing public health for sustainable development in the WHO European Region agreed at the 68th session of the Regional Committee in 2018;
- establishing the Regional Office as a European centre of public health excellence and guidance;
- energizing the life-course approach;
- investing in people e.g. through summer schools on health financing and migration and health;
- delivering a number of public health related European strategies and action plans e.g. and action plan mental health, sexual and reproductive health and men's health;
- being creatively proactive, rapidly responsive; and,
- following through on all commitments.

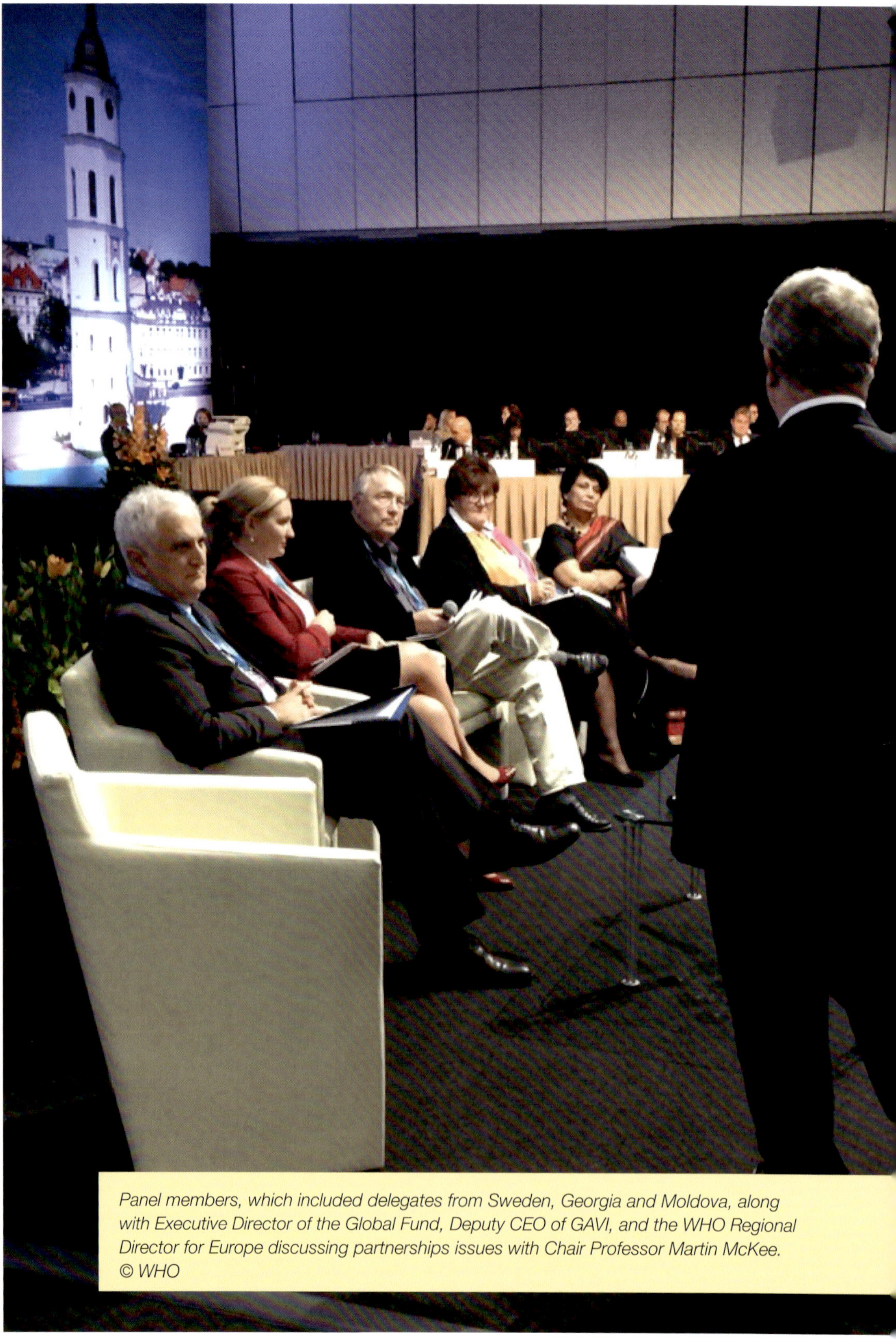

Panel members, which included delegates from Sweden, Georgia and Moldova, along with Executive Director of the Global Fund, Deputy CEO of GAVI, and the WHO Regional Director for Europe discussing partnerships issues with Chair Professor Martin McKee.
© WHO

5. Strategic partnerships

We understood early on that engaging with partners would be key to Health 2020 implementation and progress. Partnerships can create an enabling environment for public health policies. They can facilitate whole-of-government, whole-of-society and intersectoral collaboration for health, develop broad international, national and local constituencies, and create policy coherence among different actors, and more efficient use of resources. How to realize these benefits for ourselves and our Member States has been our challenge.

Finding effective ways to develop, implement and monitor performance of partnerships has therefore been a key strategic direction for the Regional Office as we have initiated new and strengthened existing collaborative work with our UN family, the EU and its institutions, global health partnerships, networks and NGOs. We have worked hard to be receptive, flexible, open and creative in forming partnerships that allow all parties to utilize their specific expertise, stay true to their mandates, fulfil their governance arrangements and enhance our collective impact on people's health and well-being.

We made sure that partnerships were always on the agenda and were reviewed at every Regional Committee. A new partnership strategy – Partnerships for health in the WHO European Region – was adopted by the 67th session of the Regional Committee, which took place on 11–14 September 2017 in Budapest, Hungary.

5.1 The United Nations

I believe that the old 'silo' approaches that WHO and other agencies within the United Nations System used to adopt will not work in today's complex interdependent global reality. Organizations cannot just focus on their own mandate, governing bodies and a narrow sectoral focus on activities and implementation. Such 'silo' approaches have been targeted for change within the United Nations reform programmes.

Regional UN agency cooperation

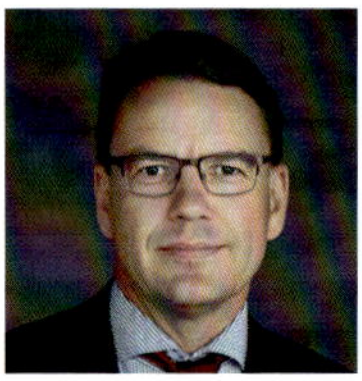

During the period of Zsuzsanna's tenure, UN agency cooperation has been greatly strengthened and expanded. In some Regions, there have been difficulties bringing together all the UN partners under existing regional coordination mechanisms. In Europe, however, we have in practice merged our Regional level UN Development Group (UNDG) and our regional coordination mechanisms. This has been a very progressive development.

I would say the WHO Regional Office for Europe as represented by Zsuzsanna is one of the real driving forces of our much stronger coordination at the European level.

Christian Friis Bach, Former Executive Secretary, United Nations Economic Commission for Europe (UNECE)

The SDGs have given a new frame and emphasis to the United Nations reform process and have encouraged us to intensify our coordinated partnership work, on both Regional and country levels, with the United Nations and the UN system, with the aim of strengthening policy coherence for health across the Region. WHO is a full part of this work in countries, working closely with UN Country Teams and UN Resident Coordinators, and using common UN instruments such as CCAs and United Nations Development Assistance Frameworks (UNDAFs), now renamed 'UN Sustainable Development Cooperation Frameworks'.

Delivering as one UN

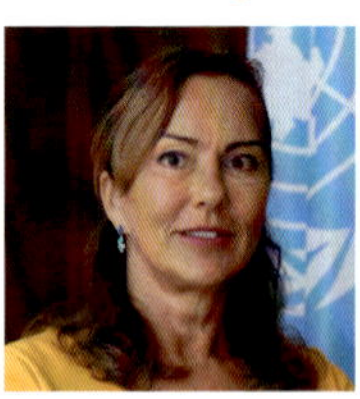

I chair the UN Regional Coordination Mechanism (RCM).

In Europe we do regular joint meetings with the Regional UN Development Group (R-UNDG) and coordinate our activities well. In fact, this has been recognized as an example of good practice by the UN Secretary General and is in line with Agenda 2030 which calls for such cooperation to 'deliver as one UN'.

We are the only Region to have developed so-called issue-based coalitions. We have six of them, where we work jointly; for example, on gender, youth, statistics and well-being and health. This has been a really successful approach and looks at issues such as how to plan joint work, how to approach countries, and how to coordinate activities on issues that affect the mandate of more UN agencies.

Olga Algayerova, Executive Secretary, United Nations Economic Commission for Europe (UNECE)

As Regional Director I have been promoting active engagement by all our staff and Offices in the UN coordination mechanisms for Europe and central Asia *(87)*. I have personally been a very active member of the Regional Coordination Mechanism (RCM) and the Regional United Nations Development Group (R-UNDG). Both the RCM and the R-UNDG provide excellent entry points for United Nations coordination and for creating synergies and policy coherence. I was honoured to serve as Acting Director of the Regional UNDG in 2018.

I am pleased to say that in 2014, inspired by Health 2020, and following the 2014 UN High-Level meeting of the General Assembly on the comprehensive review and assessment of the progress achieved in the prevention and control of NCDs *(146)*, the RCM and all UN regional directors agreed to establish the UN Regional Thematic Group on Noncommunicable Diseases and Social, Economic and Environmental Determinants of Health led by WHO. The Thematic Group sought to implement the WHO Action Plan for implementation of the European Strategy for the Prevention and Control of Noncommunicable Diseases 2012–2016 *(12)* and address other relevant aspects of Health 2020. The work of the Thematic Group not only was important to align UN work at Regional level but also supported the implementation of the Action Plan at country level. It has been seen as a good example of UN collaboration to deliver jointly at Regional and country level. While the Thematic Group itself has not continued, it served as a model for the later developed issue-based coalitions.

The UN Issue-based Coalition on Health and Well-being for All at All Ages (IBC-Health), was endorsed by the R-UNDG in 2016 *(88)*. The IBC-Health is one of the six IBCs that have been established under the UN coordination mechanism for Europe and central Asia. I have been honoured to lead IBC-Health, which works as a pan-European enabling mechanism to facilitate and promote the implementation of SDG 3 and its targets, as well as the health-related targets of the other SDGs. It aims to coordinate activities of the relevant UN funds, programmes and specialized agencies and other intergovernmental organizations and partners, with a focus on leaving no one behind.

In our first three years (2017–2019) IBC-Health has focused on areas where there is existing cooperation, a degree of urgency for further action, high political importance, high burden of disease, or high unmet population needs. Four work streams were implemented, including: maternal and child health; HIV, tuberculosis and viral hepatitis; access to medicines and health products; and migration. After the Astana Conference on Primary Health Care (see Section 9.3.4.6), a fifth work stream has been added on primary health care, led by UNICEF and WHO. The WHO Regional Office for Europe also participates in the IBC–Gender, IBC–Equity and IBC–Data groups.

A different way of working

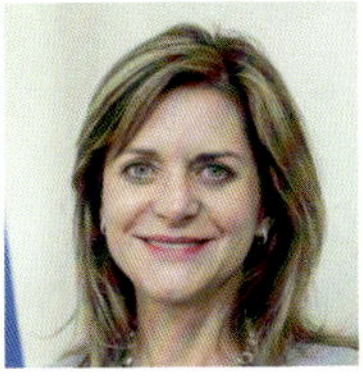

Our R-UNDG meets twice a year and provides an opportunity for all of us to talk about the key issues. The WHO Regional Director for Europe is the chair of the Issue-based Coalition on health (IBC-Health), a mechanism through which we all meet around health topics. We came up with a joint action plan, which provides the basis for our excellent partnership.

This issue-based coalition approach is really one of the ways that our Region has taken the lead in trying to drive the UN reform changes the Secretary General wants to see.

We are really working in a different way now. When one agency, for example, goes to a country we are not just there as WHO or the United Nations Population Fund (UNFPA), we are there for health, or we are there for reproductive health, or we are there for youth. In this way we bring colleagues together and decide what are the major issues. It is no longer 'per agency'.

We now work more as joint advocates. We've even come up with position papers to guide us all on what the key messages are when it comes to specific issues, whether it is population dynamics, social protection, or health for all. We deliver these common messages whenever any of us has an opportunity to meet with government officials and others who can influence policy development and implementation

It is a different way of working and the Secretary General mentioned in his report on UN reform that the Eastern Europe and Central Asia Region is leading the pack when it comes to promoting collaboration among the agencies.

Alanna Armitage, Regional Director, The United Nations Population Fund (UNFPA) Eastern Europe and Central Asia

The Regional Office, the UN Population Fund Regional Office for Eastern Europe and Central Asia, and the United Nations Children's Fund Regional Office for Central and Eastern Europe and the Commonwealth of Independent States continued their close cooperation under the Joint Action Framework, signed in 2013.

In the Action Framework, the three agencies are committed to consolidating their work to improve the quality of health care delivery for women and children, and to ensure UHC, for underserved and vulnerable populations with a focus on strengthening collaboration at country level.

Strategic partnership to achieve health for all

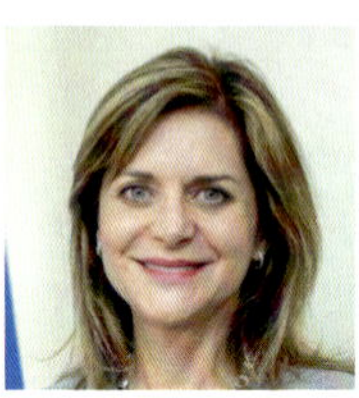

From our perspective we will never achieve health for all without partnerships. They are critical for the work we do because health is much more than a medical issue. It is very much related to social determinants and to the environment. In order to achieve health for all, or the SDGs, we must work in partnership.

At UNFPA, we are very much committed to working in partnership; most of what we do is in partnership. We are the coordinators of the International Conference on Population and Development agenda (the ICPD agenda) but we are certainly not the only custodian of that agenda. Our goal is to work with that agenda and our partners to push it forward and implement the commitments for action made at the ICPD.

Alanna Armitage, Regional Director, The United Nations Population Fund (UNFPA) Eastern Europe and Central Asia

WHO and UNICEF partnership

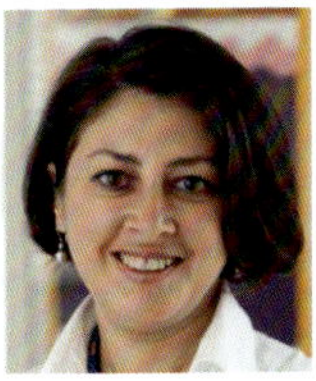

As a specialized agency with a strong Regional multi-disciplinary presence, coupled with its readiness to work closely with UNICEF which offers a strong multisectoral presence around implementation at the country level, WHO provides a structural readiness for institutional collaboration. The development of shared goals and vision, some derived from global agendas but most born or contextualized to address Regional priorities, has supported the partnership and coordinated actions.

There was excellent cooperation and coordination in responding to the polio outbreak in central Asia in 2010 and the joint polio outbreak response in Ukraine in 2015 (see Developmental reflections 6 and 10). Both agencies work jointly to support governments to respond to ongoing measles outbreaks across the Region. WHO and UNICEF are the major partners of GAVI and work together to improve and maintain high, sustainable immunization coverage.

Responding to the migrant and refugee influx to Europe, joint immunization and nutrition guidance were developed together with WHO, and both agencies collaborated to ensure vaccination and health screening of migrants arriving in Greece.

UNICEF collaborates with WHO and other partners for the development of integrated early childhood services which comprise comprehensive care of mothers before, during and after pregnancy; parenting and caregiver support; childcare; integrated services for nutritional support; access to early learning opportunities; and services for children with special needs.

In the area of HIV/AIDS, the agencies work together towards elimination of mother-to-child transmission through evidence generation, capacity-building to improve prevention/treatment, testing and counselling, strengthening monitoring system and addressing stigma and discrimination.

Adolescent health is another important area of collaboration between UNICEF, WHO and UNFPA. Several countries in the Region have been jointly supported to generate evidence on adolescent health and development, establish youth-friendly services, develop and support implementation of quality standards for health service provision to adolescents and youth.

Work on mental health has recently been initiated in central Asia and builds on initiatives around suicide prevention.

The agencies have also worked together to address persistent and emerging maternal and child nutrition problems. These include micronutrient deficiencies and stunting which are increasingly coupled with the opposite problem: growing rates of overweight and obesity particularly among urban children and adolescents.

Joint UNICEF and WHO efforts resulted in several maternities in the Region being designated as baby-friendly hospitals by promoting breastfeeding.

Afstan Khan, Regional Director for Europe and Central Asia (ECA), Special Coordinator for the Refugee and Migrant Response in Europe, UNICEF

5.2 Global health partnerships and governmental organization partners

In our work to establish and maintain effective collaboration to strengthen Regional work, including in the provision of technical assistance to countries, the Regional Office has strengthened many global health partnerships over the last ten years with, for example, Gavi, the Vaccine Alliance (GAVI) and the Global Fund to Fight AIDS, Tuberculosis and Malaria; as well as other governmental organization partners like Organisation for Economic Co-operation and Development (OECD).

GAVI is an important partner of the WHO Regional Office. It was established as a Global Health Partnership in 2000, with the aims of accelerating access to vaccines, strengthening countries' health and immunization systems, and introducing innovative new immunization technology. It has subsequently supported the immunization of some 326 million children and prevented a potential 5.5 million deaths *(95)*.

WHO is one of four permanent members of the GAVI Board and alternate Chair (with UNICEF) of GAVI's Executive Committee. WHO provides support to vaccine-related research and development, standards setting and regulating vaccine quality, as well as the development of evidence-based policy options to guide vaccine use and maximize country access. WHO also contributes to cold chain and vaccine management, training and post-introduction analysis of vaccines.

The Regional Office for Europe and the WHO country offices support the coordination of GAVI activities in countries in the European Region. WHO helps countries draft applications for GAVI support, as well as plans of action for introducing vaccines. WHO also provides technical support to the implementation of immunization programmes, including storage and logistics, as well as to monitoring and evaluation measures.

A core element of GAVI's current development model is to work together with countries in scaling up domestically funded immunization efforts. As countries develop economically, GAVI requires them to take on more of the costs until they 'transition' fully out of GAVI support.

We also work closely with the Global Fund Secretariat and provide technical assistance to countries under the Global Fund's New Funding Model. This includes technical assistance to countries in the development of concept notes.

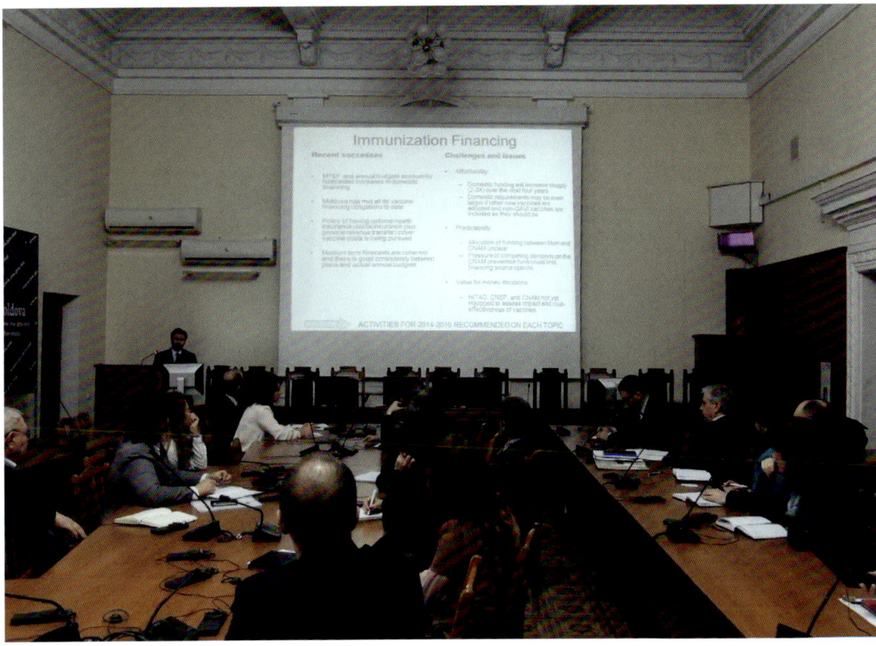

Experts from WHO and GAVI meeting with government and institutional stakeholders on 10 –14 February 2014 to provide technical support in light of the Republic of Moldova's upcoming "graduation" from GAVI support for its immunization programme.
© Ministry of Health, Republic of Moldova.

Global Fund partnership and impact

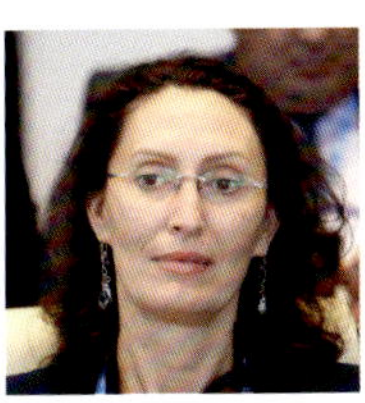

I represent the Global Fund, and our keyword is partnership. Since it began, the Global Fund partnership has had extraordinary impact. In the countries where we invest around the world, more than 27 million lives have been saved and the number of people dying from AIDS, TB and malaria has been slashed by one third. The Global Fund delivers this impact together with a diverse range of partners including bilateral partners, multilateral and technical agencies, private sector companies, foundations, implementing countries, civil society groups, and people affected by the diseases.

In the European Region, it has been a natural course of action to team up with colleagues at WHO Regional Office for Europe, both at the Regional and country level, and work with them to ensure that additional financial resources both domestically and internationally are mobilized and deployed to support well developed, technically sound, ethically based programmes for HIV, TB and malaria, and to achieve impact. Since 2010 when Dr Jakab's term started, we've had a real activation and a very committed joined up approach to addressing the challenges of HIV, TB and malaria in the Region. The two organizations signed a memorandum of understanding in 2011 which charted the course of our joint work forward.

During the last 15 years, countries in the eastern Europe and central Asia region have made significant strides in the fight against HIV, TB and malaria. We have highlighted remarkable accomplishments, with a number of countries in south Caucasus and central Asia defeating malaria. With the active engagement of civil society and joint work with governments, evidence-based HIV prevention work, including harm reduction, has been scaled up across the region to prevent generalization of the epidemic. We have jointly witnessed big strides in the fight against TB with decreasing TB incidence and mortality rates, faster and more accurate diagnosis of MDR-TB cases and expanding access to life saving MDR-TB treatment. These achievements prove that global commitment, impact-focused partnership and smart health investments can achieve remarkable success against the world's deadliest diseases.

On the road to these accomplishments, the WHO Regional Office for Europe has supported national stakeholders in the design of technically sound, evidence-based programmes to address HIV and TB challenges, country by country. WHO has also focused on addressing implementation challenges, supporting capacity strengthening in multiple countries, and providing technical guidance. For instance, the WHO Regional Office for Europe was the first to establish a Regional Green Light Committee which has become a critical pillar to support the MDR-TB fight in the Region. Supporting the development of resilient and sustainable systems for health has also been a priority area of joint work.

Still, there are continuous challenges and emerging threats in the fight against HIV and TB in the Region and we will need to further mobilize our efforts and step up the fight. To end the epidemics and achieve the SDGs, we need to jointly drive increased domestic financing, efficient investments, accelerated innovation, the reduction of human rights and gender-related barriers, even more effective partnerships with a relentless focus on impact.

Maria Kirova, Department Head, Asia, Europe, Latin America and the Caribbean, The Global Fund to Fight AIDS, Tuberculosis and Malaria

OECD and WHO Regional Office for Europe established a framework for mutually agreed health priorities in 1999 and 2005, particularly in relation to health and development. Our long-standing relationship focuses on issues of improving the collection, harmonization and dissemination of health data and indicators, issues in health systems and environment and health, and NCDs. In 2012, I signed a Joint Action Plan with Yves Leterme, Deputy Secretary General of OECD, to intensify collaboration in the European Region in developing reliable health information and analyzing challenges to health systems and policy responses.

Work on health information therefore continues to be at the core of the collaboration, especially on defining indicators and joint datasets. There is also active collaboration in devising indicators for well-being as part of Health 2020 monitoring.

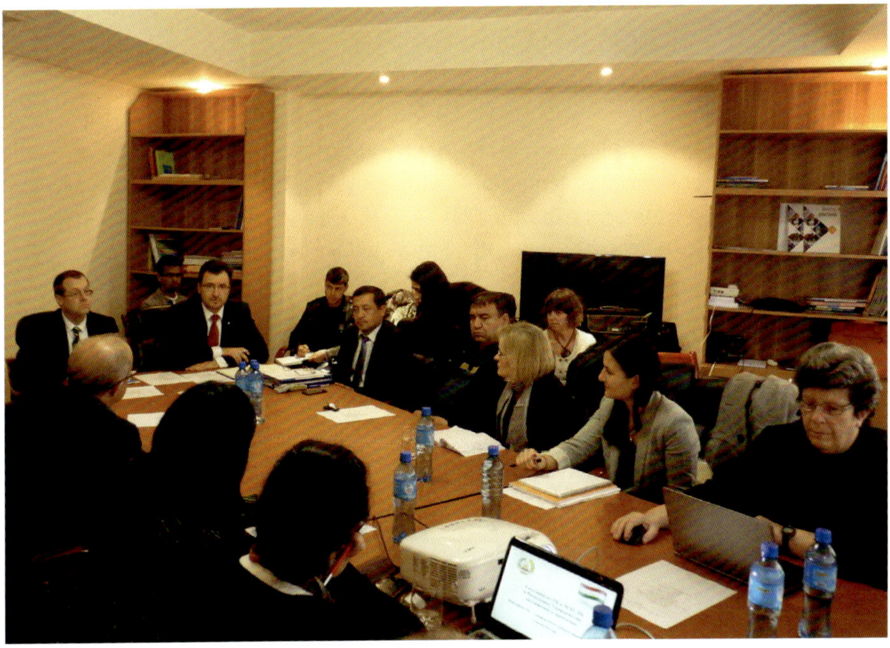

Hans Kluge, Director of the Division of Health Systems and Public Health, WHO Regional Office for Europe, meeting with national and development partners including the WHO Country Office in Tajikistan and the Global Fund Portfolio Manager, on 4 April 2014 to discuss the sustainability of the national tuberculosis (TB) programme (NTP) and overall health system strengthening within the area of TB/MDR-TB control and prevention. © WHO/Tahmina Alimamedova

In the area of health systems, successful collaboration and joint meetings have been held that are linked to the Oslo and Tallinn meetings on austerity and health systems, respectively. We have also had a close collaboration with the Senior Budget Officials of the OECD. In 2016, WHO became an official Observer in the OECD Health Committee.

5.3 The European Union

The relationship with the European Union (EU) is of profound importance for WHO as a whole and for the Regional Office for Europe in particular. The mandate of the two organizations are different but mutually supportive. I have always seen the EU mandate as being complementary to that of WHO. The EU mandate is very strong in legislative issues, for example how to improve and reduce pollution in the environment or how to label food products. They have the mandate and have more control than WHO in this area.

But, on the other hand, WHO's strength is to use strong public health evidence and build consensus around these types of issues.

Making partnerships work

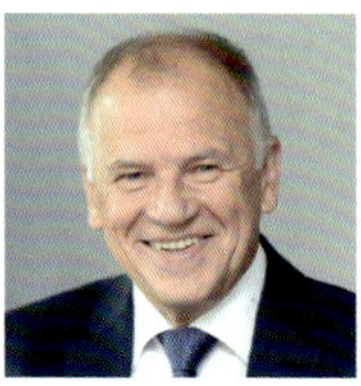

I see a fortunate combination of personal constellations and structural factors as key reasons for the success of the partnership between the Commission and WHO.

I would like to underline how much I have personally enjoyed the pleasant and productive collaboration with Dr Zsuzsanna Jakab, in her capacity as WHO Regional Director for Europe, during the last five years of my mandate as the European Commissioner for Health.

I observe the same openness and will to collaborate among the colleagues at technical level in both organizations. This mutual trust is also present in the regular meetings that we have to discuss our collaboration in specific priority areas, at high-level meetings of senior officials and in international meetings and conferences.

This positive spirit and the strong collaboration builds on the awareness in both our organizations that we share the same objectives, namely to support the EU and WHO member countries in achieving better health for their citizens, and that we complement each other as organizations: it is the WHO's mandate to set health norms, provide guidance and technical expertise. The Commission is strong in providing networks and financial support for the implementation of the set targets and objectives.

Vytenis P. Andriukaitis, EU Commissioner for Health and Food Safety

I am very supportive to a strong continued EU mandate on health issues. I have always believed that if we respect each other's mandate, work together and support each other, we can go much further than without each other. We give this message every time any of our staff go to Brussels – that health is a very important part of development and unless we invest in health, now and in the future, it will be difficult to make progress.

Until 2015, the framework for this collaboration was a joint declaration between the European Commission and the WHO Regional Office for Europe, presented at the 60th session of the Regional Committee in Moscow in 2010 *(100)*. It highlighted an agreement to strengthen existing areas of cooperation – health security, health information, tobacco control, nutrition and obesity, cancer and other NCDs, environment and health, and the strengthening of health systems – and extend cooperation to include e-health, health research, innovation in health and education. The 12th Senior Officials Meeting of the EC and WHO in 2015 assessed the progress of that collaboration, and a new partnership framework –'The objectives, principles and modalities for continued cooperation between the European Commission and the WHO Regional Office for Europe' – was jointly drafted and presented during the 65th session of the Regional Committee in 2015 in Vilnius.

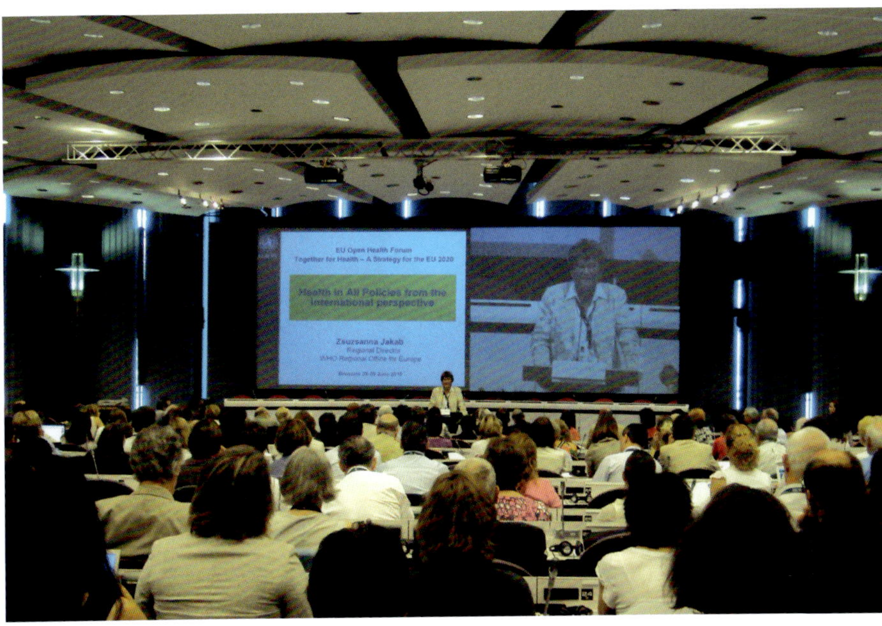

Zsuzsanna Jakab, WHO Regional Director for Europe, giving a keynote address at the European Union Open Health Forum in Brussels, Belgium, 29 June 2010 where partners discussed health in policy agendas. © WHO

PART 1

European Commission and WHO – 'close partners'

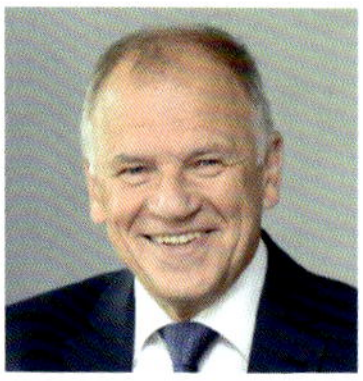

The European Commission and the WHO are close partners. It is not only reflected by the fact that the Commission is one of the biggest funders of the WHO, but also because we share the same objectives, namely to support the EU and WHO Member States in achieving better health for their citizens.

Since 2014, the Commission has contributed on average €50 million per year to the WHO budget. In 2017, it gave €81 million in voluntary contributions. It was the fourth highest contribution from a State actor. This signals the high importance that the Commission attaches to the partnership with the WHO, in Europe and globally.

The Commission builds its own work and policies on guidance issued by the WHO, i.e. its guidelines, recommendations, objectives, targets, rules, scientific evidence, and advice on health topics. In fact, the Commission is involved, with EU Member States and other countries, in their development. It pays high attention to the fact that its initiatives, such as the European One Health Action Plan on Antimicrobial Resistance from 2017 or its Communication on Strengthened Cooperation against Vaccine Preventable Diseases from 2018, are in line with the relevant WHO strategic documents and health policies. Also, in its approach to NCDs, the Commission relies on WHO targets instead of developing a separate set.

The partnership agreements and collaboration with the WHO provide valuable support for the Commission in all these activities. The so-called 'Vilnius Declaration' from 2015 established a strengthened framework for collaboration between the Commission and WHO in Europe. One example of a practical outcome is that we have improved the exchange of information on health alerts between our organizations through a renewed Early Warning and Response System. Information on dangerous infectious diseases is exchanged in a timely fashion and the response to the threats is triggered with the aim of protecting EU citizens against health emergencies.

Vytenis P. Andriukaitis, EU Commissioner for Health and Food Safety

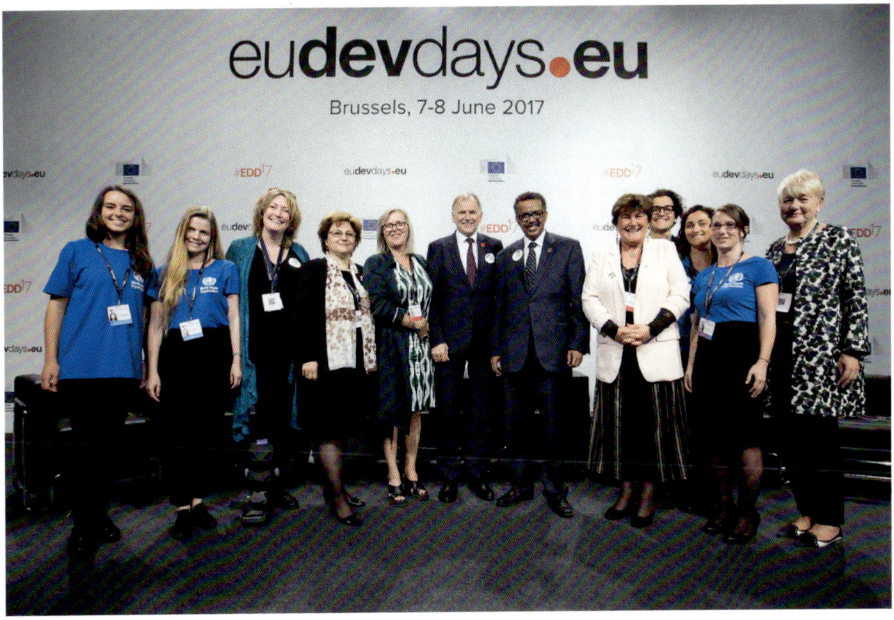

EU Development Days 2017 (EDDs 2017), Brussels WHO session on 'Reducing health inequalities through global partnership and collaboration'. © WHO/Erik Luntang

In addition, the Regional Office has continued to work with the countries holding the Presidency of the Council of the European Union to ensure coherent follow-up of priorities in the Region, to sound out the provision of support on health issues to countries holding the Presidency and to support the Presidency in its involvement with WHO governing bodies.

The Regional Office has expanded and consolidated its collaboration with the European Parliament and its Committee on Environment, Public Health and Food Safety, as well as other committees and parliamentary groups, and provides evidence-based information and WHO strategies and policies.

The Regional Office also has joint work plans and common guiding principles with the European Centre for Disease Prevention and Control, the European Food Safety Authority, the European Environment Agency (EEA), and the European Monitoring Centre for Drugs and Drug Addiction.

Collaboration with ECDC

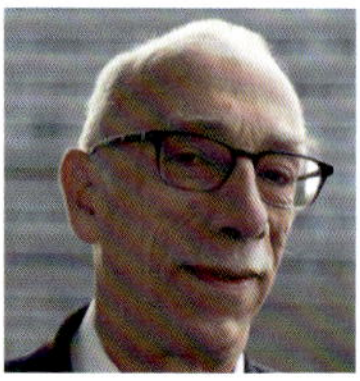

While ECDC was growing there were difficulties in finding a smooth way of collaborating with WHO. In its first years ECDC had to get itself recognized by the rest of the world as a centre of scientific excellence. Once that was accomplished, and especially since Zsuzsanna Jakab has moved from ECDC to WHO, we have entered a period of real collaboration. Among many other things, Zsuzsanna knew the added value of each organization. Current collaborations increase the efficiency of both. Regional surveillance of tuberculosis and AIDS is an example, with ECDC collecting data for the whole Region by agreement with WHO.

Another important thing from my point of view, is what at ECDC we call 'the rapid risk assessment'– it is an example of ECDC bringing added value to the WHO Regional Office for Europe because WHO assessments usually come later than the EU's.

However there continue to be reporting and turf issues that are difficult to solve. One example has been the notification of public health threats. At EU level there is the Early Warning and Response system which is a legally based system requiring EU Member States to notify such threats. On the other hand, we have the International Health Regulation (IHR) which also asks for formal notification of Member States. Member States have always asked to avoid double notification in cases of public health emergencies or threats. After discussion between the Regional Director, the European Commission and Member States' voices in governing bodies, a solution was found. A unique system of notification was established through which the same event does not need to be notified twice. It is now working quite smoothly.

Daniel Reynders, Chair ECDC Management Board,
Head of International Relations Unit, Belgian Federal Public Service (FPS)
of Health, Food Chain Safety and Environment, Belgium

It is also a matter of personal relationships

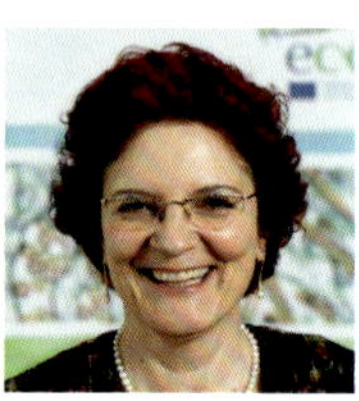

The starting point for both WHO and us is that we both have a legal mandate and there is an overlap. Both of us, for example, have certain obligations to collect data, to give advice, to do surveillance and so forth. These overlapping responsibilities gave us an incentive – both for our own sake and that of Member States – to come to an agreement on how we would like to work together.

Member States of both the EU and the WHO, for example, have to supply information to both institutions and often it was the same… causing double work … so we agreed to share the work. Now Member States report all the data on agreed diseases to us, and whatever they also need to report to WHO, we provide to WHO. In this way we were able to create an efficient allocation of WHO and ECDC resources, and also eliminate the double reporting and extra burden of work for Member States.

This agreement took some time as WHO and ECDC are not independent organizations. We are part of larger institutions with different rules; for example, on data protection. The EU data protection requirements would only let us provide data to WHO if they agreed to certain data protection requirements. WHO could not agree as their data protection requirements were different. In the end we found a way how to meet the requirements of both institutions.

This kind of creative problem solving is facilitated between organizations whose directors have good formal and informal working relations like Zsuzsanna and I. We both have affirmed our belief in such cooperation and we want to make it work. Even if there is no legal obligation, we both believe in and feel strongly a kind of ethical obligation to not cause double work. We are covering similar areas, so we work together.

Our formal agreement of cooperation is very helpful, and its policies and procedures help us work together more smoothly. It has, for example, created coordination meetings that allow us to plan our joint work programme more efficiently and transparently for the experts in Member States. But in the end, our partnership and cooperation are manifest and realized best through our personal professional relationships.

Andrea Ammon, Director, European Centre for Disease Prevention and Control (ECDC)

5.4 Non-State actors

WHO collaborates with many non-State actors, including NGOs, philanthropic foundations, academia and the private sector. These partnerships became even more important in the context of Health 2020 to ensure whole-of-society engagement. In addition, the Regional Office has a wide network of collaborating centres which implement several activities to support WHO programmes (see Section 4). Since 2016, the Framework for Engagement with non-State actors (FENSA), adopted by the 69th World Health Assembly, has been used to help facilitate these engagements *(90)*.

In 2017, at its 67th session, the WHO Regional Committee for Europe endorsed a new procedure to accredit European non-State actors (NSAs) not in 'official relations with WHO', to enable them to participate in future Regional Committee sessions *(203)*. The arrangements for 'official relations' were long-standing but had been criticized for being bureaucratic and unfriendly. These arrangements were also targeted and tailored for big global umbrella organizations. Many agencies that we were working with at the European level, therefore, couldn't really apply for that status. The objective of this Regional accreditation procedure was to enable Regional or subregional NSAs which are not in 'official relations' but work closely with WHO to participate as observers, without the right to vote, in Regional Committee sessions and to submit written and oral statements. We had the 'first wave' of 19 accredited European organizations join the Regional Committee meeting as observers in 2018.

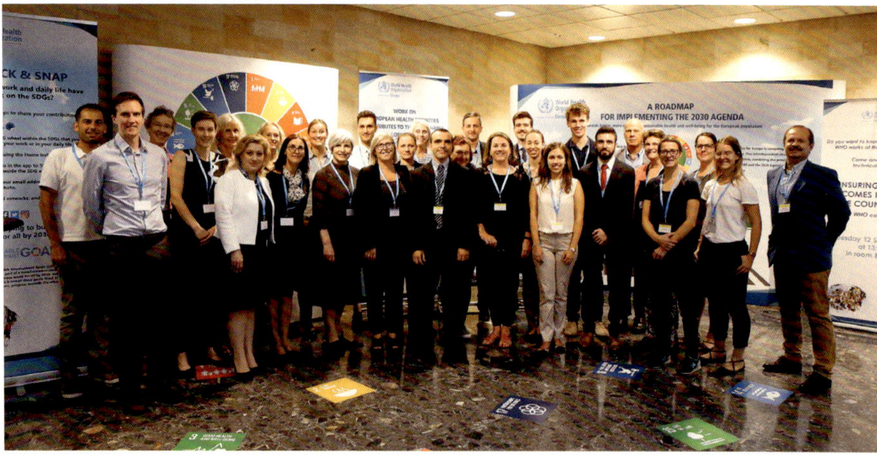

Leen Meulenbergs, Director Strategic Partnerships and WHO Representative to the EU with representatives from NGOs to discuss issues on the agenda of the 67th session of the WHO Regional Committee for Europe prior to its opening. The 67th session of the Regional Committee endorsed a new procedure to accredit European non-State actors, not in 'official relations with WHO', to enable them to participate more fully in future Regional Committee sessions. © WHO/Franz Henriksen

It is a very smooth partnership

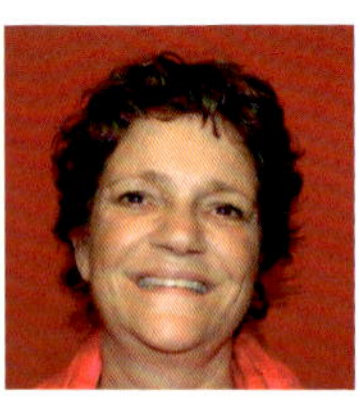

The collaboration between the WHO Regional Office for Europe and NGOs has increased in the last ten years. NGOs are more regularly invited to specific meetings and the WHO Regional Office for Europe is really targeting specific NGOs that could contribute to the Regional objectives. The WHO Regional Office for Europe is more approachable and inclusive, and it is just really pleasant to work with them.

Health 2020 has made a big difference. The WHO Regional Office for Europe has stepped up activities to involve the whole of society. This means a lot to us as they now do not just involve representatives of ministries of health – but are also actively engaging with NGOs and civil society.

Last year, for example, they asked us to help them get insights and data on actions being taken (or not taken) by NGOs related to SDGs in Member States. We conducted a Region-wide survey with our European Public Health Association (EUPHA) members in 45 countries and gathered information on perceived SDG implementation challenges and actions. We shared the results with WHO and they really appreciated that as it added value to other information collected from ministries of health, government agencies and other 'official sources'.

Since 2018, the WHO Regional Office for Europe has opened up official relations with a number of regional NGOs. This has increased our visibility and allowed for more networking between NGOs. For example, in 2018, EUPHA took the initiative of contacting all the NGOs 'in official relations with the WHO Regional Office for Europe' before the Regional Committee meeting and organized 'joint statements' on its agenda items. This resulted in more collaboration between NGOs, and that is very beneficial to all of us.

Dineke Zeegers, Director, European Public Health Association (EUPHA), Netherlands

The Regional Office engages in intensive collaboration with NGOs in many technical areas, including consultation in the drafting of policy documents and in policy implementation and advocacy. Regional and international health-related umbrella NGOs provided inputs during the preparation of Health 2020 and now support implementation of the policy framework.

5.5 Networks

Working together for improving health and well-being requires sharing this goal with new and evolving types of country, regional organizations and partnership networks for health across the Region. Examples include intercountry networks such as the South-eastern Europe Health Network (SEEHN), the Small Countries Initiative, the Visegrad Initiative for Health, the Commonwealth of Independent States (CIS), the Eurasian Economic Community, and the Northern Dimension Partnership. Other networks include setting and policy networks such as the European Healthy Cities and Regions for Health networks; and WHO's health promotion networks, including healthy schools, workplaces, hospitals, prisons and cities.

The South-eastern Europe Health Network (SEEHN) is a multigovernmental political and institutional forum for regional collaboration on the health and well-being of Albania, Bosnia and Herzegovina, Bulgaria, Israel, Montenegro, Republic of Moldova, Romania, Serbia and North Macedonia. It was established in 1999 by the international community in the frame of the Stability Pact for south-eastern Europe, as a conflict-prevention and reconstruction process in the region (see Section 1.2.2).

In 2001, a health component was added to the Pact's social cohesion initiative, to bring people together across borders to improve health in the whole region. SEEHN has received political, technical and financial support from 10 partner countries and five international organizations. From the period of its establishment, SEEHN has grown and has now incorporated membership of countries with a strong will and dedication to improve public health in their territories.

WHO has supported the SEEHN from its foundation in 2001 to today, by providing technical assistance and strategic advice and by helping strengthen national capacities. With our assistance, these countries have strengthened their health systems, discussed the environmental health challenges and impacts of climate change, and also discussed and ensured the procurement of vaccines and drugs to adequately combat and treat communicable diseases. They have been trained in emergency preparedness, and also had capacity-building on global health diplomacy and communication together. They have also become a strong and recognisable voice in our governing body meetings.

The Chisinau Pledge 2017 marked yet another milestone in SEEHN history. It acknowledged and ensured further implementation of the Health 2020 European policy for health and well-being, as an important driver for policy change and as a means towards achieving the SDGs.

As a pinnacle of collaboration between SEEHN and WHO Regional Office for Europe and given the universality of the United Nations 2030 Agenda for Sustainable Development, which calls for all countries to fully engage in its implementation at all levels, the SEEHN Secretariat and the WHO Regional Office for Europe have jointly developed and signed in July 2018 a subregional strategic document, which aims to support achievement of United Nations SDG 3 and other health-related SDG targets, especially the key target of UHC, in the member countries of SEEHN.

The South-eastern Europe Health Network

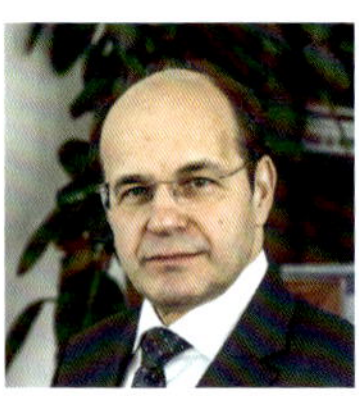

Bosnia and Herzegovina has been a proud member of the South-eastern Europe Health Network (SEEHN) since its establishment, and is partner to regional countries in the process of strengthening the responsibility for regional cooperation in the field of health, health systems and public health.

We strongly believe that collaboration is an essential part of developing good neighbourly relations, stability, prosperity, and the improvement of health in the region through the implementation of national research projects in public health.

In the past years it has been shown that SEEHN has been the undisputed vehicle of health development in the areas of mental health, communicable diseases, food safety and nutrition, blood safety, tobacco control, information systems, maternal and neonatal health, public health services and health systems. Regional cooperation in the public health field remains the highest priority in supporting political cooperation and economic development in south-eastern Europe, facilitating confidence building, and as an instrument of support for the process of European and Euro-Atlantic integration.

Adil Osmanovic, Minister of Civil Affairs, Bosnia and Herzegovina

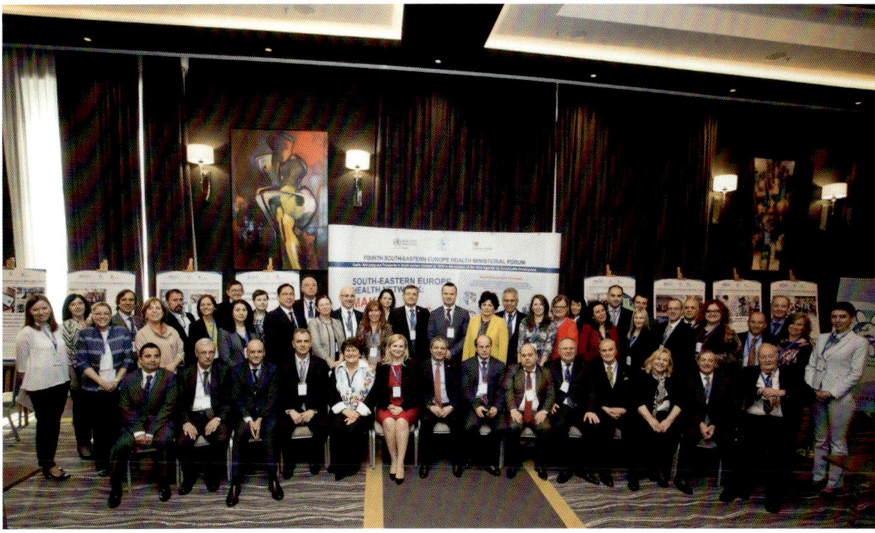

South-eastern Europe Health Network (SEEHN) at the 4th South-eastern Europe Health Ministerial Forum, Chisinau, Republic of Moldova, 3–4 April 2017. The meeting focused on the theme 'Health, well-being and prosperity in south-eastern Europe by 2030 in the context of the 2030 Agenda for Sustainable Development'. © WHO

The Small Countries Initiative was started in 2013. Small countries face common challenges such as isolation, fragmentation, vulnerability, international dependence, limited influence on the global agenda, and becoming the recipients of policies decided outside their territories. The new initiative has stimulated creative and forward thinking and has led members to develop stronger social cohesiveness, successful collaborations between policy-makers and the communities they serve, and a high degree of coherence across policies. They have been strong catalysts of Health 2020 implementation with an influence beyond their territorial borders.

Small to small support

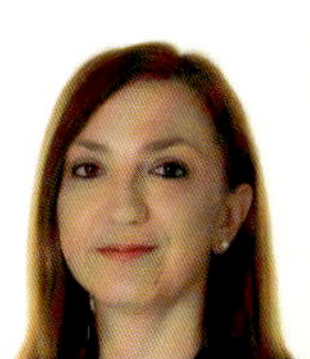

© Brian Cassar

The Small Countries Initiative has allowed a country like Malta to look at other small countries for inspiration, support and advice. Recently, for example, we've been engaging with Iceland for support on a couple of initiatives. We are finding it so useful, because immediately the two countries understand each other and come up with policy solutions that fit. And Malta has been asked by Montenegro to support them in something else.

None of this would have happened without the Small Countries Initiative. It is a very practical example of the way in which WHO, sometimes using very modest funding, demonstrates foresight and support.

Natasha Azzopardi Muscat, President of the European Public Health Association (EUPHA), Malta

Small to big Support

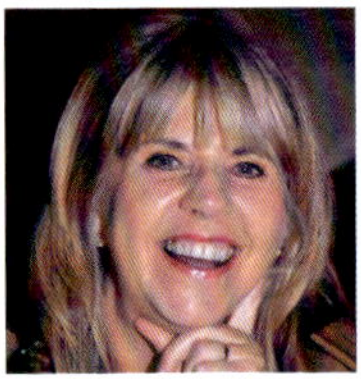

I think we have lots of examples where the small countries are doing much better than the bigger countries. With encouragement from WHO, we are now willing to tell stories from our own countries, so that other bigger countries can learn from us.

Vilborg Ingólfsdóttir, Former WHO National technical focal point, Former Director of Department, Ministry of Welfare, Iceland

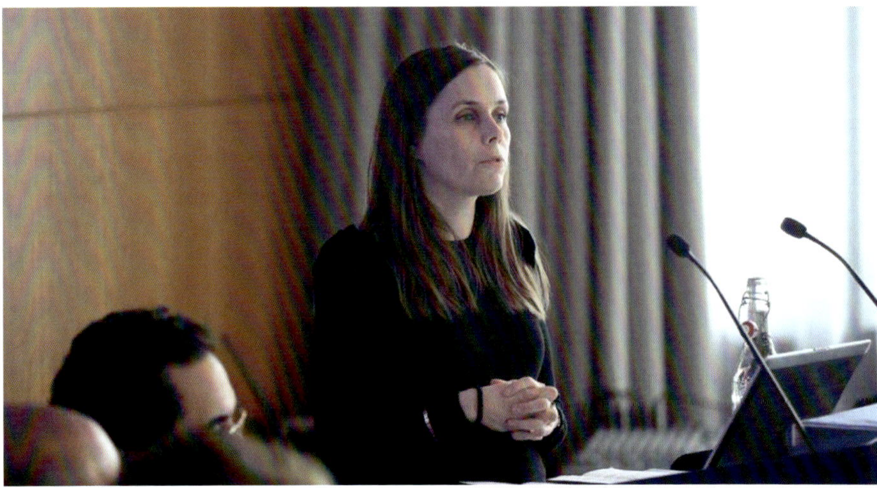

Iceland's Prime Minister Katrín Jakobsdóttir addresses the 'Fifth high-level meeting of small countries: working together for better health and well-being for all', Reykjavik, Iceland, 26–27 June 2018. © WHO

Small Countries Initiative – flexible, quick and effective

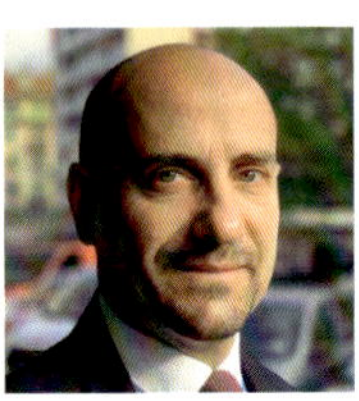

We were pleased to welcome three new members to our small country network at our Sixth High-level Meeting of Small Countries, hosted in March 2019 in San Marino. Our 8 original members – Andorra, Cyprus, Iceland, Luxembourg, Malta, Monaco, Montenegro and San Marino – were joined for the first time by Estonia, Latvia and Slovenia.

Under the theme 'Equity and sustainable development – keeping people at the centre', we shared experience on ways we have been building on the Health 2020 policy framework in our individual country efforts to achieve the SDGs. In San Marino, for example, we have created and adopted a master plan for sustainability, known as 'San Marino for all'. We have also established an intersectoral, intergovernmental commission to align all our policies with the SDGs. Our small countries have the ability to be flexible, resilient and innovative; and to set and implement policies quickly and effectively *(91)*.

Franco Santi, Minister of Health and Social Security, Equal Opportunities, National Insurance and Social Affairs, San Marino

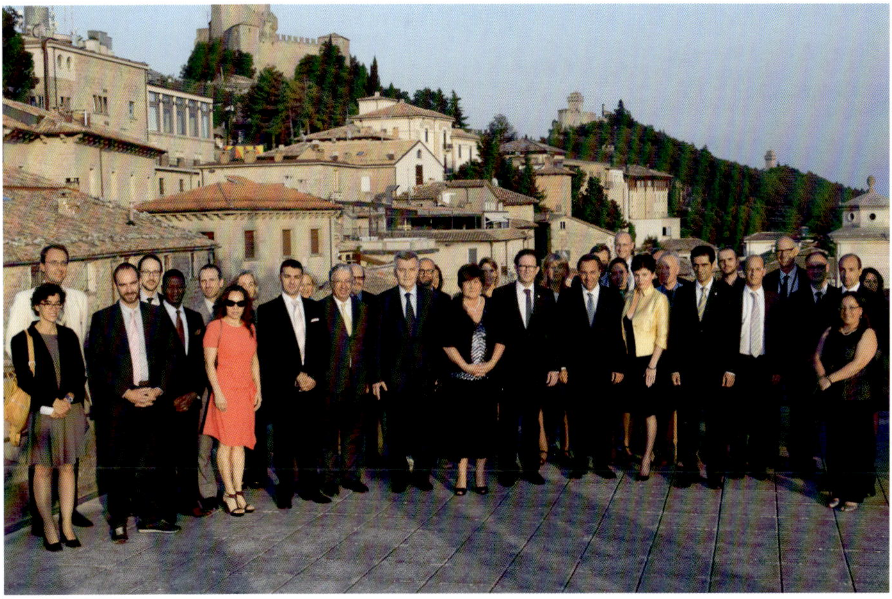

First high-level meeting of small countries of the WHO European Region on the implementation of the Health 2020 vision, San Marino, 3–4 July 2014. © Filippo Pruccoli

The WHO Regional Office for Europe and the Interparliamentary Assembly of Member Nations of the Commonwealth of Independent States (IPA CIS) have strengthened collaboration in recent years, and in 2018 signed a memorandum of understanding on broader cooperation. This includes WHO providing technical assistance in preparing and localizing model laws relevant to health. An important advance came when I addressed the Assembly in 2018 prior to their agreement to support the ratification of the WHO Protocol to Eliminate the Illicit Trade in Tobacco Products by national parliaments. As of today, more than 50 countries across the world have ratified the Protocol. Yet although all CIS countries are Parties to the WHO FCTC, to date none have ratified the Protocol on illicit tobacco trade.

Reaching out to parliamentarians – support to CIS Interparliamentary Assembly

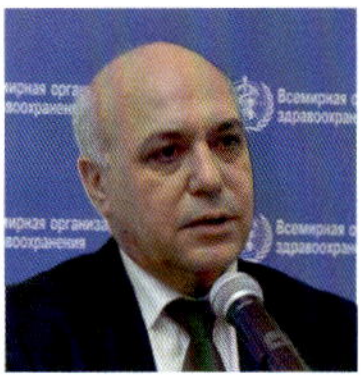

In 2014 Zsuzsanna Jakab asked me to help find ways to strengthen Regional Office engagement and support to parliamentarians, especially in the eastern part of the WHO European Region. In the EU, the Office had already enhanced their work with the European Parliament; especially in legislative research and advocacy support through our Brussels Office and in partnership with various EU and other agencies. The challenge was to find ways to extend this type of work into non-EU Member States of the European Region.

While parliamentarians are a logical and necessary target group for the Regional Office's Health 2020 whole-of-government and health-in-all-policy approaches, as a former Minister of Health, I knew that direct contacts between international agencies and parliaments were a sensitive arena in which to be operating. Supporting Health Ministries in their policy development work was standard operating practice but independent contact with legislatures wasn't.

So, our challenge was to find a mechanism to work with parliamentarians in ways that Ministries of Health would perceive as supportive. We focused on developing links with interparliamentary mechanisms that were already supporting national governments. There is, for example, the Interparliamentary Assembly of Member Nations of the CIS based in St. Petersburg. We reached out to this Assembly and over the last three years we have been able to develop relationships that now include attending each other's meetings, a formal signed memorandum outlining cooperative activities and advocacy opportunities.

One important area of work of the Interparliamentary Assembly is the development and adoption of model laws. While they did not include many health laws in the past, attention to this area is now growing. These model laws are well received by countries and often form the basis for national laws. Through our new cooperative relationships and technical assistance, we are able to help make these laws more consistent with global technical and normative standards. This could also lead, we believe, to more unified and consistent laws in countries facing similar challenges in different areas.

We have now agreed with the Interparliamenatary Assembly to support this process in three ways. First, we are reviewing the already adopted model laws; how they have been adapted for use at national level; and how this can be further supported. Second, for model laws already in process of drafting we are supporting them technically and helping to align them with international evidence and WHO policies. Third, we agreed that we may suggest (and in fact have already done so) new model laws which we think are important for CIS countries (and global health).

Other important ways we work is to raise awareness and commitment in countries for relevant global health laws. The Protocol to Eliminate Illicit Trade on Tobacco Products to the WHO Framework Convention on Tobacco Control (FCTC) is a good example of that. All CIS countries have already ratified the FCTC, but none have yet adopted its first Protocol adopted in 2012 (and ratified by more than 50 countries worldwide as of mid-2019). We asked the Interparliamentary Assembly to agree on a special resolution urging national parliaments to ratify the Protocol. This has now been accomplished and the Assembly has indeed formally encouraged national parliaments to ratify. This gives WHO and partners a strong platform upon which to follow up with Ministries of Health and other relevant sectors.

Our partnership with the Interparliamentary Assembly has also allowed for some advocacy informational opportunities. In 2019, for example, we organized an information session for the Interparliamentary Assembly on the WHO Healthy Cities approach. We made presentations and moderated a discussion on why and how the Healthy Cities movement should and can be more promoted, advocated and developed in CIS where currently it lacks strength compared to other parts of the Region.

All this is a very useful and innovative development for WHO as it gives us new ways to help countries adopt national laws and programmes based on evidence-informed international approaches. It is also an approach that could be replicated in other areas where there are intergovernmental unions and assemblies; like the south-east Europe and Black Sea areas in the European Region and in other WHO Regions.

Haik Nikogosian, Senior Fellow, Global Health Centre, The Graduate Institute Geneva; Former Minister of Health, Armenia; Former Head of the FCTC Secretariat, Former Special Representative of the WHO Regional Director of Europe.

The WHO Regional Office for Europe has established a close collaboration with the Eurasian Economic Union (EAEU) through the Eurasian Economic Commission (EEC), its executive and regulatory arm. EAEU as an international organization for regional economic integration was established by a treaty that entered into force on 1 May 2015. The EAEU's five members are Armenia, Belarus, Kazakhstan, Kyrgyzstan and the Russian Federation.

Although health is not directly part of the mandate of EAEU, the Commission nevertheless provides the Regional Office with an opportunity to address health in the countries concerned by influencing or assisting with the requirements for establishing a common market for medicines and medical products, and common sanitary regulations (including in the veterinary-sanitary and phytosanitary fields).

Since May 2017, the Regional Office has been working with EAEU on pharmaceutical regulations, prevention of NCDs and epidemiological surveillance. Collaboration with EAEU is particularly valuable with regard to the intersectoral and cross-border aspects of public health, and the inclusion of health in the regional integration agenda in the eastern part of the WHO European Region.

In the area of NCDs a joint workshop of the WHO, the EAEU and its Member States on efforts to develop and implement food policies for the prevention of NCDs was organized on 25–26 February 2019 at the headquarters of EEC in Moscow. This joint WHO-Eurasian Economic Commission workshop in Moscow brought together policy-makers and regulators from EAEU Member States, the EEC and WHO experts in order to discuss food policies for the prevention of NCDs.

The Northern Dimension Partnership for Public Health and Well-being is a policy framework for cooperation involving the European Union, Iceland, Norway and the Russian Federation. It aims at providing a common platform for promoting dialogue and concrete cooperation as well as strengthening stability and promoting economic integration, competitiveness and sustainable development in northern Europe. Health is one of the key priority themes for dialogue and cooperation. The European Region has extended its relationship with the Partnership around Health 2020, strategies on HIV/AIDS, tuberculosis and alcohol, AMR, tobacco control, NCDs and PHC.

Through working with policy networks WHO finds opportunities to connect to localities and institutions where 'things get done'. An example is the WHO European Healthy Cities Network, affecting policy decisions that impact on people living in cities. Together the cities in direct cooperation with the Regional Office and national networks cover some 1400 municipalities. These networks are vital resources and strategic vehicles for innovation and new evidence, not only as partners in implementation at a local level but also as conduits and amplifiers at national level. These cities are part of a global movement working to put health higher on the social, economic and political agenda of local governments.

Since 1993, the WHO European Regions for Health Network (RHN) has helped regions to accelerate the delivery of improved population health. Working with WHO, RHN aims to create synergy between regions and stakeholders in the field of health issues; strengthen cooperation and collaboration between international, regional and local actors in health; promote the contribution of regions and local authorities, and particularly, health authorities to the international policy-making process; and increase the understanding of regional and local health systems.

To have access to 'on-the-ground' information on the international level is very precious. Often in the Regional Office we seem far away from where citizens and populations live, love, work and play. It is crucial to be able to have the experience of local understanding of the enablers, obstacles and impacts of policies discussed and considered at a national and international level.

Guidance and contact platform

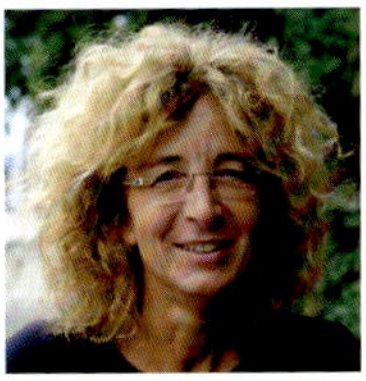

Our city of Utrecht became a member of the Healthy Cities Network in December 2016. In deciding to join the network, we asked ourselves what does an inhabitant of Utrecht gain from the fact that we are part of this network, and part of WHO, and this global movement? Our understanding from the beginning has been that it gives us an international platform that provides us with guidance and contacts that can make our local voice and capacities stronger.

Miriam Weber, WHO Healthy Cities Network Coordinator, Utrecht, Netherlands

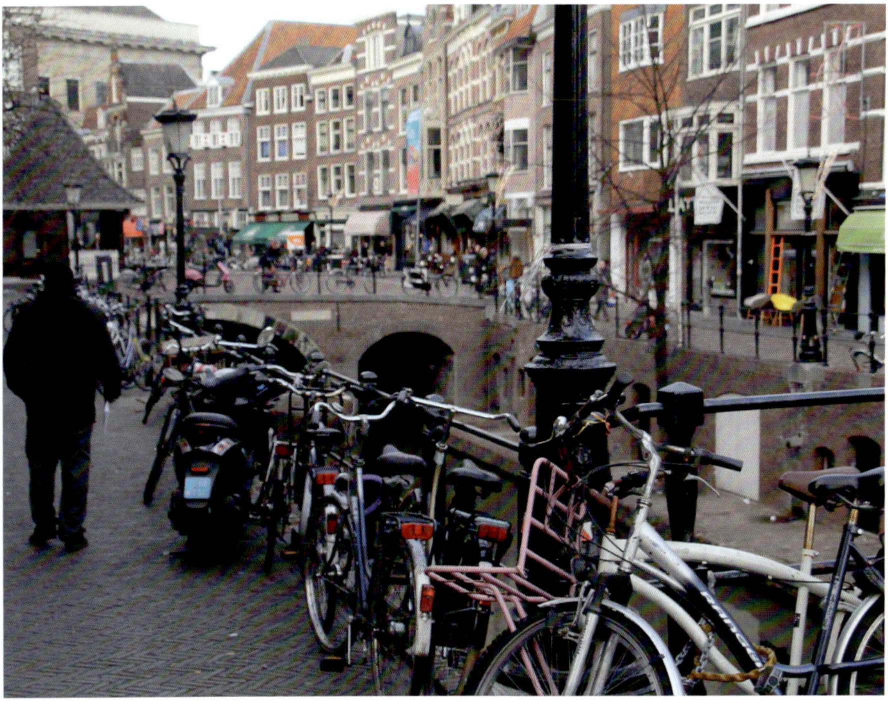

Street view in Utrecht, Netherlands, with shops, bicycles, bridge and canal. © WHO

PART 1

Healthy Ireland and Healthy Cities and Counties

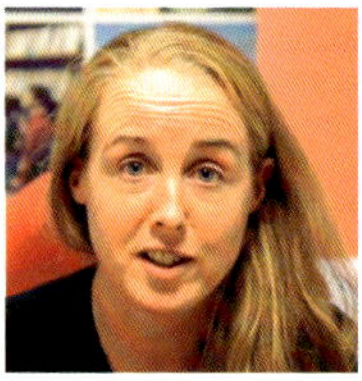

One of the good and valuable things about Healthy Cities is that it has been around since 1987. It has been long established and is credible. In Ireland, based on our population, our quota for the number of cities in the WHO Healthy Cities Network is three. In 2009, we understood that to share ideas and promote cooperation we needed to develop a national network.

Working with the existing three cities (Galway, Cork and Waterford) we set up a group to develop a National Network. We were making very little, if any progress.

Then in 2013 Healthy Ireland was launched. This is our Government's version of Health 2020. Ireland took Health 2020 and made it into a national cross-party, cross-governmental framework. We took this chance to offer the WHO Healthy Cities approach, with over 30 years of learning, as a way to implement national policy at the local level. Connecting the WHO Healthy Cities to Healthy Ireland was helped by the fact that there are strong connections between Healthy Ireland and WHO. Margaret Chan attended the launch of Healthy Ireland.

Healthy Ireland provided the national framework and mandate to promote health and well-being. The WHO Healthy Cities approach provided the system through which to implement it. We could see the value of connecting the national framework with this existing system. That sounds very simple; but it took three years.

We quickly learned that we had to make adjustments to the existing Healthy Cities concept. For example, Healthy Cities is all well and good, but Ireland is 70% rural. We have counties, so in Ireland, Healthy Counties speaks to a lot of people. Language is really important, so now we speak about Healthy Cities and Healthy Counties and that's really important. So Healthy Ireland is at a national level, but I am from Wexford, so Healthy Wexford means something more to me. Every county and city (31 in total) have their own brand but connected to the national brand.

Leveraging the Healthy Ireland brand, which aims to bring consistency and connection across health and well-being campaigns and initiatives to strengthen their impact, was very deliberate and a key strategic move to reinforce the Healthy Cities and Counties as the system to implement Healthy Ireland.

Since 2017 over ten million euros have been invested in supporting the implementation of Healthy Ireland at a local level with each county and city receiving funding.

This is a game changer. It has moved action outside the health sector into partners who deal with the wider determinants of health. Importantly, about 70% of what we are doing is really strengthening initiatives and programmes which already exist; 20% is about making connections with what already exists and 10% is about new activities, which we call social innovation. For example, the Healthy County and Healthy City plans are making connections and aligning to the SDGs.

The time invested in aligning Healthy Cities and Counties to the national health and well-being framework, Healthy Ireland, has been critical and is the foundation for sustained political support and investment to improve the health and well-being of all across Ireland.

Fiona Donovan, WHO Healthy Cities and Counties Coordinator, Ireland

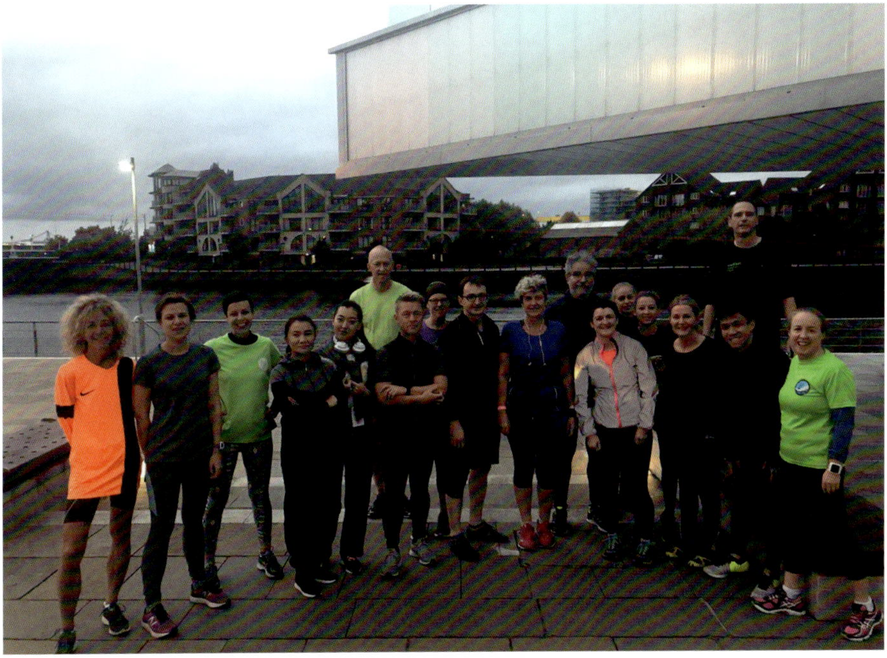

Participants gather for a morning run as one of the physical activity sessions at the WHO International Healthy Cities Conference, Belfast, United Kingdom, 1–4 October 2018. *© WHO*

5.6 'Hosted partnership'

We have also strengthened our collaboration with the European Observatory on Health Systems and Policies, the only WHO 'hosted partnership' in the European Region *(204)*. The Observatory has supported and helped us promote evidence-based health policymaking through comprehensive and rigorous analysis of the dynamics of health-care systems in Europe and direct work with policy-makers and experts throughout the Region.

'Hosted partnership'

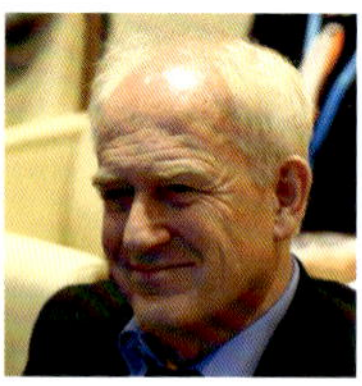

Zsuzsanna has been very good at embracing the Observatory partnership and embedding it within the work of the Office, without compromising its role or independence. This has been conceptualized as a 'hosted partnership'. WHO lends its administrative, legal and fiduciary framework to the Observatory secretariat while it participates in its leadership as an equal partner. To lead and manage the Observatory in this way shows vision, courage and commitment.

Embracing the principle of partnerships is easy but putting them in place is a far more complex task fraught with competing interests and ownership issues. Understanding the advantages of sharing ownership and that the sum of the total is higher than that of the individuals is not something everyone embraces.

Under Zsuzsanna's leadership the WHO Office has provided management support and strategic leadership to the Observatory, keeping the partners involved and supportive, while working with the Observatory's Steering Committee to ensure that the Observatory's evidence is fully relevant to the work of the Office. This approach has greatly helped to shape the Observatory's agenda over these last ten years. For example, we have contributed by developing evidence to inform Health 2020 such as with intersectoral approaches to health policies, the economics of prevention or financial incentives. In the same way the Observatory has provided evidence support to the seminal work of the Tallinn Conferences on health systems and on the three guiding principles of inclusion, investment and innovation. In this way the Regional Office has been able to work with the Observatory very positively and constructively.

Josep Figueras, Director of the European Observatory on Health Systems and Policies

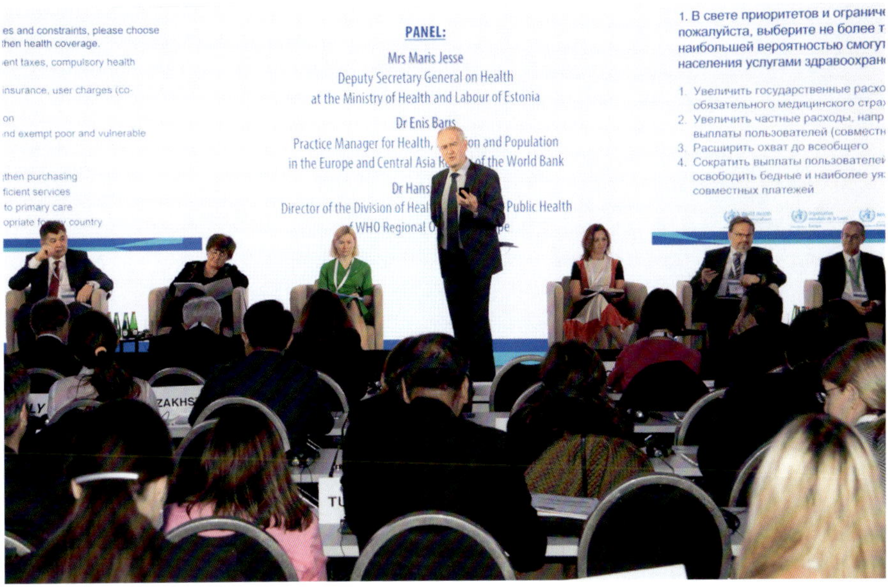
PANEL:
Mrs Maris Jesse
Deputy Secretary General on Health
at the Ministry of Health and Labour of Estonia

Josep Figueras, Director of the European Observatory on Health Systems and Policies, moderating panel at the WHO high-level regional meeting, Health Systems for Prosperity and Solidarity: leaving no one behind, Tallinn, Estonia, 13–14 June 2018. © WHO/Erik Peinar

Complementarity of partnership

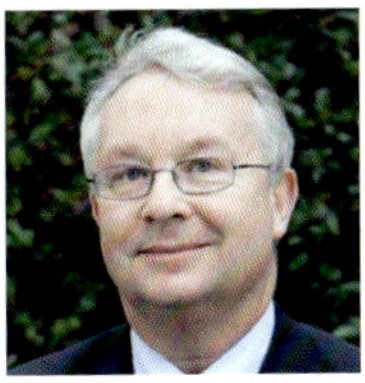

I think Europe is way ahead of the game compared to the other regions in its willingness to tolerate and, indeed, to encourage partnership. Its work with the European Observatory on Health Systems and Policies is an outstanding example that has attracted global attention.

Here in WHO Regional Office for Europe we have seen a willingness to take on some of the tough issues; for example, the work done on patient-centred care and tuberculosis within the Tuberculosis Regional Eastern European and Central Asian Project with a very nice partnership of universities. Such partnerships help us realize the great strength of complementarity. There is cross-membership of the groups and people share data and results. I think that's good.

Martin McKee, Professor of European Public Health, London School of Hygiene and Tropical Medicine (LSHTM), United Kingdom

Summary reflection

Strategic partnerships

Message 4: Collaboration beats competition

We have learned how we can enhance resources, policy coherence and impact through partnerships. Today's health challenges are complex both in nature and resolution, and all those agencies and institutions involved in their resolution must work together. The sometimes-seen old ways of competition for attention and resources must give way to inclusive cooperation. The Regional Office has therefore actively engaged in forming strategic partnerships with many other stakeholders to jointly improve health and well-being in Europe and beyond. This has involved establishing new partnerships and networks e.g. the Small Countries Initiative, the IPA CIS, the SEEHN; enhancing collaboration with the EU, OECD, ECDC, and the Global Fund; extending collaboration and joint working with UN partners; establishing new ways of collaborating with partners; and moving beyond competition and finding truly mutually beneficial collaborative practices based on sharing information and resources. It has also required a new culture of listening, engaging and understanding the perspectives that all the parties bring to an issue, with a problem-solving approach that transcends the differences they bring.

6. Strengthening the European contribution to global health

6.1 Global Policy Group (GPG)

The Global Policy Group (GPG) of WHO is an internal advisory mechanism for the Director-General to ensure coherent development and implementation of decisions, policies and strategies across all levels of the Organization. Established by Margaret Chan, over the years it has gone from strength to strength and become an increasingly important global body advising the Director-General and ensuring coherent implementation of joint decisions.

GPG – a space for collective strategic thinking

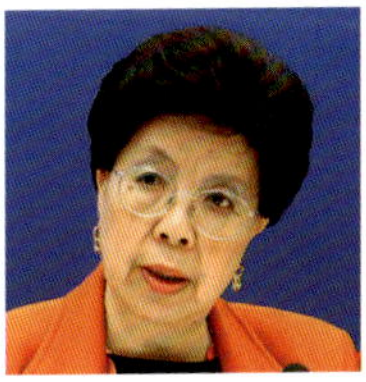

One of the initiatives that made me very happy, as the then WHO Director-General, was to build up our Global Policy Group, which consisted of all the six Regional Directors, my Deputy Director-General and myself.

One thing I quickly understood was that we were seven elected officials in the group and we all had our political and technical roles. I learned that some decisions, while technically appropriate, might sometimes not exactly fit what each of the Regions wanted or needed.

My approach was first to listen to all concerns and make sure that I found the most valuable solution for public health and then to see how I could help each and every Region to do some give and take.

I tried to make the GPG a space where we could put aside our daily chores and put ourselves into a mode where we just could talk, reflect and develop our collective strategic thinking. We would talk about all our issues and challenges including management, strategic and finance aspects. The GPG functioned very well. Zsuzsanna and other RDs told me many times how useful and collegial a group it was.

Margaret Chan, WHO Director-General, 2006–2017

Dr Tedros has given it his full support and strengthened it even further. All decisions are made on a more or less collective basis, so there is a lot of lively debate.

GPG leadership

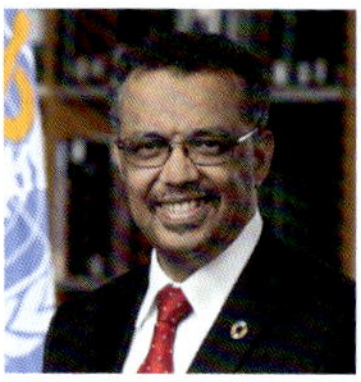

Dr Jakab has been a critically important member of, and contributor to, the work of the Global Policy Group across a range of strategic, technical, political and managerial issues. She brings a unique perspective to the GPG in view of the broad socioeconomic, demographic and political dynamics of the Region she represented. Her insights provide a vital viewpoint on key health issues, including cross-sectoral collaboration to achieve the health-related SDGs, evidence-based tools, approaches and interventions to strengthen health systems towards universal health coverage, and revitalizing primary care.

Issues of particular significance to the Region, including the health of refugees and migrants, as well as emerging areas such as the future of digital health systems, are some examples of the Regional perspectives that are invaluable to the work and deliberations of the GPG.

Tedros Adhanom Ghebreyesus, WHO Director-General

GPG collaboration

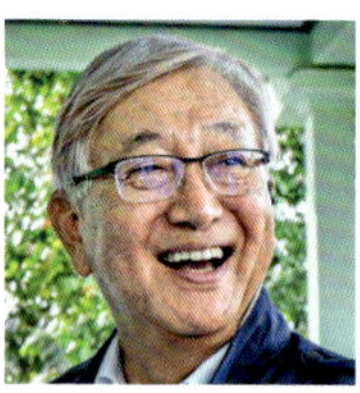

Zsuzsanna and I worked together for almost 9 years in the GPG of Regional Directors with the Director-General. Zsuzsanna and I became Regional Directors about the same time. The GPG became an important forum that helped, for example, inform the new Director-General about some of the complexities of our Regional engagements and our unique history of working in a highly decentralized way. Zsuzsanna is the person I would call before meetings to discuss issues and make our case in the GPG. And she also consulted me. We developed quite a respect and friendship with each other.

Young-soo Shin, Regional Director,
WHO Regional Office for the Western Pacific, 2009–2019

The GPG has worked to globalize different Regional Initiatives. Health 2020, for example, was used as an inspiration for the Organization as a whole, to work with countries to develop, renew and update their national health policies and strategies.

6.2 WHO Reform and Transformation

The WHO Regional Office for Europe, in the development of Health 2020 and its Regional governance and administrative reforms, has been fully supportive of the WHO Reform process started by Dr Chan in 2011 and now continued as the process of WHO Transformation introduced by Dr Tedros. Both processes have made major contributions to global health governance.

Improved technical capacities in the Office have allowed for both better support for the implementation of international instruments and for preparing the Regional contribution to international discussion, particularly around the United Nations 2030 Agenda for Sustainable Development and the SDGs.

The work of the Office has been aligned with many international agreements, focusing on their translation at Regional level, including the WHO Framework Convention on Tobacco Control, the Doha Declaration on the TRIPS Agreement and Public Health (related to intellectual property), and the outcome documents from the 2011 United Nations General Assembly High Level Meeting on Noncommunicable Diseases (see Section 9.3.2).

WHO Regional Office for Europe Health Reform health reform leadership – governance and management

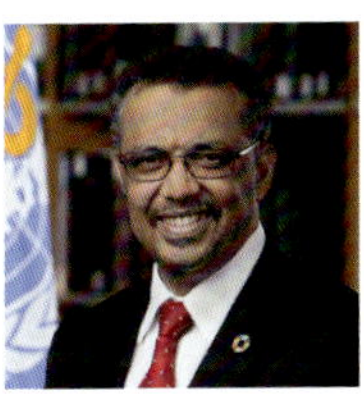

The Regional Office for Europe under the leadership of Dr Jakab has been in the forefront of WHO Reform globally. It has been a major innovator of processes and policies and a leader of several important global initiatives. For instance, the Regional Office advocated turning the Programme Budget into an accountability tool, where Member States could clearly understand, track and measure what the Regional Office will deliver during a biennium. This also included introducing a results chain in 2012–2013, which later inspired the results chain of GPW12 and is now an integral part of WHO's planning framework.

The first compliance unit was established in the WHO Regional Office for Europe to carry out checks and analyses of administrative processes, and was identified as best practice in subsequent audits. This helped to implement a culture of zero tolerance for non-compliance in the European region, strengthened donor confidence and built trust. Now all Regions have similar compliance units in WHO.

During Dr Jakab's time the WHO Regional Office for Europe introduced several innovative policies, including on travel and forward planning of meetings, which were taken up globally and now form integral part of WHO's world-wide policies.

Together with Dr Asamoa Bah, Dr Jakab also co-led a working group on reforming resource mobilization in WHO. Many of its recommendations are reflected in the current transformation of resource mobilization.

Tedros Adhanom Ghebreyesus, WHO Director-General

PART 1

6.3 Health 2020, the United Nations 2030 Agenda for Sustainable Development and the SDG global narrative

In the Regional Office we were pleased to see how well Health 2020 fitted into and was aligned with this new global approach. For us it was really good news that the SDGs and Health 2020 were completely consistent. Clearly the Regional Office was on the right track with Health 2020. By embracing Health 2020 values and principles and starting implementation, WHO European Member States ensured that they were better prepared and had a head start in tackling the SDGs.

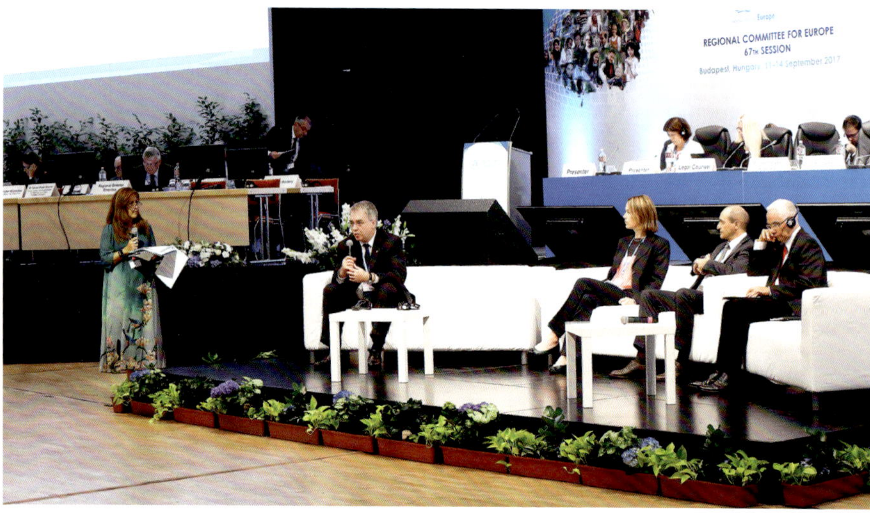

Lucianne Licari, Director, Country Support and Communications moderating a ministerial panel which discussed experiences of increasing governance for health in the SDG era, at the 67th session of the WHO Regional Committee for Europe, Budapest, Hungary, 12 September 2017. © WHO/Franz Henriksen

Since the adoption of Health 2020 and the SDG Roadmap see (Section 2.7), support has been provided to Member States, when requested, in the development, revision and implementation of national development plans, in particular through a one-UN Mainstreaming, Acceleration and Policy Support (MAPS) assessment and as part of 'voluntary national reviews'. Country initiatives supported have included:

1. Albania and Serbia – support to the EU accession process.
2. Belarus – promoting a specific approach in focusing on youth and promoting the fight against NCDs.
3. Georgia – to strengthen whole-of-government approach towards the SDGs.
4. Kyrgyzstan – to strengthen health systems.

5. Romania – support to high-level policy dialogues were carried out with the President of Romania and within the Romanian EU presidency.
6. Turkmenistan – scaling up investments in primary health care and NCDs reduction.
7. Ukraine – developing and implementing an integrated, coherent, and adequately funded National Health Programme to improve health and well-being for all.
8. Uzbekistan – to support the new national health policy development for achieving the SDGs.

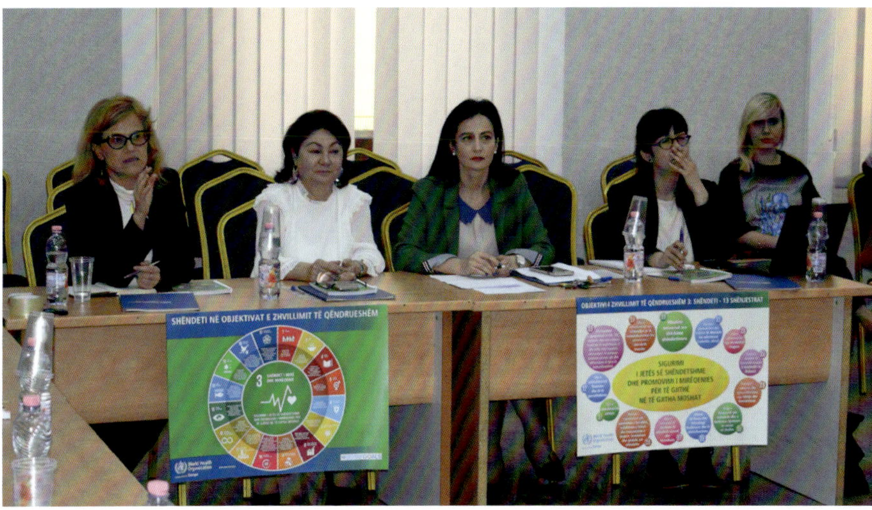

Representing the United Nations Issue-based Coalition on Health, WHO Regional Office for Europe joined efforts with other UN agencies and the Albania United Nations Country Team to support the Government of Albania in adapting the SDGs to national needs and context in 2018. They did so using the MAPS (Mainstreaming, Acceleration and Policy Support) approach. © WHO/Nazira Artykova

We have also supported National Health Policy (NHP) development. In 2017–2018, for example, the Regional Office worked on NHP in 21 countries[8]. Health 2020 has encouraged Member States to take active steps to align their policies with its broader goals, and many have even endorsed their Health 2020 national health policies, strategies and plans *(92)*. Health 2020 core values of 'fairness, sustainability, quality, transparency, accountability, gender equality, dignity and the right to participate in decision-making' have been put at the centre of public health policy-making *(93)*.

[8] Albania, Bulgaria, Czechia, Estonia, Georgia, Greece, Hungary, Ireland, Israel, Kazakhstan, Kyrgyzstan, Malta, Montenegro, North Macedonia, Portugal, Republic of Moldova, Slovenia, Tajikistan, Turkey, Ukraine and Uzbekistan.

6.4 Identifying and championing new initiatives and approaches

Having a value and evidence informed policy such as Health 2020 in place has given us a clear framework and point of reference to think out and try new ideas. We have, for example, taken new initiatives in identifying more effective ways to respond to determinants, promoting the environment and health process, strengthening health systems to make them more coordinated and people-centred, building on the links between health systems and the management of NCDs, and developing migration and health policies.

Regional leadership

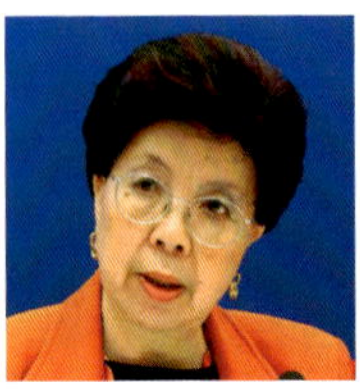

During my tenure as Director-General, I experienced many instances and examples of European Regional leadership in global Health issues. Chancellor Merkel of Germany and Prime Minister Erna Solberg of Norway, for example, together with the then President of Ghana John Dramani Mahama, wrote me a letter in 2015 about the need for strengthening the WHO emergency programme. This letter catalysed action.

Zsuzsanna Jakab and the Regional Office for Europe helped us organize a key GPG retreat in Venice, Italy, where we developed plans for our new Emergency Programme. We crafted a plan that would allow the Organization to become more of an operational agency, in addition to playing its normative and technical coordination roles. This plan was presented to and approved by the World Health Assembly in 2016.

During my tenure there were many more examples of European forward-thinking and leadership on key global issues like the development of the SDGs, AMR, (United Kingdom, Belgium and Denmark), health and development (Germany), health system reform (e.g. Estonia), migrant health (Italy), the rights of women and sexual and reproductive health (Nordic countries), NCDs (Russian Federation) and foreign policy and health (France and Norway).

Zsuzsanna and the Regional Office have also been instrumental in enhancing our WHO partnership with the European Union and ECDC. Under Zsuzsanna's leadership the European Office moved into the UN City building in Copenhagen. This has led to greater UN coordination and cooperation and is facilitating synergies.

Margaret Chan, WHO Director-General, 2006–2017

A little machine outside

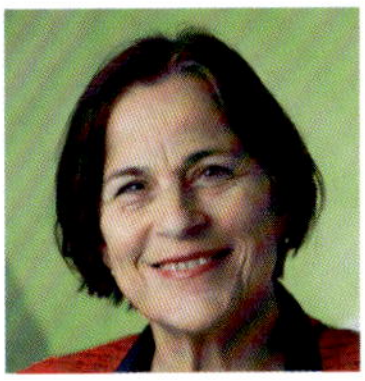

In certain areas the WHO Regional Office for Europe has been more advanced than WHO Headquarters. As such the Regional Office has developed many issues that have been inspirational for Headquarters. Many products have found their way into Headquarters, on nutrition and NCDs in general, as well as health systems work.

WHO Headquarters has found that the WHO Regional Office for Europe could serve as a little outside development machine for all kind of issues.

Annemiek Van Bolhuis, Director of Public Health and Health Services, National Institute of Public Health and the Environment (RIVM), Netherlands

6.4.1 Case study: migration and health

Migration is high on global political agendas. The United Nations General Assembly high-level summit to address large movements of refugees and migrants, and agreement to the New York Declaration for Refugees and Migrants, held in New York in September 2016, were watershed events in strengthening the governance of international migration. Subsequently work proceeded on the development of two global compacts: a UN Global Compact on Refugees *(201)*, and a Global Compact for Safe, Orderly and Regular Migration *(94)*.

The WHO Regional Office for Europe has taken a leading role in assisting Member States globally in promoting and protecting the health of refugees and migrants since 2011.

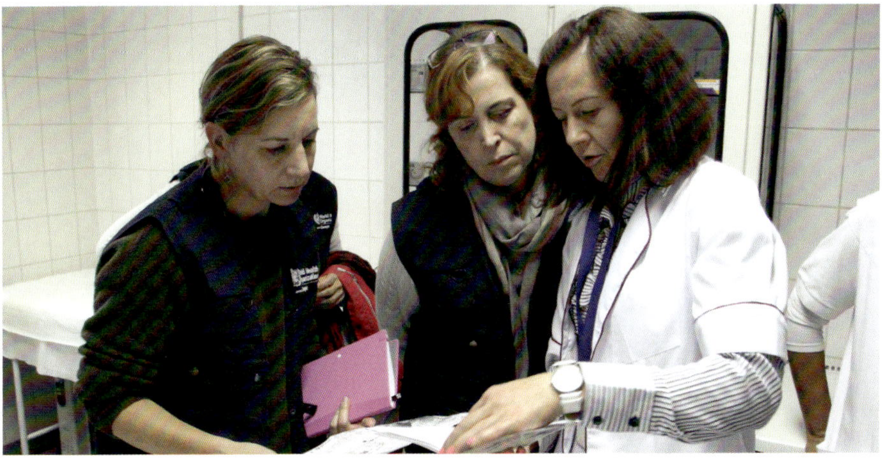

Nedret Emiroglu, Director of Division of Health Emergencies and Communicable Diseases and Director of Programme Management, WHO Regional Office for Europe, speaks with staff at a health centre to analyse the public health implications and capacity of the Hungarian health system to cope with large arrivals of refugees and migrants, Hungary, 2015
© WHO/Sara Barragán Montes

There when you need them

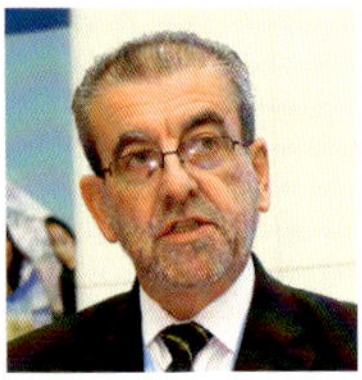

In 2011, during the Libya crisis, Malta received about 60 000 migrants in one week. That is 15% of our whole population! We needed urgent help to process and address the needs of this massive and sudden influx. Political considerations were complicated. The WHO Regional Office for Europe was swift to respond and quickly arranged for experts to come to assess and advise us on how to strengthen our limited human resource capacities. The Regional Office also helped us engage other agencies like the Red Cross. All this led to Zsuzsanna's call to Ministers of most affected countries in 2012 and the migration and health process which followed and continues to this date. The Regional Office has taken a real leadership role in this area. Activities have included the Regional Committee declaration and development of tools, guides and provision of ongoing training through the WHO summer schools. I give the Regional Office under Zsuzsanna Jakab's leadership very high marks here for fast, effective, persistent, reliable and creative problem solving assistance in this area. Importantly, this was one of many initiatives of the Regional Office that has had tangible impacts and helped set global standards that others have followed.

Ray Busuttil, Former Director General, Public Health Regulation Department, Ministry for Health, the Elderly and Community Care, Malta

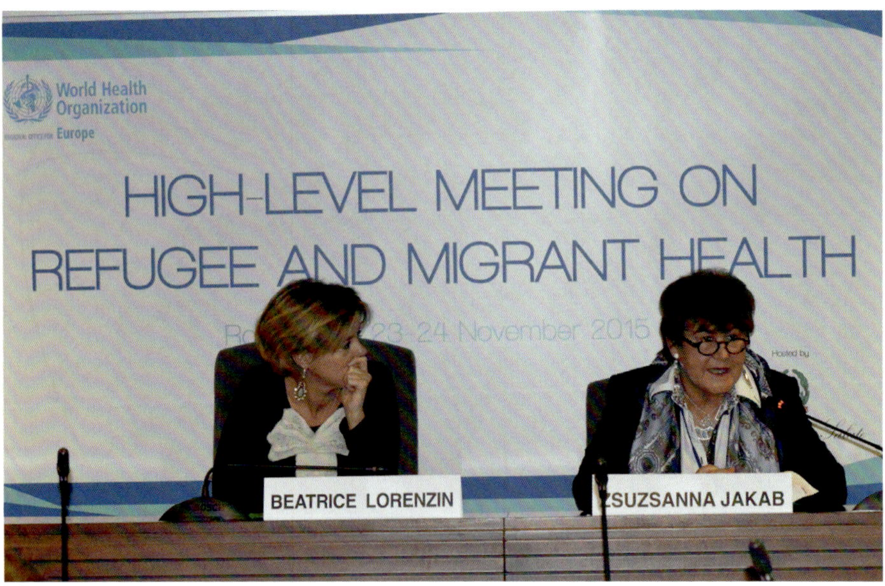

Press conference with Zsuzsanna Jakab and Beatrice Lorenzin, Minister of Health of Italy, at the high-level meeting on Refugee and Migrant Health in Rome 23–24 November, 2015.
© WHO/Roberto Urbani

Global migration and health leadership

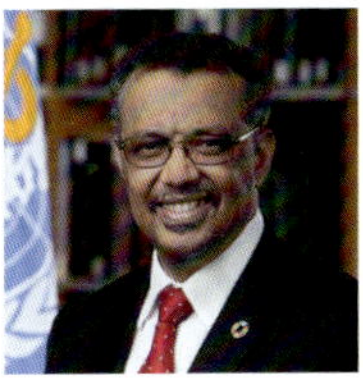

The WHO Regional Office for Europe has taken a leading role on migration and health at a global level. It has provided continuous support and assistance to HQ and made migration a key priority for the Organization.

In 2015, a high-level meeting on refugee and migrant health was organized in Rome, which laid the groundwork for the first WHO strategy and action plan for refugee and migrant health in the WHO European Region in 2016 *(95)*. That strategy served as a reference for a resolution on 'Promoting the Health of Refugees and Migrants' endorsed by the World Health Assembly in 2017 *(96, 97)*.

The Regional Office for Europe provided further support and assistance to WHO headquarters in developing a global action plan on the health of refugees and migrants, adopted in 2019.

In collaboration with the Regional Office for the Eastern Mediterranean and the Regional Office for Africa, the Regional Office for Europe has also been instrumental in implementing projects in migrant detention centres, by facilitating coordination with national health authorities and NGOs working on the ground.

Tedros Adhanom Ghebreyesus, WHO Director-General

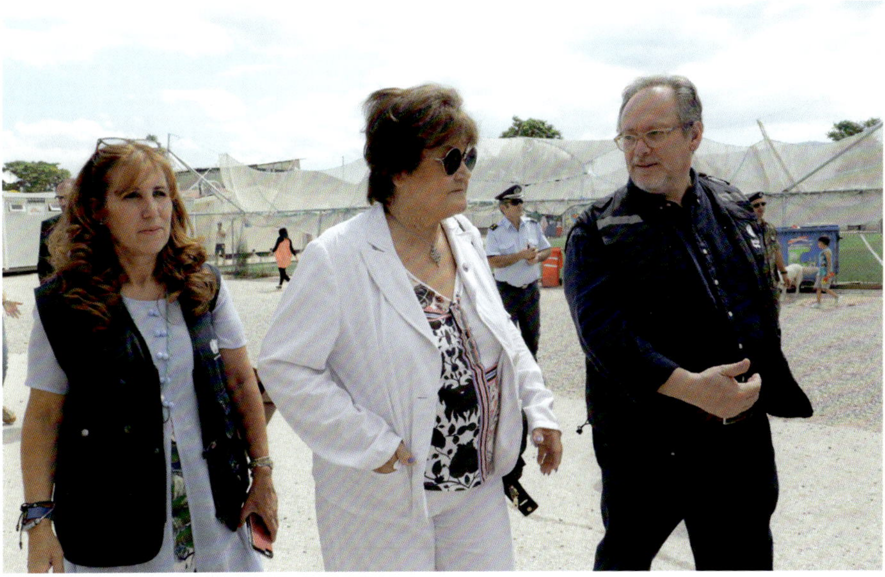

Lucianne Licari, Director, Country Support and Communications, Zsuzsanna Jakab, WHO Regional Director for Europe, and Santino Severoni, Coordinator, Public Health and Migration, Division of Policy and Governance for Health and Well-being, visiting Eleonas Camp, an open accommodation centre for asylum seekers in Greece, 2018.
© WHO/Lefteris Partsalis

In 2012 the Regional Office established a Public Health Aspects of Migration in Europe programme (PHAME). Given the growing number of arrivals throughout the years and the increasing number of European countries exposed to large-scale population movements, the activities of the PHAME project rapidly expanded, setting the basis for the establishment of the first Migration and Health programme at the WHO Regional Office for Europe and the establishment of a second three-year project (PHAME2) allowing the continuation and scale-up of the work in this area.

The Migration and Health programme has been built up on four areas of work: technical assistance; health information and evidence; advocacy and communication; and policy development. Since its establishment, the programme has provided continuous support to Ministries of Health. Health systems assessment missions have been conducted in several countries.

Sharing 'ground' experience

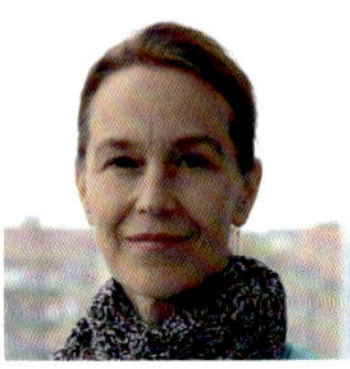

We have been collaborating with the WHO Regional Office for Europe in recent years in its Migration and Health programme because we have good 'ground' experience-based knowledge. We have welcomed a lot of migrants over the last few years. Our collaborations have been on how to work with the health and the health system challenges this raises in the acute, short-term and long-term phases. How to assure, for example, equal health care and safety, as well as preventing diseases and promoting health.

We have been participating in a subgroup that has prepared policy guidance in this area. And we helped to prepare a high-level conference on how to work with migrant health issues, and develop systems that provide quality, equity, and accessibility for migrant populations.

Olivia Wigzell, Director General, National Board for Health and Welfare, Sweden

The Regional Office has provided support and policy advice on contingency planning, technical assistance and guidance, public information tools and training modules on refugee and migrant health for health and non-health professionals (see Developmental reflection 2). The research agenda is a top priority area of work and the capacity of the Regional Office has been expanded by nominating three WHO collaborating centres on refugee and migrant health, which are supporting evidence and research activities.

A collaborating centre on Migration and Health has been established in Pécs University, Hungary; the Public and Patient Involvement (PPI) Research Unit, at the University of Limerick, Ireland, has been nominated WHO collaborating centre for migrant's involvement in Health Research; and a WHO collaborating centre on Health and Migration Evidence and Capacity Building has been established at the National Institute for Health, Migration and Poverty in Rome, Italy.

Enhancing cultural competence

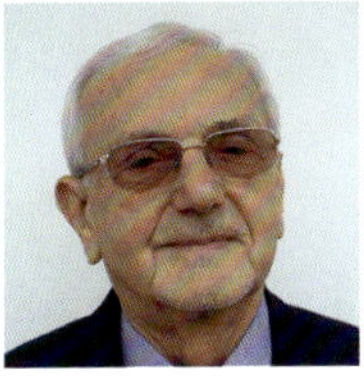

In 2011, we started to work with WHO on their new Migration and Health programme. Initially we were given the responsibility of publishing a quarterly electronic newsletter to create an evidence-exchange platform for migration and health issues. We were the designated editorial office with an editorial board with 20 excellent scientists from across Europe and beyond *(98)*.

Since 2007 our medical school has provided courses for medical students on migration and health topics. They are very popular and regularly enrol 330–400 students a year from more than 50 countries. Ironically, these students are all migrants themselves of one sort or another. We are now starting a postgraduate course on 'Specialist in Migration Health'.

In 2017 we were designated as a WHO Collaborating Centre for Migration Health Training and Research, and have participated in a wide variety of conferences, meetings and visits.

Our centre is now focused on developing a migration-health database. Migrant sensitive health care systems need evidence for their development and currently data is not consistently available across the European Region.

We believe that stronger data will help gather stronger political support. To convince the European governments to support our programmes, we have needed data to show that our work addresses public health security related to migrants. This issue is at the top of the government's policy agenda and we can show we can help.

PART 1

All WHO reports underline that migrants do not mean a special health hazard for hosting countries, however in general, one cannot say that migration has no health and public health impact. We approach the governments from the point of view that our work in training medical and health professionals with additional knowledge on migrants allows them to better protect the health of both migrants and host populations. We also enhance our student practitioners' cultural competencies.

Istvan Szilard, Co-chair WHO Collaborating Centre for Migration Health Training and Research, Pécs, Hungary

A Knowledge Hub on Health and Migration has also been established as a joint effort between the WHO Regional Office for Europe, the Ministry of Health of Italy, the Regional Health Council of Sicily and the European Commission.

Three successful summer schools on refugee and migrant health were organized in 2017, 2018 and 2019. The first two in collaboration with the International Organization for Migration, the European Commission, the European Public Health Association and the Italian National Institute for Health, Migration and Poverty and supported by the Italian Ministry of Health and the Sicily Regional Health Authority.

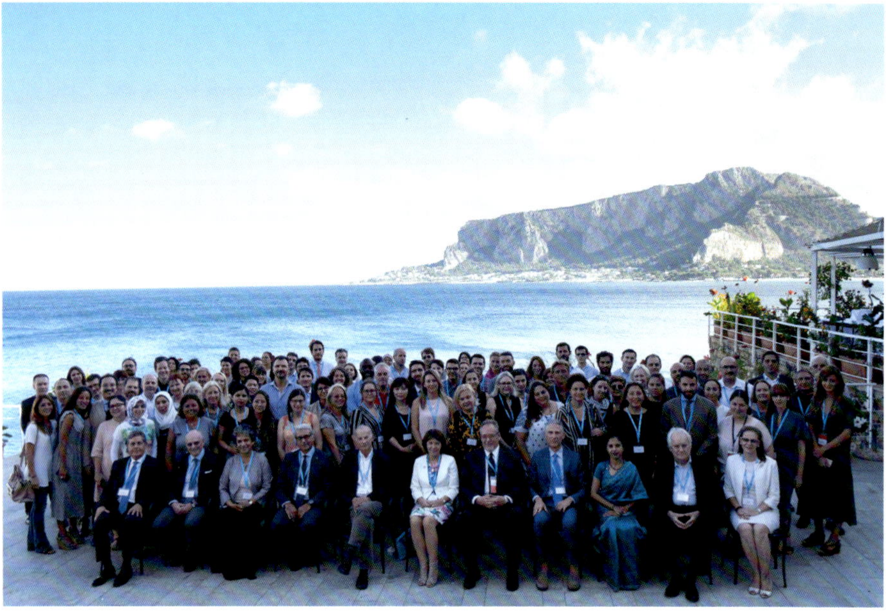

'Second edition' WHO Regional Office for Europe Summer School on Refugee and Migrant Health, 24–28 September 2018, Palermo, Italy. © WHO/Francesco Bellina

The 2019 school was in collaboration with the International Organization for Migration and the European Public Health Association and supported by the Ministry of Health of Turkey.

In December 2018, the Regional Office published the *Report on the health of refugees and migrants in the WHO European Region*, the first of its kind aiming to support evidence-informed policy-making to meet the health needs of both migrant and host populations *(15)*. The Regional Office has also published several WHO Health Evidence Network (HEN) reports on migrant health.

Developmental reflection 2
Protecting the health of migrants
Health 2020 in action

Our work on migration and health is a wonderful story of innovation and different country initiatives applying Health 2020 approaches. It all started in a quite singular manner, in February 2011 when migrants started to come from north Africa during what has become to be known as the 'Arab spring'.

Our Office was at the time very focused on determining the impact of the ash of the Iceland volcano on the health of Europeans. And what was going on in Africa was at first considered an episodic situation. Staff sought my advice about the situation and raised concerns that that this human crisis could become a public health issue of relevance for Europe. After reviewing these reports my leadership team and I thought that this risk needed to be quickly researched. Our idea was to go to the 'frontline' to see the reality for ourselves.

We contacted countries in the southern part of the Region, which were receiving the bulk of the new arrivals, to see if we could assess the situation and their systems to receive, process, settle and/or relocate migrants, so that we could identify ways to support them. For example, we could help with coordination, if the assessment revealed a need for health and medical interventions.

I wrote to Ministers of Health in Italy, Greece, Malta, Spain, France, and Hungary (which held the Presidency of the European Commission at the time). Italy was the first one to respond. The Italian Minister came to Copenhagen on the next Sunday to meet with our team. We had a meeting in the Regional Office that day with the Minister, the Italian Ambassador to Denmark and our migrant health coordinator. The Minister let us know very clearly that the health sector was feeling unprepared and challenged by the current situation. He pointed out that health is not usually too involved with migration policy and services which are usually managed by the Minister of Interior through their work on border control and crossings.

We agreed to start our work in Sicily, and with Lampedusa. Soon after, Malta and Greece also requested our assistance.

Assessments were conducted in these countries and resulted in the development of guidance on the real health needs of migrants. They were found to be very useful for informing and empowering Ministers of Health and their representatives in their respective councils of Ministers discussions on migration-related interventions.

What we were finding in this first 'lab stage' of our work was evidence of potential actions the health sector could usefully take to address migrant needs and challenges, and to use this data to reach out to other sectors to be involved in the decision-making and planning processes. Typically, this topic was considered to be the domain of other UN agencies and the role of the public health sector was not well developed or articulated. So, our assessment initiated a process of learning.

One of the first lessons we learned was that our task was not only to protect refugees and migrants, but also to protect the health of the resident population. It quickly became clear that we cannot separate public health and health for migrants from the health of the rest of the population. We realized that we could not and shouldn't separate this into a 'silo' programme for refugees and migrants. We also realized that it was inextricably linked to our core work and the principles including health for all, UHC, inequity reduction, etc.

It was a extremely fascinating time, and initiated a lot of internal discussion across the whole Office on the best ways to address entry points with Member States, and to find ways countries could engage with these health issues in non-political ways; clearly separating politics from the public health dimension.

We worked on developing very solid health arguments that, in spite of strong political polarization and sensitivities, nobody could disagree with, based on the relevance and objectivity of the health issues. To inform this process, we again contacted the six Ministers of Health and arranged a meeting, hosted by Italy and the European Commissioner for Health and Food Safety.

The Ministers noted that health interventions were considered as a side-effect of the situation and then only if an outbreak developed. We shared with them our preliminary findings and concerns about impacts on health systems. They all wanted to address the short- and long-term effects on their systems in a pragmatic way; to learn more about how they could promote structural interventions or structural system adjustments to address the needs of refugees and migrants. After the meeting, Italy provided the office with funding to develop some assessment and action guidance in this area.

We called it Public Health Aspects of Migration in Europe (PHAME). We could see that despite having tons of assessment tools, none of them was suitable for this purpose. We put together an expert group and started work on designing our own assessment tool, then pilot-tested it by conducting assessments in Member States, including Albania, Bulgaria, Cyprus, Greece, Hungary, Italy, Malta, Portugal, Serbia, Spain and North Macedonia. By developing the toolkit in collaboration with the Office of the United Nations High Commissioner for Refugees (UNHCR) and the International Organization for Migration (IOM) we obtained the blessing of the expert specialized agencies.

This initial phase allowed us to start to work in countries and assess the situations. We were not in a position to give financial or technical assistance but more to offer tools and useful approaches that Ministries could take. We could see early on how important it was to start to build a sense of ownership by the Ministers of Health, and their critical role in helping other sectors see the health impacts of their work. We worked on this for about three years and used our experience to draft the first toolkit for assessing the health of migrant or assistance needed within the first 30 days of their arrival *(99)*. These activities defined our work from 2011–2015.

Then things changed. With the 'Big walk across the Balkans' in 2015 we started to see for the first time, more generalized negative sentiments towards migrants. From a kind of humanitarian perception, countries started to turn towards focusing on how to manage or stop the situation, and how to protect themselves. Again, we discussed what to do, and called for a Ministerial lunch on health and migration, at the Regional Committee in Lithuania in 2015. For most of the Ministers and delegates, this was a completely new topic. It was interesting to see how concerned the Ministers of Health were already. They really didn't know how to handle this new challenge and immediately called for a high-level meeting that Italy offered to host in Rome.

It was held within 6 weeks! It was the first Ministerial level conference on the topic. Its aim was to decide whether and how the WHO Regional Office for Europe was to be involved in this topic. The Office very quickly identified guiding principles, priorities and a rationale for an intervention. The discussions were very open, and Ministers expressed real concern that the health sector should be actively engaged. They adopted an outcome document which was reflected, two years later, in the New York Declaration which has led the process of global engagement. Retrospectively, we can appreciate that the WHO Regional Office for Europe set up a really powerful process, with its consensus paper and outcome document.

We then had a policy framework and we began working hand-in-hand with Member States, supporting confidence building in the issue and more of a sense of ownership. This process of trust-, confidence- and capacity-building, led to unanimous adoption of the first-ever strategy and action plan with a complete solution at the Regional Committee in Copenhagen in 2016 *(16)*.

Unanimity was based on two factors. An intensive consultation process – I think we had 15 or 16 one-to-one and small and large group consultations over an 18–month period with partners, stakeholders and Member States. Secondly, our clarity about not challenging the management of migration policy, but simply discussing public health protection for all.

Following the adoption of the Strategy and action plan for refugee and migrant health in the WHO European Region in 2016, the Migration and Health programme was established at the Regional Office. This programme was established to support Member States in their efforts to strengthen the health sector's capacity to provide evidence-informed responses to the public health challenges of refugee and migrant health. The programme operates under the umbrella of the Health 2020 European health policy framework, providing support to Member States under four pillars: technical assistance; health information, research and training; partnership building; and advocacy and communication. The programme promotes a collaborative intercountry approach to migrant health by facilitating cross-country policy dialogue and encouraging homogeneous health interventions along the migration routes to promote the health of refugees and migrants and protect public health in the host community.

Everything we produced was accompanied by solid evidence. Evidence was the keyword as we focused on countering false rumours and fake news. When we spoke about enhancing access to TB treatment for migrants, for example, we provided the evidence that their TB was not a threat if you have a prepared system.

Since the Strategy's adoption in 2016, we have seen strong and lasting commitment in Member States; no political controversy or manipulation or media coverage has been able to stop the process. By 2018 about 50% of the countries of the region are engaged in capacity-building, and action-planning on national, regional or local levels, including those where migration is most affecting politics.

Other Regions have recognized our leadership here and are asking for our help. When the New York Declaration was adopted in 2016 the decision was made to go for two compacts, one on migration, and one on refugees. Because migration still carries a negative narrative, we wanted to be there deciding what the compacts should look like. The one on refugees recognizes that they are people in need of support within a stronger international legal framework, so the process was smoother than the process for a global compact on migration.

This work developed through very intense intercountry negotiation. We stepped in because, as we had seen a few years before in the Region, countries were not really recognizing the role of the health sector. The global compact was focusing on security, on crisis, on the legal framing of the process of migration; health was a side-effect that might be considered later. We engaged in a very intense negotiation and lobbying with Member States and the global framework. The work done with WHO became the official reference of the global compact, for the health dimension. I like to call it Health 2020 in action, really operationalizing Health 2020 on this multi-faceted, complex topic.

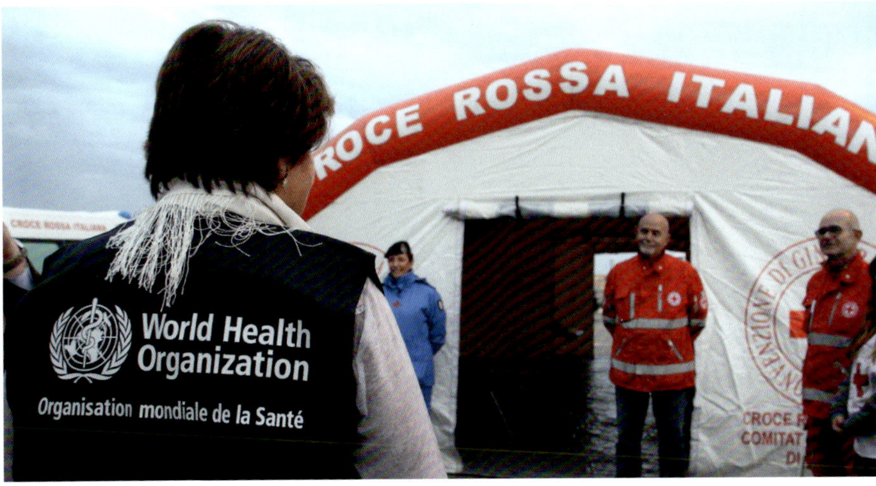

Zsuzsanna Jakab visiting medical tents where migrants and refugees are treated on arrival in Trapani Harbour, Italy, 14 November 2016. © WHO/Sara Barragan Montes

Summary reflection

Strengthening the European contribution to global health

Message 5: Think Globally act Regionally

In strengthening the European contribution to global health, the WHO Regional Office for Europe has been repositioned as an initiator, tester, and driver of global health approaches. Many technical policies and programmes initiated in the Region have 'gone global'. New relationships between Regions and WHO Headquarters have been developed and 'One WHO' approaches embraced more strongly. Examples include new all-determinant approaches to health and development; the promotion of whole-of-government, whole-of-society and health-in-all-policies approaches to the promotion of health and well-being; a stronger focus on the social determinants of health and equity; development and implementation of Health 2020 as a forerunner of the United Nations 2030 Agenda for Sustainable Development and the SDGs; introduction of governance for health in the 21st century concepts and approaches; expansion of networks such as Health Cities; elaboration of necessary skills and capacities for todays' public health; 'catching the moment' and taking quick action when required e.g. on migration and health; 'addressing 'difficult' issues' e.g. developing strategies for sexual and reproductive health, child abuse and maltreatment, and mental health in institutions.

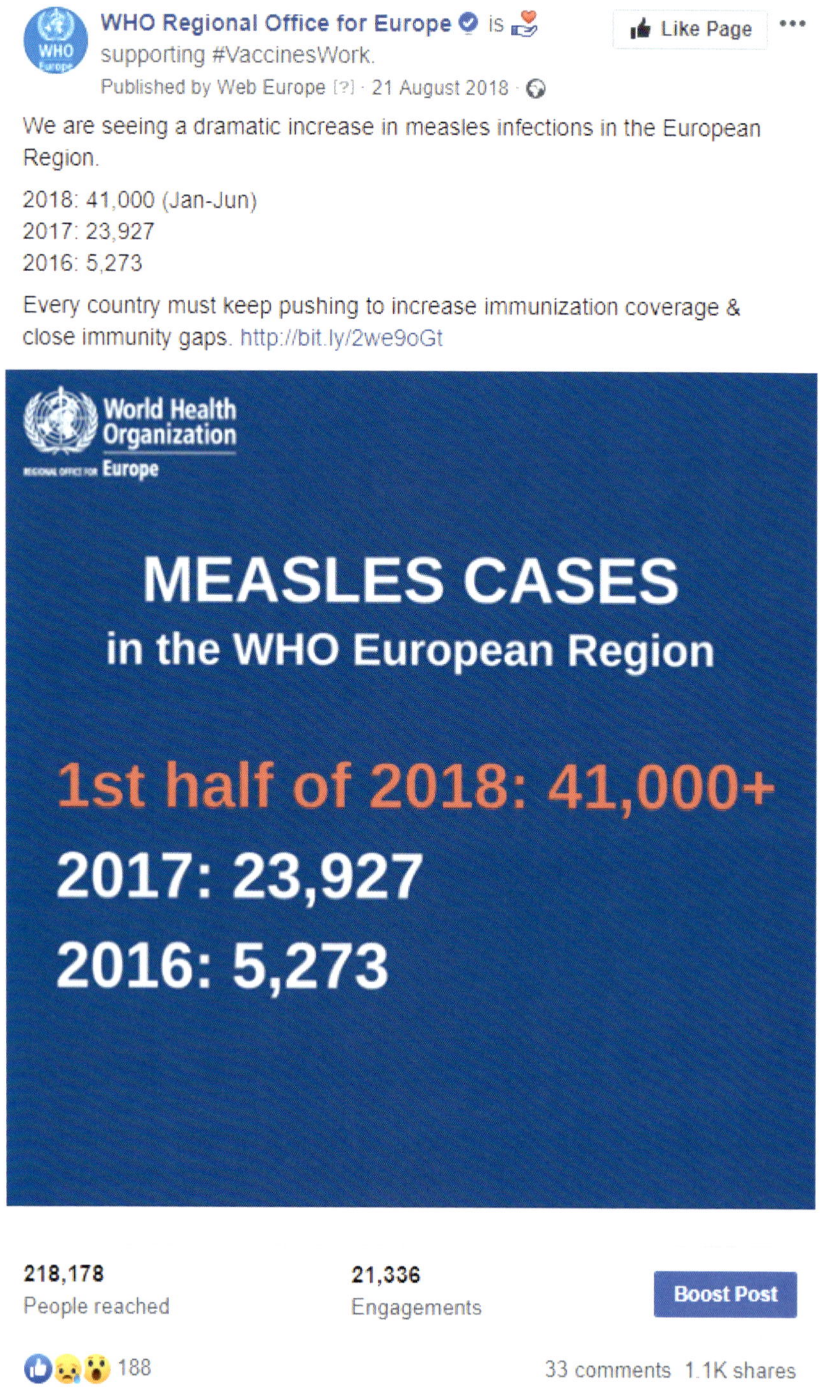

Example of WHO Regional Office for Europe Twitter message, 21 August 2018. Source: WHO

7. Reaching out through information and communication

In these last ten years, the Regional Office has used a variety of innovative and impactful information and communication initiatives to make evidence-informed materials more easily accessible and useable to all public health stakeholders.

7.1 Information

The importance of information and evidence was acknowledged early on in the Health 2020 process. A key conclusion of Health 2020 is that while health policy-making in Europe should be informed primarily by evidence, it is essentially a political process in which scientific evidence has to compete with beliefs, personal interests, political considerations and priorities, traditions, past experience and financial constraints.

Inequalities and information

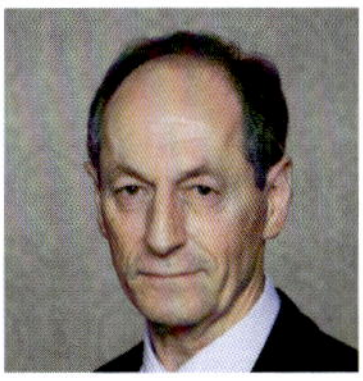

To address inequalities in health in Europe, our first step must be to address the inequalities in health information. All too commonly where health is poorest, health information tends to be poorest.

Health information is absent or incomplete just where we need it most. Health information is crucial in all countries, rich or poor.

Sir Michael Marmot, Director, University College London, Institute of Health Equity, United Kingdom

To address these challenges we have moved from relying on solely quantitative evidence into a completely new era of using both quantitative and qualitative evidence. For the very first time we are describing and measuring well-being; we are using and measuring the concepts of Health 2020 such as community empowerment, resilience, the whole-of-society approach, the life-course approach.

All this requires new framing related to health information; a framing that is consistent with the kinds of conceptual changes inherent in our shift from health governance to governance for health. We have moved from having a health information department to now having an information systems for health department. Much of our 'health-related' information now comes out of other systems: for example, transport, education, environment and social work. This is a unique shift that is taking place for the very first time in the history of WHO. And we are doing this consistently and systematically.

Over the last 10 years we have developed and implemented initiatives to strengthen evidence-informed policy-making using these new perspectives, as well as addressing competing constraints. These initiatives have included the establishment and management of several support networks and partnerships; identification and implementation of innovative ways to incorporate qualitative data; other novel approaches to evidence gathering for policy processes; active translation interventions; and new joint reporting mechanisms.

The 2010 Strategic Partnership mandated the Regional Office and the European Commission to work towards a single health information system for Europe as a key milestone to strengthening the use of evidence. This focused on information sharing and avoiding duplication of reporting *(100)*. This also opened the door for closer working relations between our two institutions and initiated an ongoing process of joint problem-solving and development.

The vehicle developed to achieve goals was the European Health Information Initiative (EHII) launched in 2012. This network is committed to improving the quality of information that underpins health policies in the European Region. It has five main pillars *(101)*:

1. development and harmonization of indicators for health and well-being;
2. enhanced dissemination of health information;
3. capacity-building;
4. strengthening of health information networks; and,
5. support for health information strategy development.

The stakeholders include Member States, WHO collaborating centres, health information networks and associations such as the European Association of Public Health (EUPHA) and charitable foundations such as the Wellcome Trust. The Organisation for Economic Co-operation and Development (OECD) is also an active participant.

European health information initiative (EHII)

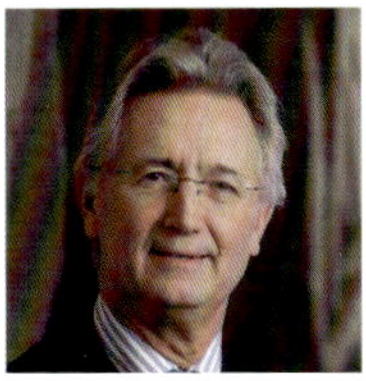

In 2012 Zsuzsanna Jakab and I signed a memorandum to start the EHII. Our aim was to create a network committed to improving health by improving the information that underpins policy.

Our Ministry of Health, Welfare and Sport of the Netherlands, within which I directed RIVM at that time, provided seed money.

We were well aware that that we needed a broad involvement of other countries and agencies. This, I am pleased to report, quickly developed as many other agencies; including the EU, OECD, several WHO collaborating centres from the United Kingdom and the Russian Federation, as well as Public Health England, the European Public Health Association (EUPHA), the Commonwealth and the Wellcome trust and many countries got interested and involved. We also benefitted from early links with the EU funded Bridging Information and Data Generation for Evidence-based Health Policy and Research (BRIDGE) Health project consortium.

I think one of the keys to EHII success was that this was not an initiative of public health experts alone but also directly engaged with policy-makers.

I think the idea of WHO Autumn School for Health Information and Evidence for Policymaking was a very good thing. In this school we created a kind of masterclass for policy-makers and top experts interested in systematic health information. The school has become a platform where experts and policy-makers can help each other develop concepts further.

I think EHII was a wonderful development and has really got good results. It has helped public health policy-makers have good information, good indicators and to better know how they compare. It has worked well across the whole of the European Region and I think the model could work around the world.

Andre van der Zande, President of the International Association of National Public Health Institutes (IANPHI)

PART 1

Over these last years we have continuously improved the development and harmonization of the information and analytical resources of the Regional Office. The Health for All family of databases remains our most comprehensive source of health statistics for monitoring and assessment in key health policy areas. We have made great efforts to harmonize data collection definitions, processes and quality with the statistical office of the European Union (Eurostat) and the Organisation for Economic Co-operation and Development (OECD). We have published annually core health indicators and have carried out extensive work on the development of health and well-being indicators for Health 2020 target monitoring (see Box 5). The Regional Office has collaborated on this with the Institute for Health Metrics and Evaluation (IHME) in Seattle, United States of America.

Experts from the Netherlands National Institute for Public health and the Environment (RIVM) have collaborated with WHO to design a new 'one-stop webportal' for health information hosted at the WHO Regional Office for Europe. This European Health Information Gateway has enhanced access and dissemination of health information and allowed us to provide a wealth of health-related information in real time *(102)*. We have developed new search tools to make access, navigation and graphic generation even easier through the Gateway. The *Health for All Explorer,* for example, now provides integrated access to all indicators and allows open access to users to dynamically compare and explore data, and create customized graphics *(103)*.

Three health information networks have already been established in the Region monitoring Health 2020 targets and indicators – Central Asian Republics Information Network (CARINFONET), the Small Countries Health Information Network, and the South-eastern Europe Health Network, which proposed the creation of a health information network during the Albanian Presidency in 2015.

A repeated request from Member States has been about the burden of reporting to different policy framework indicators. All Member States of the WHO European Region are committed to report on Health 2020, the Global Action Plan for the Prevention and Control of Noncommunicable Diseases (NCD framework), the SDGs, and targets of the United Nations 2030 Agenda for Sustainable Development.

While different governing bodies produced these frameworks independently, there are considerable similarities between them. To take advantage of opportunities for joint reporting our Division of Information, Evidence, Research and Innovation undertook an assessment of indicators across the three frameworks. This mapping exercise showed that *(104)*:

1. there is 76% alignment between Health 2020 and SDG indicators; and
2. almost 6 out of 10 (56%) NCD framework indicators are also SDG indicators, as are one third of Health 2020 indicators.

Eliminating duplicate reporting

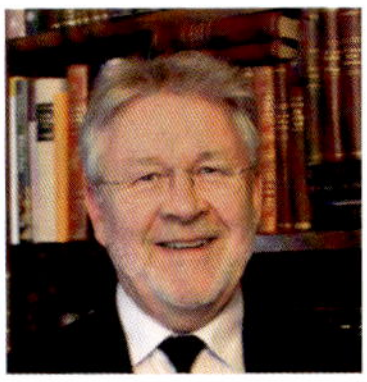

A Joint Monitoring Framework (JMF) was adopted at the 68th session of the Regional Committee in Rome. This framework was developed to address countries' burden of reporting. In my home country Iceland, as in many other Member States, there was the feeling that key European health agencies like WHO, ECDC and OECD were not exchanging data, and all three were asking the same questions, and feedback from some of them was quite limited. When you spend a lot of time collecting and submitting data, it is very important that you see the data used sometime later in a publication or report. We have been pushing all these agencies to work more in partnership and collect data together. This new JMF really does this and is a great accomplishment, especially for databases which relate to sustainable development agenda, Health 2020 and NCD reporting.

I was in a WHO Regional Office for Europe-convened group of 12 scientists, data specialists and other stakeholders who took on the task of developing this JMF. WHO had to build a group that had competence. Experts needed to be found from across the Region because data registers are not everyone's game. Every country has a limited number of well trained people within their data registries; people who know what is a strong indicator and what is a weak one, etc. So it was a very mixed group of people who were brought together from across the Region.

The group decided what we did and didn't need. We started by reviewing various data requests and throwing out a lot of repetitions. These were not complicated decisions, but it needed to be done. There was a lot of discussion and fine-tuning. This JMF will save countries a lot of work, enhance the quality of reporting and the coordinated use of data by agencies and Member States. It has been a great partnership success.

Sveinn Magnússon, Former Director General for Health, Iceland

As we move ahead, the Office is now collaborating with different agencies and Member States in looking at ways to strengthen evidence-informed policy-making by incorporating qualitative and novel approaches into measurement tools, and ways to integrate health determinant related data from different sectors.

Integrated health information system in Finland

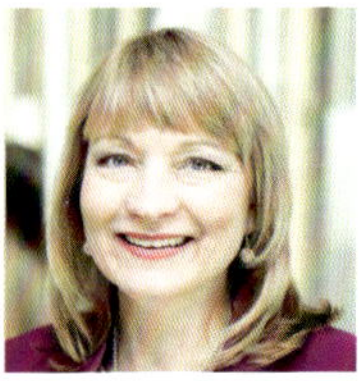

Our constitution in Finland gives everyone the right to health and social care. That makes it the responsibly of government to develop legislation which ensures that individuals will get the support and services they need. Our social security and health and social services are built on this base. Since the 1960s we have had a national identification number. We have collected data from our population to different registries and used this information to develop efficient and effective public sector processes.

There is always critical debate in the parliamentary committees to ensure that any new legislation is in harmony with individuals' rights to have support. Equality and inclusiveness are very important. Everyone in Finland gets free education and social and health services. We have universal health care and universal health coverage in Finland and in that way we have built a lot of trust in the public sector services, civil servants and our government. People are very positive about giving information for administrative purposes to ensure services for themselves, and for research purposes.

That is why in Finland we have a good basis for thinking about the new possibilities of technology, artificial intelligence and digital information. In addition, we have socioeconomic information which can be integrated with health data.

We now have a structure of municipalities providing primary health and social services and 20 specialized health care districts, including five university hospital districts responsible for the most advanced care. We have 100% digitalized patient health records and a national health data repository through which patient information and prescriptions are available for different care purposes across the country.

We are now in process of introducing social service information according to the same principles, to support the integration of social and health services. It will be particularly important for elderly care, but also for family care and prevention related to disabled people, mental health, substance abuse, etc.

And now, for the first time in the world, we are introducing legislation for the secondary use of data. That will enable the combination of data from different registers for research, development and innovation as well as for management and supervisory purposes, ensuring data security.

We value our collaboration with the WHO Regional Office for Europe in all these processes. In the WHO European Region over the past ten years there has been continuous quality improvement in governing processes, transparency, and sharing of information and good practices among countries to strengthen sustainable health systems. We highly appreciate and support the Regional Office's work on evidence and data-based decision-making not only to recognized problems but also to identify and share solutions. We are really like-minded in the ways we think and do things.

Päivi Sillanaukee, Permanent Secretary,
Ministry of Social Affairs and Health, Finland

The Health Evidence Network synthesis report series is an information service that continues to turn published evidence into policy options to improve health for vulnerable populations, and to reduce health inequalities by defining the barriers to accessing health services. One example was a very useful series on refugee and migrant health, published in 2018 *(105)*.

Capacity building in collecting, analysing, reporting and, importantly, using evidence includes the Evidence-informed Policy Network (EVIPNet) launched in the Regional Office in October 2012 as part of a global WHO initiative to assist with evidence transfer and translation *(106)*. EPIVNet is now active in 13 Member States of the European Region and aims to promote the systematic use of health-related research in policy-making.

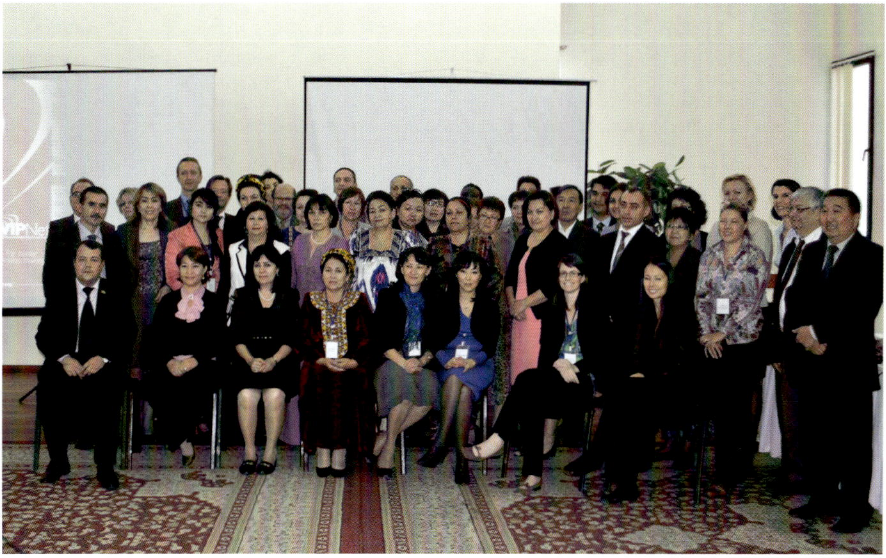

Claudia Stein, Director of the Division of Information, Evidence, Research and Innovation, WHO Regional Office for Europe with participants at the launch of Evidence-informed Policy Network (EVIPNet) Europe, in Bishkek, Kyrgystan, 10 October 2012. © WHO

In 2016 the Regional Committee developed and adopted an Action Plan to strengthen the use of evidence, information and research for policy-making in the Region with the aim of helping Member States engage with and use all these resources. The Action Plan emphasizes a systems approach to health research; aligns research agendas with public health priorities; facilitates multisectoral, interdisciplinary health research practices; and fosters the systematic and transparent use of research in local health decision-making. Such capacities are proving to be especially important in this era of 'fake news'.

Addressing fake news

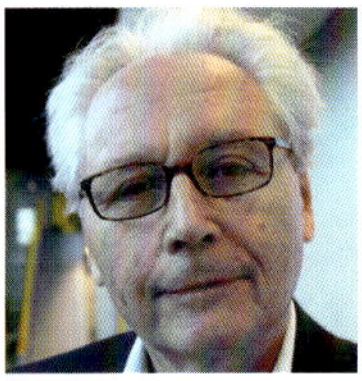

It has been reported that over the last five years information dealing with health matters on social media was 50% fake news *(107)*. This reinforces the importance of WHO's Action Plan to strengthen the use of evidence, information and research for policy-making in the WHO European Region. It is absolutely essential that when it comes to development of policies and implementation of policies all are evidence-informed.

The importance of research in the national context and the need for capacity-building, especially in countries with fewer resources has been well supported by the WHO Regional Office for Europe over the last 10 years. The EVIPNet programme, for example, has successfully been supporting countries in the European Region with capacity-building which is enabling better use of evidence in decision-making *(108)*.

Göran Tomson, Member of the WHO European Advisory Committee on Health Research, Sweden

Addressing fake news – real reliable resources

We live in a world where there is a fight about the reality of fake news and fake data.

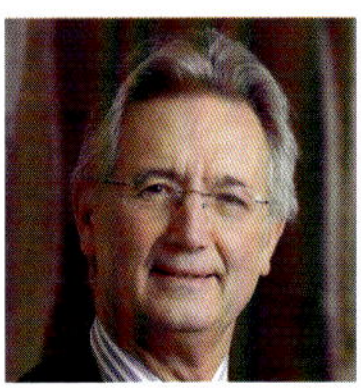

There is fake everything, so good data, good heavy data, strong data is very essential for all our work. WHO and the International Association of National Public Health Institutes (IANPHI) are in the position to develop tools like fact-checkers and other validating mechanisms, so that both politicians and citizens working in public health, can find real reliable resources, when they doubt the fake news and fake facts.

Andre Van der Zande, President of the International Association of National Public Health Institutes (IANPHI)

The Autumn School on Health Information and Evidence for Policymaking has also helped build capacity in health information and trained participants from more than 27 Member States since 2013. The Advanced Health Information Workshop has been held annually to further strengthen countries' specific capacity in health information areas that are particularly relevant to Health 2020. The Regional Office has also developed and piloted a support tool for countries to assess their health information systems, advance health information strategies, and ensure that their national health information systems are fit for Health 2020 monitoring.

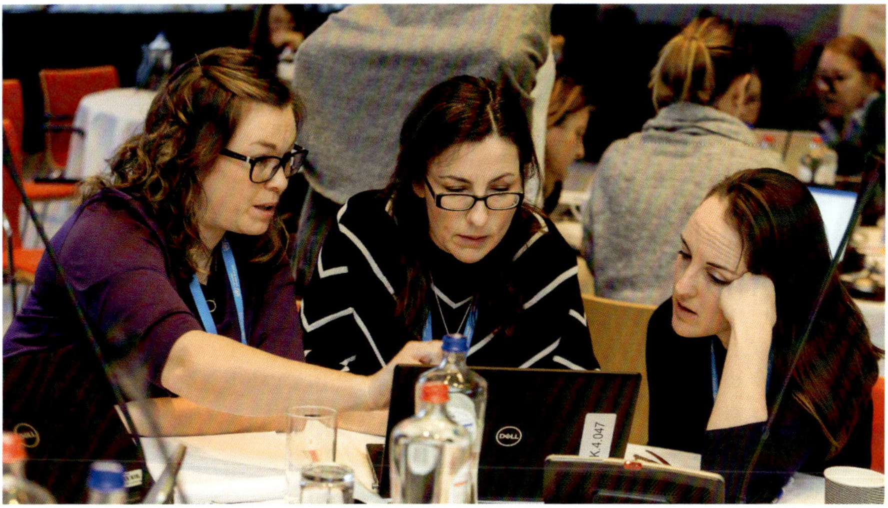

Twenty participants from 9 countries gained practical insights and solutions for improving national health information systems at WHO's Autumn School on Health Information and Evidence for Policy-making, The Hague, Netherlands 29 January – 1 February 2019.
© WHO/Koen Peters

One of the most exciting areas of technological innovation is the use of IT and electronic data to support health assessment and health care delivery. A Regional report on the implementation of e-health strategies that support Health 2020 was published to catch this tide in early 2016.

PART 1

The Office has also developed a wide variety of digitally delivered newsletters to support communities of practice in different public health areas (see Box 14).

Box 14. The WHO Regional Office for Europe – digitally delivered newsletters *(109)*.

1. *WHO/Europe news highlights (110).* Monthly newsletter with public health news, publications and events highlights from around the WHO European Region.
2. *European Environment and Health Process Newsletter (111).* This newsletter provides regular updates and developments in air pollution, cities, chemical safety, climate change and water, sanitation and hygiene, waste and contaminates sites, and environmentally sustainable health systems following the Declaration signed at the Sixth Ministerial Conference on Environment and Health held in Ostrava, Czechia, 13–15 June 2017.
3. *Flu Focus (112).* Newsletter covering recent developments, research, reports, materials and resources on influenza.

4. *Health systems newsletter (113).* News, events and publications about health systems and public health issues in Europe.
5. *HEN News (114).* Updates on new publications and other news from the Health Evidence Network.
6. *Joint TB, HIV and viral Hepatitis (JTH) newsletter (115).* This newsletter, informing on TB, HIV and viral Hepatitis in the WHO European Region, replaces as of now the previous TB and M/XDR-TB newsletter and reflects the Regional Office's new coordinated and integrated approach towards reducing the burden of these three related diseases.
7. *Noncommunicable diseases newsletter (116).* News, events and publications about NCDs and risk factors in Europe.
8. *Observatory e-Bulletin (117).* Information about the newest publications and activities of the European Observatory on Health Systems and Policies.
9. *Publications news (118).* Updates on new publications from WHO Regional Office for Europe.
10. *Public Health Aspects of Migration in Europe (PHAME) newsletter (98)*. Quarterly newsletter with news, know-how and best practices on migration, produced in partnership by the Regional Office and the University of Pécs, Hungary.
11. *Public Health Panorama.* Published four times a year *(119).* It features good practices in policy and research in public health from around the European Region. It is published online and in print in English and Russian.
12. *Regions for Health Network newsletter (120).* Information about the activities, events and publications of the Regions for Health Network.
13. *Roma inclusion newsletter (121).*Quarterly newsletter with information and resources related to improving the health of Roma living in the WHO European Region.
14. *Vaccine-preventable diseases and immunization (VPI) news (122).* Updates on news, events and publications from the Vaccine-preventable diseases and immunization programme of the Regional Office.

7.2 Communication

'From one voice to many voices' encapsulates how our communications have developed over the past decade. Communications have always been and remains an essential component of WHO's public health work. What we say and the actions we recommend – on issues as diverse as the formulation of baby foods to the number of measles cases in our Member States – have an impact on the lives of over 900 million people in the WHO European Region, and indeed beyond.

What has changed, as we all know, is the environment in which we communicate, and the powerful digital communications tools we have at our fingertips (see Box 15). I have long thought that WHO must anticipate and capitalize on the opportunities that technological and societal developments offer us, to ensure that our work remains relevant, visible and valued. On becoming WHO Regional Director for Europe, one of my seven strategic action priorities was to identify innovative ways to analyse and disseminate health data, information and advocacy messages.

Box 15. The Regional Office's social media channels

In 2010, at the beginning of my mandate, the Regional Office began engaging on social media, opening accounts on both Twitter (in English) and Facebook.

By August 2019, these accounts were already a reliable, daily source of relevant public health information for our Twitter account's 72 000 followers, 143 000 Facebook fans and 27 000 Instagram followers. Twitter accounts have also been opened in German and Russian, as well as for the Healthy Cities and Regions for Health networks, the WHO Office in Brussels, and the vaccination and immunization programme.

Our outreach and engagement at country level has increased, with opportunities to share information in national languages thanks to 11 Facebook pages, 2 Twitter accounts and 1 Instagram account managed by country offices.

The diverse content – messages, images, video, infographics – shared on our social media platforms makes an impact. A single tweet, for example, related to measles cases in the WHO European Region in August 2018 had nearly 140 000 impressions, while a Facebook post had a reach of more than 200 000.

The communications team works to continuously update its social media tactics to stay in line with the latest social media trends and to encourage engagement, including using new features (e.g., Twitter threads, Instagram stories and Facebook Live), and carefully tracks analytics in order to gain insights into which types of content yield the best performance. The team collaborates with country offices, GDOs and technical programmes throughout the Regional Office to develop a wide variety of content covering all areas of the Regional Office's work.

Our audiences have expanded from 'those who can influence health policies' – traditionally ministers of health, decision-makers and policy-makers – to also include 'those with a stake in health' – meaning all of us, public and professionals alike. Health 2020, and more recently the United Nations 2030 Agenda for Sustainable Development and the SDGs have given us the political mandate to fully engage in and promote whole-of-society, whole-of-government and health-in-all-policies approaches to improve health and well-being for all. In working to fulfill this mandate we have become more strategic – building our communications around a Region-wide strategy with clear objectives and strengthening audience familiarity and identification with WHO through visual identity guidelines.

New technology has further facilitated the democratization of communications. Beyond the well-established WHO European Regional website, publications and outreach to journalists, we now listen to, engage with and tailor our messages to many diverse groups through social media, apps, and live webcasting. Today, I believe that WHO has several voices speaking in harmony and with aligned messages.

Giving a voice to those living with challenging health conditions, in difficult circumstances, or with unique experience of health issues has been a valuable, and well-received extension to the Regional Office's communications portfolio in recent years. The "Voices of the Region" series, for example, integrated into three Regional Committee sessions, have brought an added dimension to our governance discussions.

As audiences consume information in different ways, we have catered to this, sharing our public health expertise using visual and multimedia storytelling through video, photos, infographics and podcasts. We have been supported in these efforts by our ever expanding image library, which offers one of the most wide-ranging collections of images across WHO.

Similarly, as part of efforts to make governance processes more transparent and accessible to wider audiences, the proceedings at Regional Committee sessions and high-level ministerial conferences, have been webcast live and content shared on dedicated websites and social media. We are also making the work of the governing bodies easier through searchable on-line databases of resolutions and other documents.

One initiative that that has been welcomed by delegates attending has been an events app to help participants find details of upcoming sessions, access all documents, navigate their way around the venue and the hosting city, check weather forecasts, social events and transport schedules, and receive notifications about important changes in the programme. They can also share photos, join the conversation on Twitter, interact with other participants and more recently use the app as a communication mechanism (see Developmental reflection 3).

Developmental reflection 3
The WHO Regional Office for Europe
Mobile events app *(123)*

In 2015, I asked our Web team a few weeks before our Regional Committee session, if it was possible to develop a mobile app for RC, similar to the app built by our colleagues in Geneva for World Health Assembly (WHA). We wanted to make it easy for RC delegates to access documents and navigate their way through the annual meeting in September. I assumed, given the short time to the RC, that we would introduce our app at our 2016 meeting. To my surprise and delight, our team was amazingly quick and able to come up with a very attractive user-friendly app in just a few weeks! We launched this at the 65th session of our RC in 2015. This was very well received. And, as they say, the rest is history!

Over the following years, our events app has become more and more powerful, useful and user-friendly. It has become much more than an access platform for documents and meeting navigation. It now is really a public health communication channel in its own right: it saw adoption rate going up to 83% in 2018, which is much higher than the non-profit sector average of 48.5%. Our app now has functions that allow for real-time interactions between presenters and participants. Questions can be posed by presenters, opinions polled. Moreover, answers with cumulative scores displayed in a variety of attractive formats can be flashed on screens instantly, and the results can be used in panel discussions. General reminders and alerts about programme changes and meeting transport information can be communicated rapidly and easily to all. Participants can use the app to connect and communicate with one another. The app has now even been used as a platform for counting steps and 'heart points' competitions, in support of the global Walk the Talk initiative, and in the effort to make our meetings healthier (see Google Fit app informed by WHO *(124)*). Our events app has also served as an example for other Regional Offices (SEARO, for example) and UN agencies (FAO). The app has been an important prototype venture for the WHO Regional Office for Europe into the world of digital health communications and for all the potential benefits that area of innovation promises to bring (see Section 9.3.4.8).

Communicating what we do and its impact on health has be enhanced by focusing on our country work. Hence in our news coverage and on our website, activities and developments in countries take pride of place. To facilitate this within our Office structure, the management of country offices and communications come together under the Country Support and Communications unit.

We also established a National Technical Focal Points for Communication Network as an effective mechanism for exchanging communications intelligence, campaign materials and recent developments across Member States. We currently have plans to further strengthen our communication support to Member States by enriching the country sites with information about BCAs and their implementation in respective national languages. Country offices' capacity in communications has recently been strengthened.

Further opportunities for outreach have been taken through participation in UN communications networks, and by communications staff taking part in WHO network events, including workshops and plenary sessions for the Small Countries Initiative meetings and at Healthy Cities events, as well as strategic support to SEEHN meetings. Sharing information with non-State actors, including donors, has also been prioritized.

I am delighted that the excellent work of our professional communications team was acknowledged in 2016, when they were awarded the Director-General's Reward for Excellence. I am proud to pass on this legacy of strong communications to my successor.

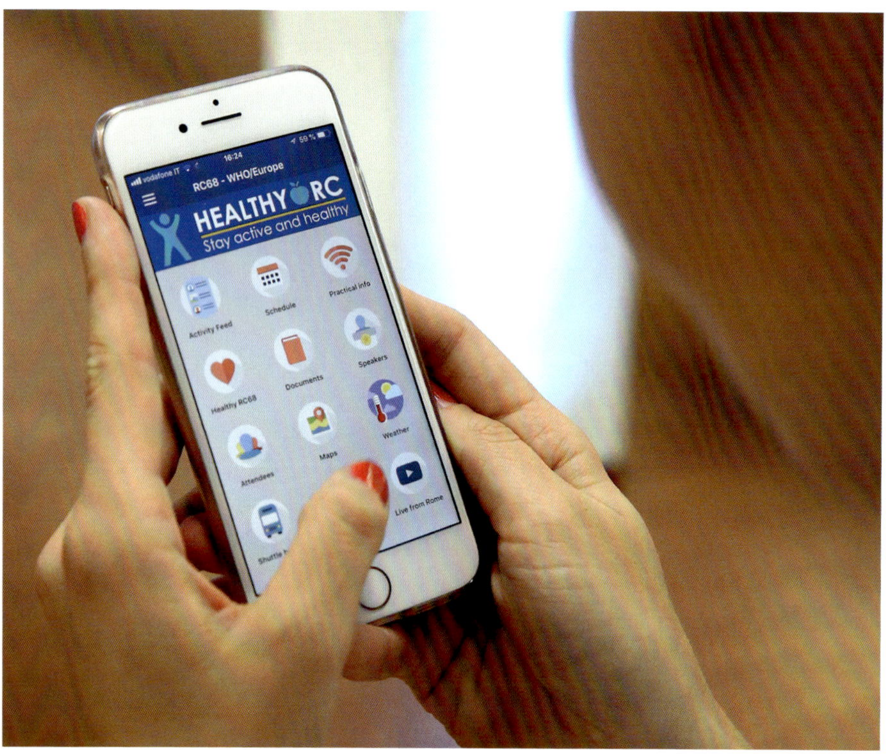

A delegate uses the app at the 68th session of the Regional Committee in Rome, Italy, 17–20 September 2018. © WHO

7.3 Emergency risk communication (ERC)

ERC is a vital public health intervention. It can save lives during emergency situations and, as such, should be considered an investment in people's health, safety and security. Under the 2005 International Health Regulations (IHRs), countries commit to measuring and strengthening their national risk communication capacities. This involves improving understanding of ERC principles and practices as well as developing, testing and implementing national ERC plans.

At present, many Member States as States Parties to the IHRs in the WHO European Region do not have an ERC plan dealing with all hazards within their IHR framework. In recent years WHO has scaled up efforts to work with these Member States to build up this critical capacity, including dissemination of training materials and guidance documents as well as the provision of workshops, trainings, mentorship and support.

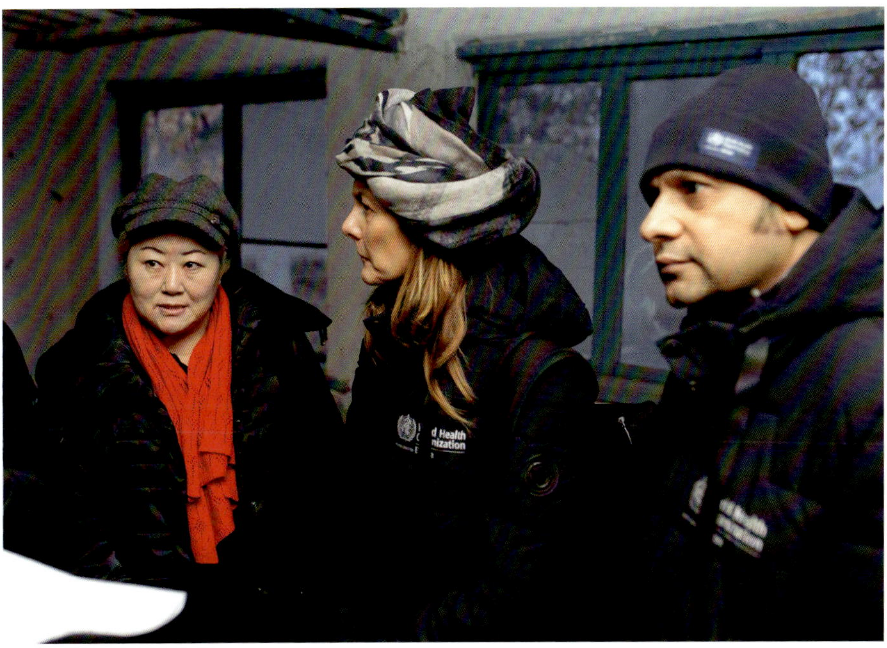

SocialNet training, Bishkek, Kyrgyzstan, 10–14 December 2018. Participants engaging with the Regional Office for Europe and UNICEF during a simulation exercise. © WHO

PART 1

Relevant to all Member States

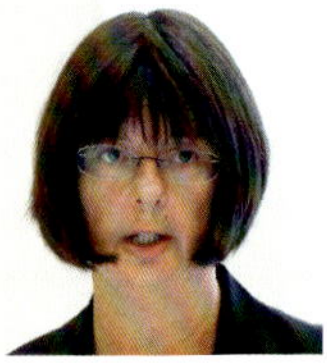

Pandemic and emergency preparedness, in spite of large efforts on national and international level, remains high on political agendas and needs further action. The Ebola outbreak was a wake-up call, letting us all know that we are only as safe as the most fragile State. We commend WHO for enhancing their Health Emergency Programme which has already demonstrated its capacities to respond quickly and effectively; e.g., during the Ebola outbreak in the Democratic Republic of the Congo in 2018. We welcome that many countries have already undergone independent voluntary joint external evaluations. We are pleased to see that the European Region is working hard to accelerate IHR implementation. The German Government is supporting these efforts with voluntary contributions; for example, supporting the development and implementation of new training tools in emergency risk communication. Such initiatives are relevant to all Member States in our mutual efforts to strengthen our IHR capacities.

Dagmar Reitenbach, Head of Division Global Health, Federal Ministry of Health, Germany

In 2018 the WHO Health Emergency programme in the Regional Office launched a capacity-building package on ERC going beyond training and supporting full multisectoral country development or strengthening of their all-hazard ERC plan within the IHR framework *(190)*. The five-step package is a unique, sustained country-tailored capacity-building approach, initially piloted in 13 European countries for one year, that is now being rolled out globally *(125)*. The five steps engage countries in an iterative process to develop, test and adopt national health ERC plans and to integrate them into new or existing national action plans for emergency preparedness and response under the IHR. The comprehensive package includes tools for multisectoral training, capacity mapping and development, testing and adoption of an ERC plan.

Experiences from ERC country preparedness and field response make the package relevant and practical. Our communication staff has also been called upon to work globally in many recent public health emergencies, such as the Ebola virus disease outbreak in west Africa (2014–2015), and the emergence of the Zika virus syndrome (2015–2016). Lessons learned are brought back to the European Region. For example, a Zika manual and an associated app have been developed to assist public health authorities in the WHO European Region to communicate in response to possible outbreaks of the Zika virus, and other mosquito-borne diseases. The main objective is to enable European countries to learn from the experience of other Regions on how to communicate about Zika and apply these lessons in a European context.

As part of ERC, Social Science Interventions (SSIs) are critical to ensure that affected populations are engaged and enabled to take informed decisions to protect themselves and their loved ones during crises. The SocialNET training, a global initiative of WHO under the Pandemic Influenza Preparedness (PIP) framework, is the first of its kind in the European Region. Started in 2018, it engages countries in integrating SSIs into health emergency response; establishing a roster of Regional experts; and outlining SSIs plans.

Summary reflection

Reaching out through information and communication

Message 6: Put evidence-informed health information within the reach of everyone in our Region and beyond

We have learned a lot over these 10 years about ways to put accessible, understandable and useful evidence-informed health information within a hand's reach of everyone in our Region and beyond. This has involved a better understanding of increasing health literacy in the population; making evidence and information more accessible and easier to understand for all; amplifying and broadening the reach of our communication through enhanced web and social media feeds; active partnerships with NGOs, universities, cities, networks, regions etc.; the role of ambassadors (e.g. HRH Crown Princess Mary, Patron of WHO/Regional Office for Europe) and high-level advocacy with presidents, prime ministers, ministers of finance and other sectoral leaders (e.g. during country visits and meetings).

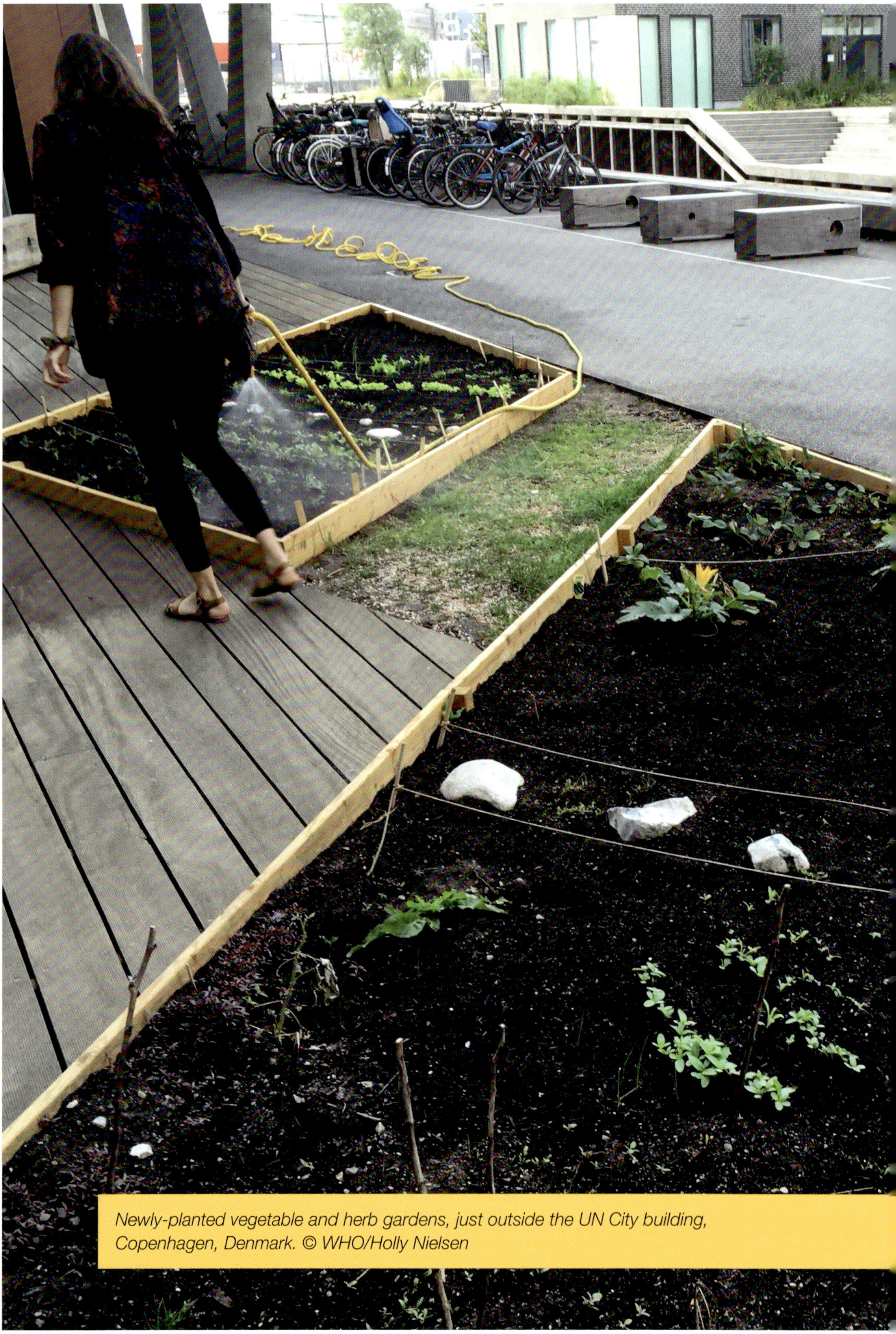

Newly-planted vegetable and herb gardens, just outside the UN City building, Copenhagen, Denmark. © WHO/Holly Nielsen

8. Creating a positive working environment

8.1 Positive working environment

I have always believed in creating a positive working environment for our staff. In April 2013, we moved our head offices in Copenhagen to the new UN CITY building, along with all other UN agencies in Denmark. We had outgrown our original offices and had experienced 3 major floods in 2011 and 2012, which disrupted work and caused extensive damage to property and archives. Besides providing excellent office space, management, catering and security services for our staff, the new premises have facilitated closer working relations with our sister UN agencies.

I would like to give thanks to Denmark which has always been a very good and generous host country for the Regional Office.

To help promote a positive working environment, the Office has established a comprehensive internal communication strategy, making optimum use of the intranet and increasing information sharing and interaction between all WHO offices in the Region. We have also introduced regular web-based meetings linking all country office staff to our general staff. All staff now has the possibility of linking with major Regional and Global meetings through web streaming.

Our recruitment and training activities have focused on ensuring that we have technically strong programmes, and staff, who are motivated, inspired and empowered. As Regional Director, I have regular meetings with the European Regional Office for Europe's Staff Association (EURSA). We review the work experiences of our staff in Copenhagen, GDOs and country offices on a regular basis. We solicit staff feedback and address their problems wherever possible. The working conditions of interns have been a specific area of concern and I am pleased that we have made changes to ensure their improvement.

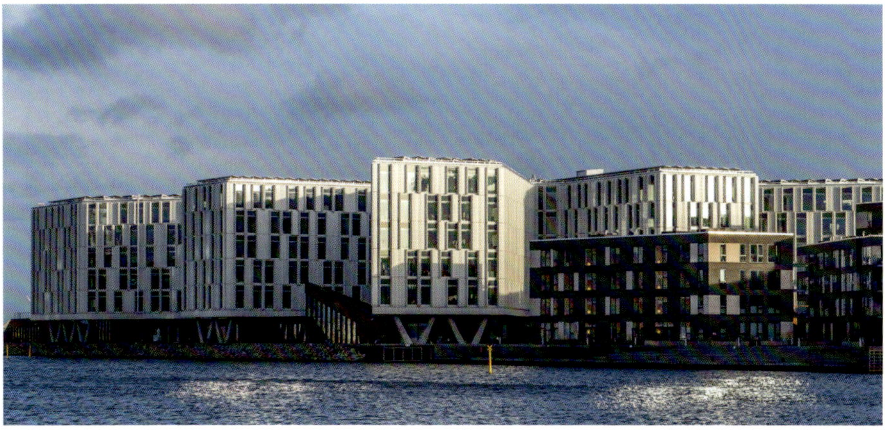

Exterior view of UN City, Copenhagen, Denmark. © WHO/Daniel Urrutia

8.2 Internalizing Health 2020

All the work of the Office has been organized around Health 2020 principles and approaches. Staff have been challenged to move out from their individual technical areas and find ways to reframe their work and vision to embrace the new integrated, intersectoral approaches necessary to implement Health 2020.

Don't just go through the motions

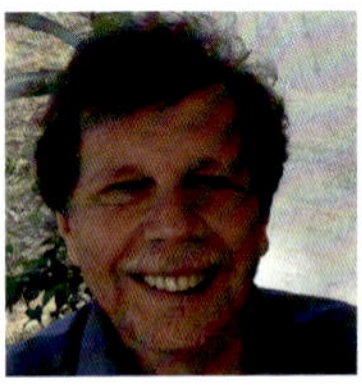

There is a misconception that everything and everyone within an organization as vast and diverse and unique as WHO, which speaks with one voice to the outside world, think and breathe in the same way. That is not true, at all. There is great diversity in the way attitudes and perspectives are expressed within WHO, and this becomes evident in various aspects of its work, much like in any other organization.

So, it was also important to get the house on board with Health 2020; to be able to get the house to support this process, not only to go through the various motions and then forget about it, but to really engage and commit to making this the main framework for the work of the whole Office. This required a strong determined politically savvy and astute leader which we had de facto with Zsuzsanna!

Agis Tsouros, Former Director, Policy and Governance for Health and Well-being, WHO Regional Office for Europe

Much progress has been made in what is an ongoing learning process. Health 2020 united the staff of the Regional Office and strengthened their effectiveness and pride in their work. It gave public expression and recognition to our vision and values, both externally and to the staff entrusted to carry out and champion its messages. It helped staff deal with the increasingly complex environment within which we work, and created an action platform for integrated working on all levels, with all sectors and with our many partners and networks.

Health 2020 also helped staff to work in closer partnership with WHO at the global level, and other UN agencies on regional levels, as well as the European Union and other public health actors.

If you think it is going to work, try it out

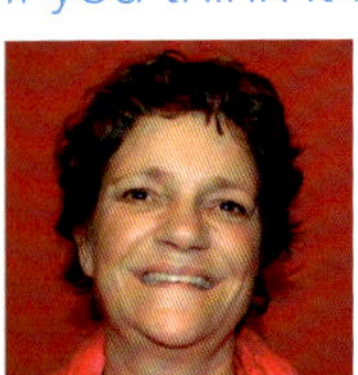

I believe the changes in relations between the WHO Regional Office for Europe and NGOs is very much down to the openness to collaborate from the highest level of management at the Regional Office. For instance, the Coalition of Partners, initiated by the Health Systems Division of the Regional Office, was a very open-minded and novel approach to working with multiple partners looking at how best to reach continued results. I think that this open-mindedness and willingness to try out new ways of engaging all actors is not just appreciated by the NGOs, but also by the Member States. Basically, I see that they have created an organization that is very open to innovation, partnerships, and initiatives that will help their Member States implement agreed strategies to improve health and well-being in Europe.

Dineke Zeegers, Director, European Public Health Association (EUPHA), Netherlands

8.3 Sustainable financing

Improving technical work without strong, enabling support functions is not possible. The proportion of administrative expenditure and the fixed component had previously been relatively high in the Regional Office for Europe, due to what has been an historically relatively small budget, and the demands of many languages, 53 Member States and 29 country offices. At the start of my tenure as Regional Director in 2010, administrative expenditure took up more than half the available corporate resources. This left little room for strengthening technical areas which do not receive funding from voluntary contributions.

We therefore decided to reallocate resources to technical areas and introduce efficiency measures to reduce the administrative burden in the Office. In this way we managed to establish a more sustainable path for the Regional Office. The goal remains to further consolidate administrative functions and improve efficiencies. We have also worked hard on fundraising to enhance support for our technical programmes (see Developmental reflection 4).

Developmental reflection 4
Donor relations and fundraising

We have changed our resource mobilization approaches over the last ten years. First, we established a team that is really focusing on it, along with partnerships, based in my office. Our basic approach was to see donors in the first instance as partners rather than just as those who give us money. In line with global approaches we work hard to establish some sort of proper partnerships and relationships with all our donors.

For example, the European Commission which is one of our very important partners is also one of our largest donors in Europe. We understand that being a trustworthy technical and political partner is an appropriate prerequisite to raising or mobilizing resources from the Commission.

So, a lot of the money we have been receiving in the last couple of years has been based on the political agreements and the joint declarations we have with different agencies. They actually provide us with funding to address some of the priority areas identified in our joint declarations.

This strategy has worked well and has helped support our technical work programmes on Regional and country levels.

The work of the European Region makes a significant contribution to WHO's global activities and achievements. The Regional Programme Budget (RPB) specifies the Region's contribution to the global Programme Budget (PB) results, notably through the Regional programmatic outputs by category and programme area. As an illustration, the RPB for 2016–2017 formed a contract for the joint accountability of the Regional Office and Member States for the delivery of PB results.

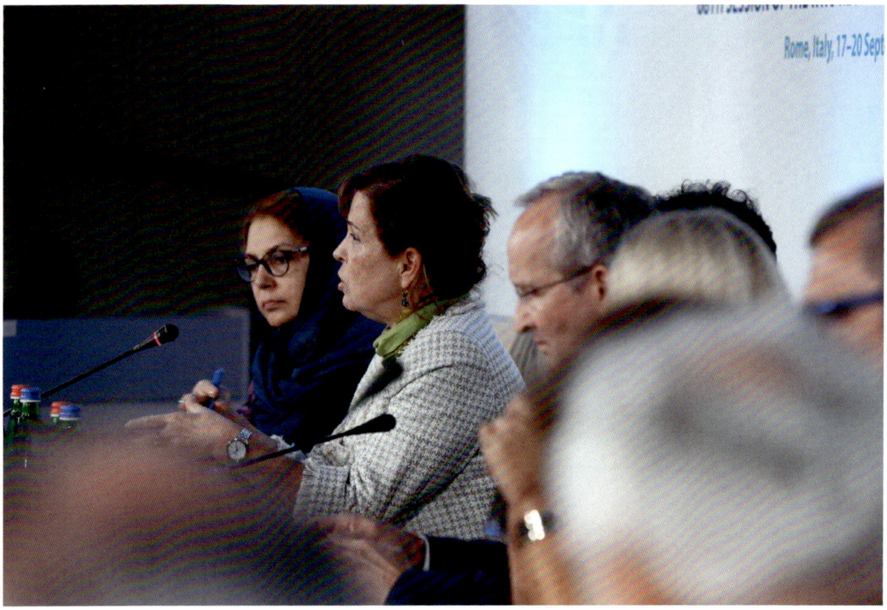

Nedret Emiroglu, Director of Division of Health Emergencies and Communicable Diseases and Director of Programme Management and Sussan Bassiri, Director of the Division of Administration and Finance for the WHO Regional Office for Europe, leading a discussion on the WHO programme budget for 2020–2021 at the 68th session of the WHO Regional Committee for Europe, Rome, Italy, 17–20 September 2018. © WHO/Franz Henriksen

Summary reflection

Creating a positive working environment

Message 7: Invest in people

We have invested a lot in promoting the Regional Office as an organization with a positive working environment and ensuring that we have sustainable funding for our work. We have learned a lot from the feedback of our staff and others whose lives have been influenced by work with the European Office.

The Office has been transformed through various initiatives taken over the last ten years, including:

- developing and implementing the Health 2020 common policy framework;
- strengthening our country offices with internationally appointed WHO Representatives working collaboratively within United Nations Country Teams;
- raising morale through positive engagement with all Member States;
- establishing the Regional Office as an important 'go to' centre of excellence in public health in Europe, including the creation of a new 'vision for public health for the 21st century' agreed by the Regional Committee in 2018;
- securing funding;
- improving internal management and financial procedures and accountabilities; and,
- motivating and retaining staff.

We have also put a lot of energy into gender balancing our staff, our intern programmes and in recruiting younger and highly motivated staff who can lead the Organization into the future.

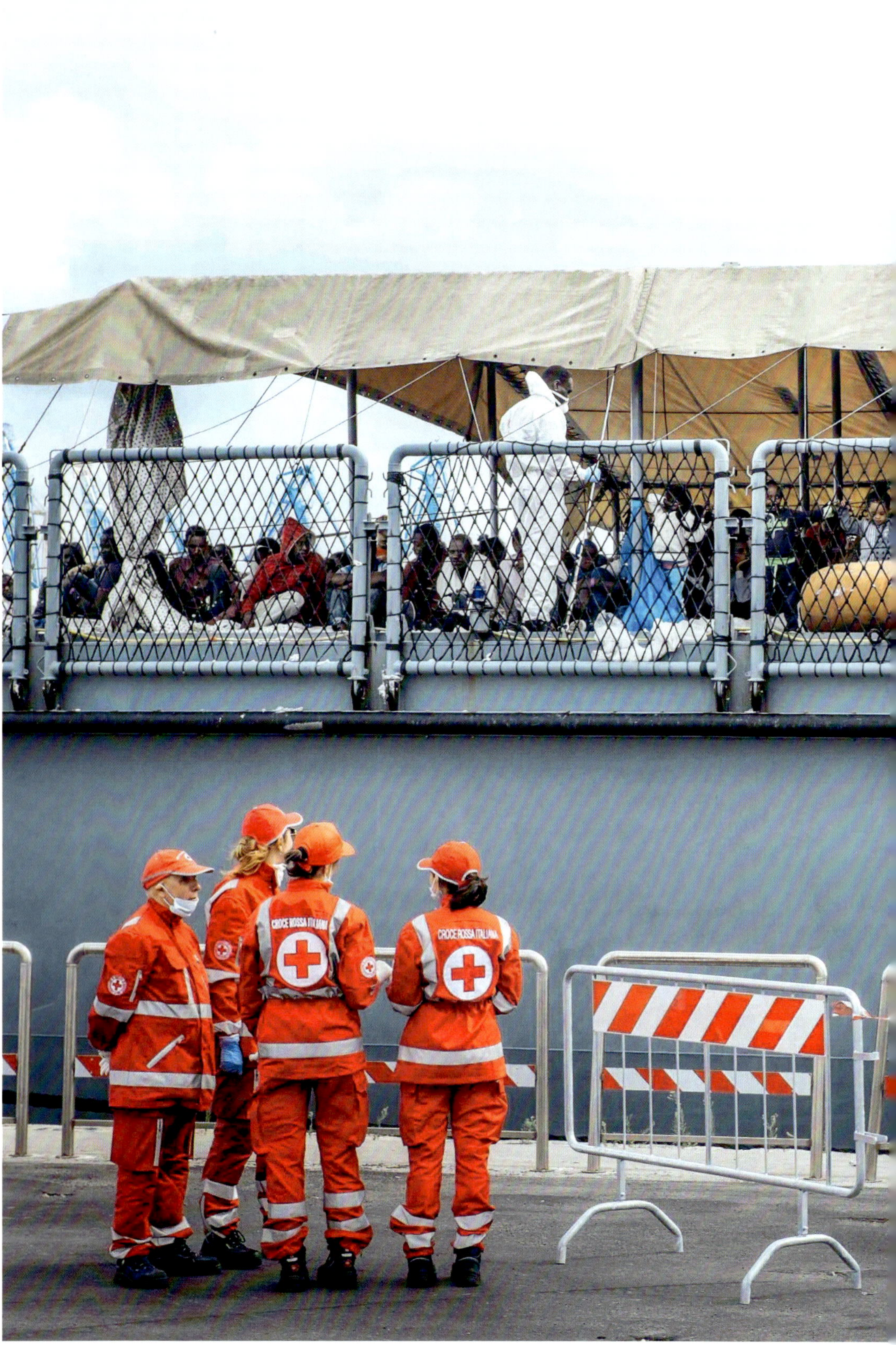
CROCE ROSSA ITALIANA
CROCE ROSSA ITALIANA

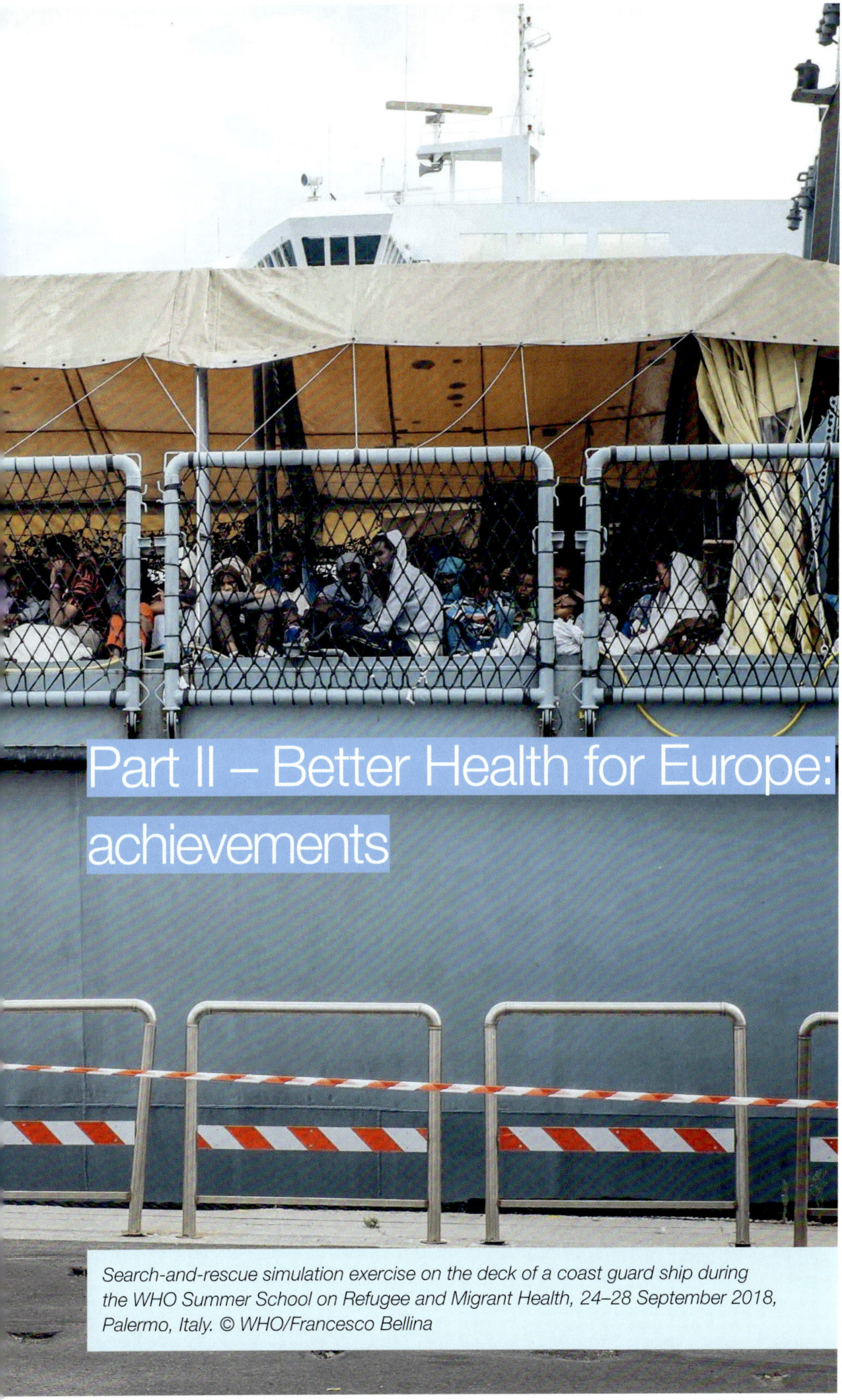

Part II – Better Health for Europe: achievements

Search-and-rescue simulation exercise on the deck of a coast guard ship during the WHO Summer School on Refugee and Migrant Health, 24–28 September 2018, Palermo, Italy. © WHO/Francesco Bellina

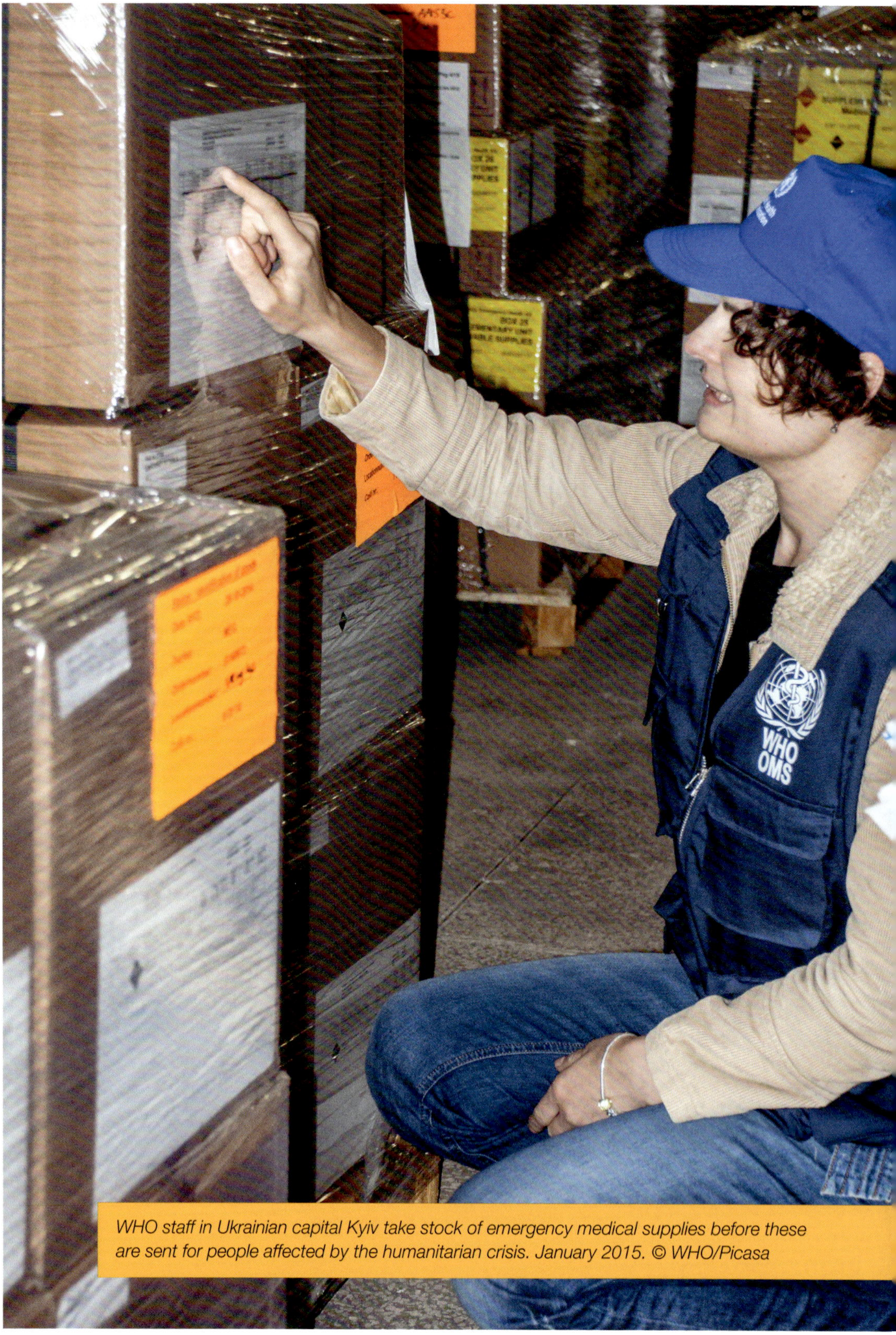

WHO staff in Ukrainian capital Kyiv take stock of emergency medical supplies before these are sent for people affected by the humanitarian crisis. January 2015. © WHO/Picasa

9. Health 2020 – Addressing objectives and priority health areas

In 2012, Member States were requested to develop and update their health policies, strategies and action plans, considering the Health 2020 policy framework, and their own circumstances and priorities. They were also asked to support Health 2020 through international health activities, through partnerships and intersectoral collaboration at the national level. Another request was to contribute to data-gathering processes that would permit the monitoring of progress. As countries started to take action and respond to these requests, the Regional Office began to systematically develop both quantitative and qualitative measurement and reporting strategies.

By adopting Health 2020, Member States explicitly put the core values of fairness, sustainability, quality, transparency, accountability, gender equality, dignity and the right to participate in decision-making at the centre of public health policy-making in the WHO European Region. As I have indicated, these commitments anticipated the value-base of the United Nations 2030 Agenda for Sustainable Development and the SDGs.

Subsequently all of the technical work of the Regional Office has been reframed around Health 2020 and its two objectives and four priority action areas (see Box 4). In this section, I will look sequentially at each of the objectives and priority action areas and reflect on achievements in the various areas. We have achieved a lot.

9.1 Objective 1 – Improving health for all and reducing the health divide

Health and well-being are public goods and assets for human development and of vital concern to the lives of every person, family and community. Pursuing health equity means minimizing inequities in health and in the key determinants of health. Inequities in health are systematic inequalities that should be considered as unfair or unjust and that could be avoided by reasonable means.

As we have seen overall across the Region, whilst health has improved and the range between the highest and lowest levels of health measured by life expectancy and infant mortality rates has narrowed, absolute differences between and within countries remain substantial. Resolving these health inequities is a priority both at human and policy levels.

Health 2020 and the pursuit of health equity have provided the basis of many national seminars and dialogues involving policy sectors across governments. National reviews of the social determinants of health and health inequity have also taken place. The findings from such national reviews have been used to develop stronger cross-sectoral policies and commitments, programmes of health reform and systems strengthening, as well as updating of public health programmes and partnerships.

Environmental equity focus

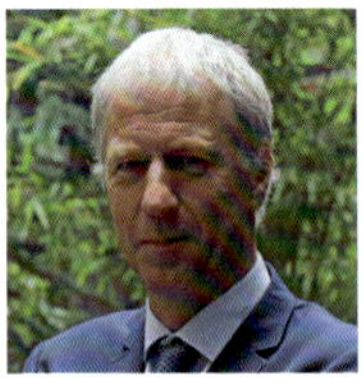

A new domain of work for us is the link between environmental exposures and the socioeconomic status of citizens. We are also looking at demographic issues related to younger and older people and making links to vulnerability. Our latest report on the inequalities of exposure to environmental hazards made a clear link with WHO methodologies and work. This report has been recognized as an agenda-setting piece of work.

Hans Bruyninckx, Executive Director, European Environment Agency (EEA)

The Office has developed, tested and made available a methodology on how to strengthen gender and human rights components in health policy dialogues. We have designed capacity-building courses that include multi-country workshops and e-learning programmes on equity in health in all policies to be rolled out on an ongoing basis.

Addressing inequalities– Ensuring rights of women and children

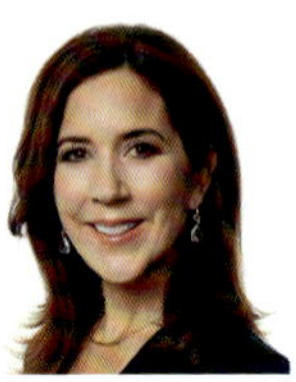

© Daniel Stjerne

It is my hope that through a better understanding of how inequalities affect the health of women and children and how we can minimize those inequalities, that we can ensure the rights of women and children are protected and respected. Understanding is the first step to creating real and sustainable change.

HRH Crown Princess Mary, Patron of WHO/Regional Office for Europe

In 2018 we launched a Health Equity Status Report initiative (HESRi) to support countries, partners and WHO to act to strengthen the equity impact of health sector and cross-sectoral policies and services *(126)*. The results of this initiative to date have been quite remarkable (see Developmental reflection 5).

Developmental reflection 5
Health Equity Status Report initiative (HESRi)
Health Equity Policy Tool

The Health Equity Status Report initiative (HESRi) was developed to provide a suite of tools that would accelerate action on health equity within all countries throughout the Region. It has brought forward innovations in the analysis of the relationships between health status and the security and quality of five conditions which are essential for every child or adult to live a healthy life in Europe in the 21st Century. These conditions include health services, income security and social protection, living conditions, social and human capital and working conditions. Never before have we had such a clear picture of the factors that drive and compound health inequities in our societies or about the incentives, policy options, and solutions that can deliver positive changes. The HESRi suite of tools can be tailored to differing country needs and reflected our prime aim to help ensure that health equity becomes a priority for policy development and implementation within all countries and partners of the WHO European Region.

We formed a new multidisciplinary Scientific Advisory Expert Group (SAGE) consisting of 30 leading international experts from institutions which are collaborating with WHO and our Venice GDO – the WHO European Office for Investment for Health and Development, who have led the initiative. We asked them to help us develop new metrics and evidence-informed solutions to reduce inequities in health. The SAGE group has been very productive. One of their first products was an interactive Health Equity Atlas. This is a comprehensive new data set covering the status and trends in health equity and underlying determinants over the last 10 years *(127)* and the progress made to implement a range of policies with a strong effect on reducing inequities.

The findings and analyses from the Health Equity Atlas have been presented widely in many country meetings and policy dialogues. With this new and innovative data, countries can get important insights into the relative influence of different determinants in explaining their current status in inequities in health. Several countries have been inspired to embark upon their own national health equity status reports. Building on their analyses of data and country-based feedback, the SAGE group and Venice GDO have developed a complimentary suite of policy and intervention tools. The European Health Equity Policy Tool, for example, identifies 51 effective measures for reducing health inequities. The HESRi has helped to reframe the prevailing mindset on health inequity as a wicked problem, that cannot easily be addressed, to a we-can-do/we-must-do investment for a healthy and prosperous society. Policy-makers are already starting to use the tool in priority setting and resource allocation decisions to identify where they can have greater impact for health equity through interventions in the health sector and with other sectors across government.

A high-level Regional conference on solutions to move forward equity in health – 'Accelerating Progress Towards Healthy and Prosperous Lives for all in the WHO European Region' –which took place in Slovenia 11–13 June 2019, was a landmark event *(128)*. A wealth of evidence-informed material, including our new *Health Equity Policy Tool,* was shared on ways to achieve the right conditions, accelerate progress and influence other sectors so that more people can prosper and flourish *(129)*.

On the panel discussing influence, for example, speakers representing justice advocacy organizations, nongovernmental organizations, governments, international banks and employee-owned businesses in the private sector called on delegates to reach out to unlikely partners – such as lawyers, academics, regional politicians, small businesses and ministries of employment – to seek dynamic alliances, work outside their comfort zones, speak the language of other sectors, tell a good story and dare to ask challenging questions to those driving the economic discourse.

Member States agreed to and expressed their strong support for the Ljubljana Statement on Health Equity which calls for the establishment of a multidisciplinary health equity alliance of scientific experts and institutions. The alliance will generate cutting-edge evidence and methods for ministries of health and governments to make the case for, prioritize and scale up scientific, technological, social, business or financial innovations that will support systematic and effective action for health equity. This will enable champions of health equity to align with other equity agendas, nurture honest dialogue and innovations, and build a common path for sustainable change. The Ljubljana Statement will be brought as a resolution to the 69th session of the WHO Regional Committee for Europe in Copenhagen, Denmark, in September 2019.

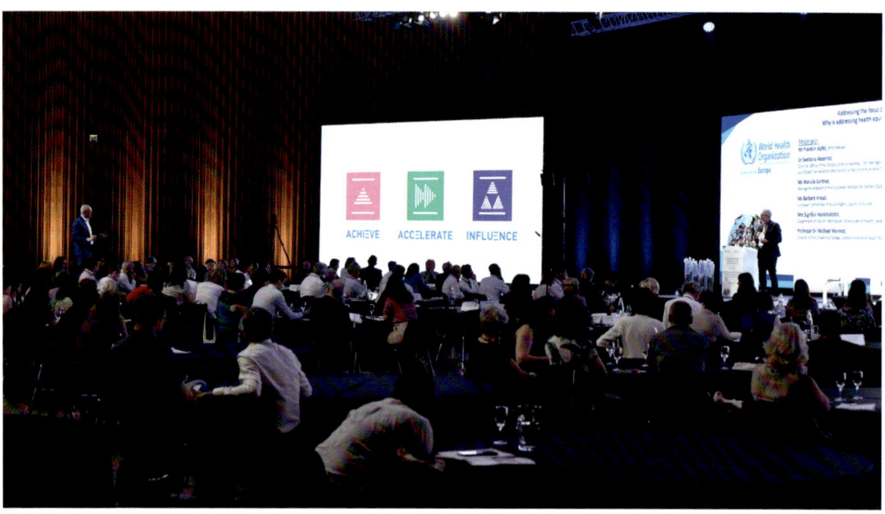

Opening plenary, High-level Conference on Health Equity, Ljubljana, Slovenia, 11–13 June 2019. ©Tamino Petelinsek/STA

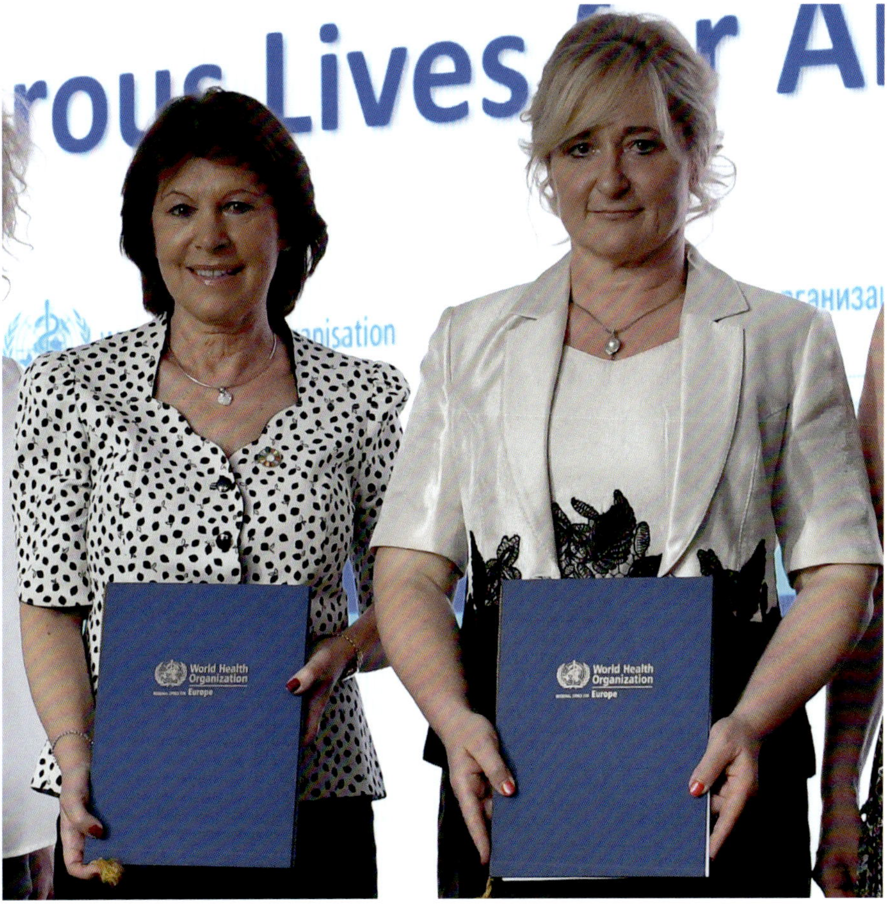

Piroska Östlin, Acting WHO Regional Director for Europe, and Simona Repar Bornšek, State Secretary for Health and Chief Physician, Slovenia, welcomed the approval of the Ljubljana Statement at the High-level Conference on Health Equity, Ljubljana, Slovenia, 11–13 June 2019. © Tamino Petelinsek/STA

PART 2

9.2 Objective 2 – Strengthen leadership and participatory governance for health

9.2.1 Leadership

Political, administrative, professional and technical leadership is crucial to promote health and well-being, and to support public health officials, workers and advocates to achieve the new skills and capacities needed to respond to today's changing complexities and challenges. Such leadership needs to support national, regional and global dialogues on societal values and goals, of which health and well-being are essential components.

In facilitating such universal ownership of the health agenda, we recognize that health needs must be expressed at the highest level of presidents and prime ministers, as well as ministers of health. Commitment to the implementation of the SDGs at the very highest levels of Government, can act as a catalyst for the promotion of health and well-being as a societal goal.

Health 2020 and its governance studies identified the leadership capacities and skills needed. These include adopting an extended understanding of health that deals with all determinants; looking outwards towards other sectors as well as inwards; abandoning linear thinking; and accepting the unpredictability and uncertainty of complexity. It requires leaders who can build trustworthy health policies and institutions that reflect better use of foresight; multi-stakeholder deliberation; the development of self-organizing networks and decentralized decision-making; and continual learning to manage risks and create more enduring policies.

All this is encouraging. Yet I must say clearly that these leadership qualities necessary to promote and develop national health policies which are multisectoral, and based upon whole-of-government, whole-of-society and health-in-all-policies approaches, are easy to describe, but difficult to acquire and deliver. Leadership for health and well-being requires new skills, recognizing the increasing global emphasis of health as a core component of development, and as an important dimension of global security, economic, environmental and trade discussions. Those concerned with promoting health need to understand and be able to operate convincingly in these areas.

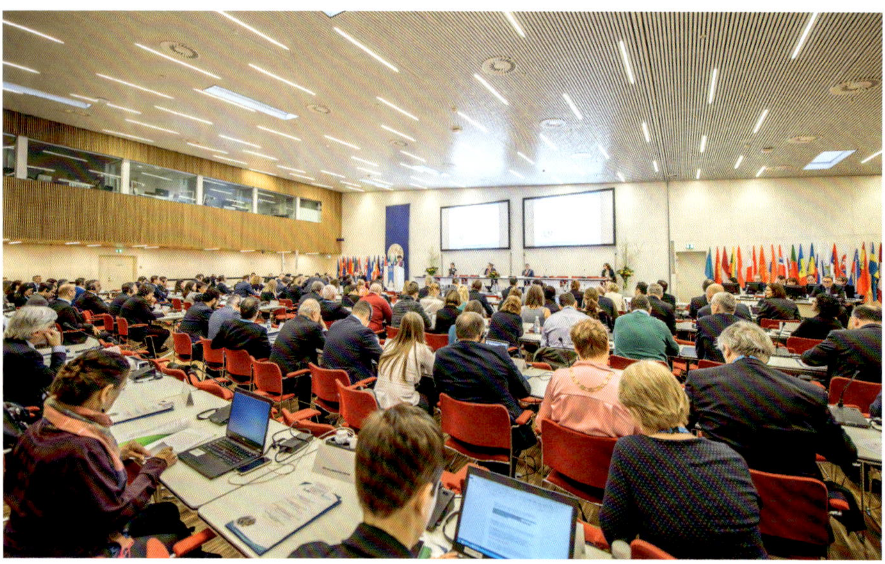

WHO European Healthy Cities Network Summit of Mayors, 12–13 February 2018, Copenhagen, Denmark ©WHO/Daniel Urrutia

Leadership characteristics

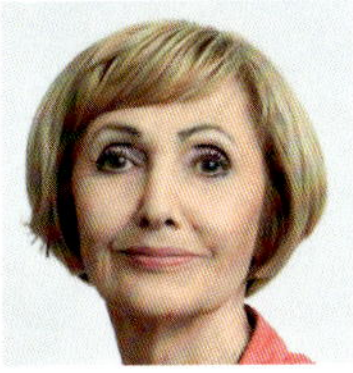

First of all, you have to be professional and a trustworthy person working for the benefit of the whole population and not having any private interests. Then, it is useful if you have professional experience in different fields.

I am lucky because I worked as a State Secretary at the Ministry of Finance for ten years. Thus, I was very familiar with public finances, which was a big advantage in health budget negotiations with both the finance minister and other ministers. The support of a prime minister is also crucial in the process and good professional staff as well.

I also worked in the insurance industry for fifteen years. A mixture of such work experience is a good basis not only for thinking strategically but also for understanding needs related to work on the operational level.

Having a good goal-oriented systematic and analytical approach is necessary but not sufficient. You also need to be persistent. When I felt that an initiative was absolutely right for the people of Slovenia I did everything to make it happen. When I did not have enough support at the beginning I presented additional evidence to achieve the goal or to find a compromise.

And last but not least, I would like to emphasize the importance of preserving a public health care system in order to ensure access to high-quality and sustainable health care for all.

Milojka Kolar-Celarc, Former Minister of Health, Slovenia

To enhance staff capacities in these areas we worked with the Graduate Institute of Geneva in conducting training in global health and health diplomacy *(131)*.

Diplomacy is about influencing power

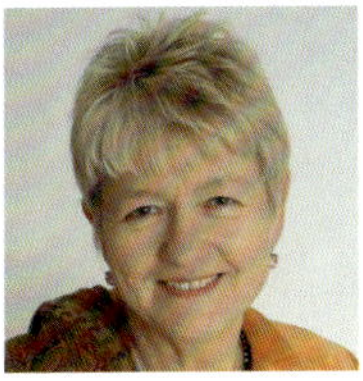

How do you get a governance decision? That is the key challenge of health diplomacy. How was the FCTC negotiated? How did the WHO AMR resolution come about?

The Regional Office understood very quickly that 21st century governance requires new public health skills and competencies including diplomatic negotiating skills. Everybody dealing with health decision-making needs to have them. It is not only about negotiating high-level resolutions or frameworks, but also building a capacity to influence decision-making in their everyday work. WHO staff, especially country-based WRs, for example, need these skills to be bridge-builders and relationship developers with the forces of power within their countries, with donors and other agencies (even within the UN system).

To address this need, we developed with the Regional Office a whole series of global health diplomacy training initiatives for country office staff that brought people together in a variety of ways, with country representatives. As a good technical person, you do not necessarily learn negotiation skills. You learn how to be a content expert but not necessarily how to explain to a minister in ways they can understand and be persuaded, for example, why a sugar tax might be important. We helped staff better understand how they can play a more active role in a political process, for example, that leads to a sugar tax. And how that requires diplomacy skills. This is different from the advocacy civil society organizations might be doing to influence a government.

Diplomacy is always about processes of power and how you deal with them, negotiate with them and how you manage to influence them.

One of the nicest things that happened was that we did two or three trainings with the SEEHN that actually led to them preparing for Regional Committees together. Now you get joint statements by the SEEHN.

Ilona Kickbusch, Director of the Global Health Centre, The Graduate Institute Geneva, Switzerland

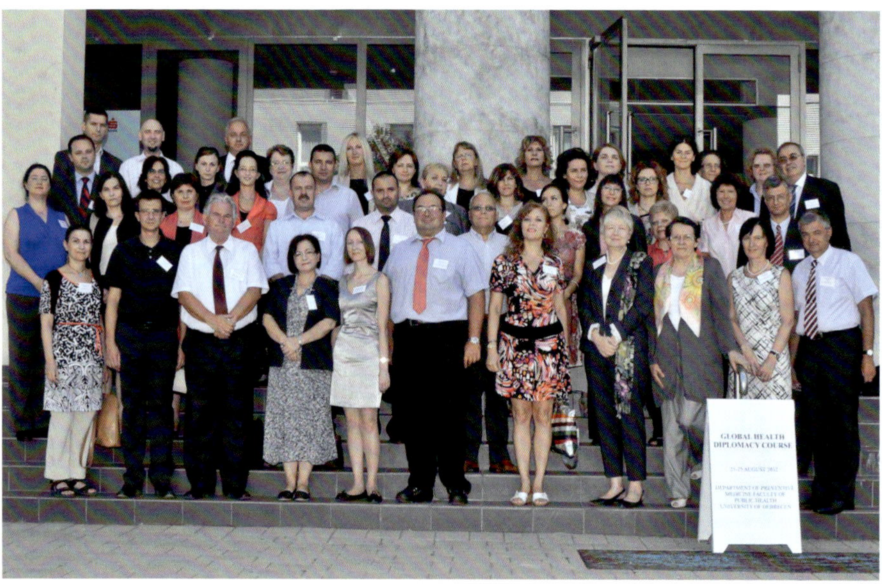

Health Diplomacy Executive Course for the SEEHN countries in Debrecen, Hungary, 2012. © WHO

9.2.2 Governance

We knew from our research that the biggest challenges in public health cannot be solved without improving and strengthening governance. In 2012 WHO European Member States recognized this by ensuring that governance for health and well-being became a cornerstone of Health 2020 *(83)*.

Our understanding of the term 'governance' is that it describes systems, including structures and processes, which shape the overall direction of policy or strategy, as well as provide supervision and accountability for development and implementation. Good governance for health is based on a values framework that includes health as a human right and a global public good, and as a core component of well-being.

In 2012 when Health 2020 was adopted, governance structures across the Region still mainly focused on health care services and were inadequate to rise to the challenge of addressing the wider determinants of health, as well as the reduction of health inequalities. So, we needed to identify ways to help people reframe the way they thought about health development and shift their thinking to a different model which gave emphasis and priority to improving health and well-being and to reducing health inequities. Health needed to move out of a model narrowly confined to, and based on, health care alone. It needed a broader perspective which better reflected stewardship for health and health improvement as a public priority and as a measure of good governance, dealt with all determinants, focused on health as an investment rather than a cost, and on health improvement as a measure of a good society.

Our research showed that the necessary governance structures to achieve these goals are horizontal, networked and collaborative. Such structures enable managing, coordinating, and supporting the implementation of action for health and well-being between diverse actors across all levels of government and beyond. Our research also showed that these structures should demonstrate transparency, accountability, participation, integrity, policy coherence and capacity *(32, 83)*.

These are complex ideas. To give these ideas substance following the adoption of Health 2020 by the European Regional Committee in 2012, WHO European Member States in 2015 adopted a decision on *Promoting intersectoral action for health and well-being in the WHO European Region: health is a political choice (58)*. This built upon the governance for health work led by Ilona Kickbusch during the development of Health 2020 and called for a new approach to governance for health and well-being, as central to the call for transformative change within the United Nations 2030 Agenda for Sustainable Development.

To take this work forward we undertook several actions, including the development of the *Assessment tool for governance for health and well-being (133)*. This tool helped countries assess their capacity to design, coordinate and implement different governance approaches for improved health and well-being. It is supported by the *Tool for mapping governance for health and well-being: the organigraph method* the first WHO tool of its kind allowing mapping of accountability and governance for health and well-being *(134)*.

Helping to shape new thinking

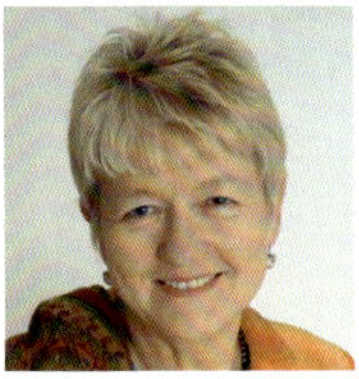

Importantly, the research we published was not a sort of "I read this, I do this" thing, but rather it was aimed more at helping people rethink the way they understood governance. And we mustn't forget that ten years ago the word 'governance' was not even used, it was considered by many as too complicated a concept. Now we use it as a 'matter of fact'.

By asking us to do this research, the Regional Office was quite innovative and contributed significantly to legitimising the new kind of thinking the term and concept of governance for health requires. We tend to forget how much changes within ten years, because we are part of the change. So many things to which we say "Oh yeah, sure" today, were quite innovative at that time.

The two publications were the result of a co-production process that involved a wide group of experts. The first was about how we understand the key challenges for governance and what the action principles of 'smart' governance are. The second focused on concrete examples of how countries did this thing, to show how countries were really working in a new way.

These publications were ahead of their time. They were never about "Oops, we are implementing this tomorrow," but they really were meant to be a catalyst to help shape thinking, so that when the right time comes you can use it.

Of course, there is a long history of that in public health development. It started with our new concepts of health promotion (Ottawa Charter), continued in the development of the settings approach (e.g. WHO Healthy Cities Network) and Health for All policies. All these started in the WHO Regional Office for Europe and then influenced WHO Headquarters. These things do not come out of the blue.

Ilona Kickbusch, Director of the Global Health Centre, The Graduate Institute Geneva, Switzerland

A 2018 review, *Multisectoral and intersectoral action for improved health and well-being for all: mapping of the WHO European Region,* considered how far we had come in achieving the multisectoral and intersectoral action for health and well-being that was needed *(135)*. The review identified regional, national and local case studies of multisectoral governance action that were influencing mainstream thinking. Key conclusions pointed to the need for high-level political support, training and skills development, including health diplomacy.

9.3 Technical work in the four action areas of Health 2020

Since 2012, the Health 2020 policy framework has provided an intellectual and policy template to guide Member States and other public health stakeholder action, and to monitor progress.

This process can be illustrated by considering some important areas of technical work in which the Office has been engaged. These are organized and presented here under the four priority action areas described in Health 2020:

1. Investing in health through a life-course approach and empowering people;
2. Tackling the Region's major health challenges;
3. Strengthening people-centred health systems, public health capacity and emergency preparedness, surveillance and response; and,
4. Creating resilient communities and supportive environments.

9.3.1 Investing in health through a life-course approach and empowering people

One of the most exciting areas of today's health science is our new understanding of the dynamic interactions between individuals' genetic make-up and all aspects of their environment over their life-course. This new knowledge has increased exponentially from a range of scientific disciplines: from genetics to epidemiology, from psychology to neuroscience, from economics to environmental, political and social sciences. The implications are potentially huge but cannot be accurately predicted. However, over the last decade we have learned enough to throw new light on strategic approaches to empowering people, promoting their health and improving their quality of life.

We now know that the trajectory of human life is affected by genetic, epigenetic and intrauterine legacies, by environmental exposures, by nurturing family and social relationships, by behavioural choices, and by social norms and opportunities carried into future generations, as well as by historical, cultural and structural contexts. Action is therefore needed across the life-course, from preconception, pregnancy, foetal development and on to the most vulnerable life stages.

Political, social, economic, gender and environmental factors drive women, men, and different social and ethnic groups to live inequitable lives. These factors differ within and between countries. Some people flourish across a long lifespan, while others die younger, suffering from diseases more frequently and earlier, with a childhood scarred by stress, neglect and abuse, having underachieved academically, affected by frequent periods of unemployment and separation, with inferior access to social support and to personal and collective coping mechanisms.

These diverse and inequitable trajectories are strongly influenced by policies, environments, opportunities and norms created by society, and for which society bears responsibility. Policy changes can create long-term sustainable opportunities for health for which governments at all levels and society bear responsibility, and on which they should act.

In 2015, as noted earlier, we convened a major international conference in Minsk, Belarus, to consider the life-course approach in the context of Health 2020. This resulted in the Minsk Declaration which set out strategies for countries to improve health and well-being across the life-course (see Box 10) *(65)*. One focus was the importance of life-course transitions, including early childhood, adolescence, adulthood, employment and unemployment status and ageing.

Amongst the many recommendations two policy areas are of particular note. The first is early childhood development where the interaction between genetic expression and the environment is at its most intense. The second is active labour market policies later in life to secure employment. Such approaches require integration between health and social welfare and close collaboration with education, social policy and employment sectors.

Let us look at two examples where application of life-course interventions in countries are leading to improved health.

9.3.1.1 Maternal and child health

The focus on preconception and conception interventions in Health 2020 such as, addressing nutritional conditions, tobacco use, genetic counselling, environmental circumstances, fertility issues, pregnancy timing, psychoactive drug use, vaccination, and violence, has produced results *(136)*. The average maternal mortality ratio in the WHO European Region has decreased. In addition, the introduction of modern, effective contraception and the promotion of sexuality education have contributed to the reduction of abortions in the WHO European Region.

Our work in this area has been amplified by our partnership with UNFPA. The Regional Committee in 2016 adopted a *WHO Regional strategy on sexual and reproductive health (137)* and a *Strategy on women's health and well-being in the WHO European Region (66)*. The Office has also supported Member States through implementation of *the Investing in children: the European child and adolescent health strategy 2015–2020 (72)*.

Partnership amplification of impact

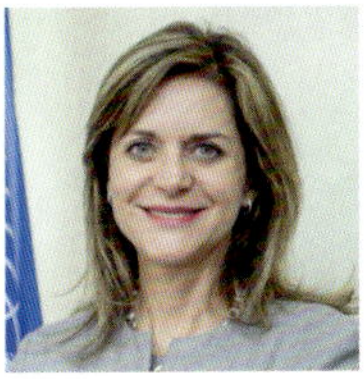

UNFPA and WHO worked very closely together on the development of the sexual and reproductive health action plan for Europe endorsed by the 66th session of the Regional Committee. UNFPA has country offices in most of the Member States, certainly in the Member States of eastern Europe and central Asia, so we utilize our technical experience at the country level. We have relatively large offices that are working directly with ministers of health, education, and women. Through these partnerships we really galvanized support for the sexual and reproductive health action plan, together with WHO. And together with WHO we have been involved in the development, in the approval, and now in the implementation, supporting Member States on designing and implementing national sexual and reproductive health action plans.

It is a very good example of the two organizations using their own areas of strength to come together to really push forward the agenda in the Region.

Alanna Armitage, Regional Director, The United Nations Population Fund (UNFPA) Eastern Europe and Central Asia

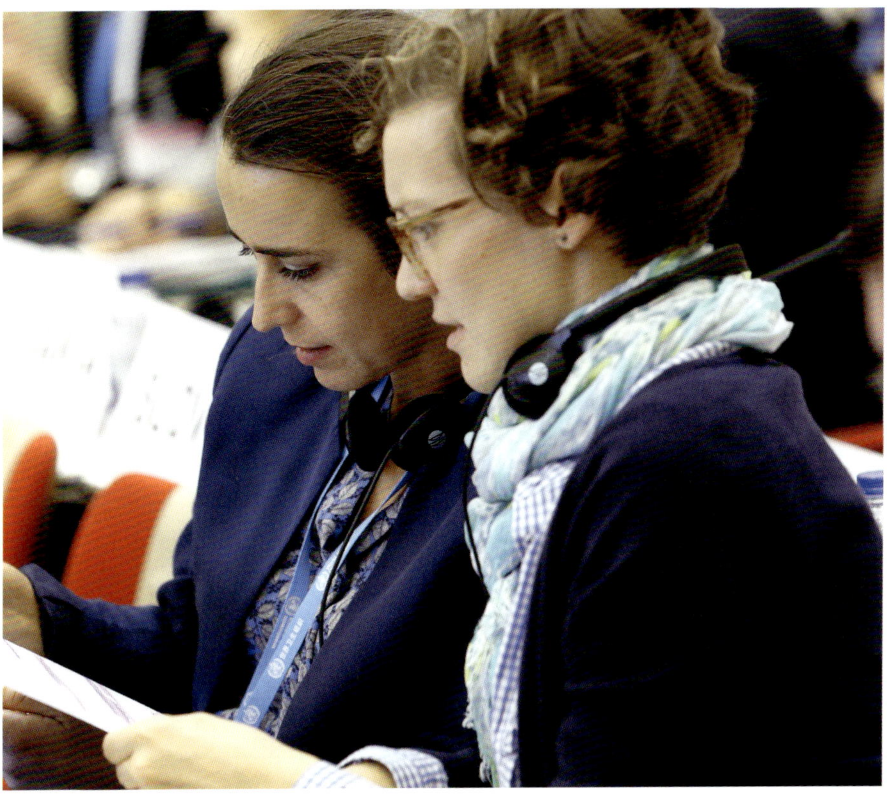

Delegates at the session on women's health during the 66th session of the WHO Regional Committee for Europe, Copenhagen, Denmark, 12–15 September 2016. © WHO/Franz Henriksen

Rapid intervention for women's health in Turkey

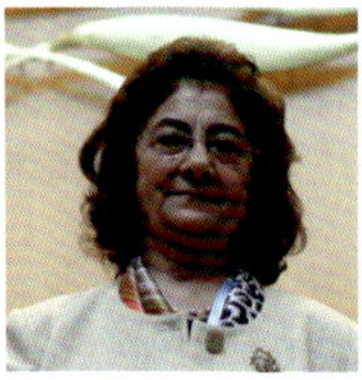

In Turkey, we passed a law in 1983, legalizing induced abortion up to 10 weeks on request. After its legalization maternal deaths due to unsafe abortion decreased markedly. However, 'abortion' is a sensitive issue, here as in many countries, and very often used or abused for political purposes. In 2012, there were strong, sudden and surprising moves made on the highest political to repeal or restrict our 1983 law. We were shocked and did not know what to do. We made every effort to stop what seemed like a strengthening political movement.

At that point the most influential interventions came from Dr Zsuzsanna Jakab. I will never forget her timely actions. I sent her an urgent email. She answered me immediately and at the same time she called our Minister of Health. Later she told me that she had a very long conversation on the phone about the ongoing events related to abortion in Turkey.

She also sent a group of experts to the Ministry of Health to help them tackle the issue. These timely interventions – the call and expert visit – solved our very important women's health issue in Turkey. Since then, so far no one has touched our 1983 law on family planning. I am very thankful to Dr Jakab and the WHO Regional Office.

Ayse Akin, Professor Public Health, Maternal and Child and Reproductive Health, Baskent University, Ankara, Turkey

Sexual and reproductive health

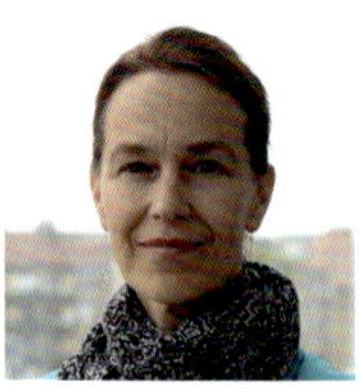

Reaching an agreement on the sexual and reproductive health action plan in the WHO European Region in 2016 was very gratifying. Not only for me personally, since I firmly believe that the right to health includes SRHR, but also for Sweden, since it resonates with the values of our feminist foreign policy and the work we do on a national level.

Ensuring that women and girls can enjoy their fundamental human rights is both an obligation and a prerequisite for reaching health, wealth and sustainable development – all of which the Europe of today is built on. I am proud that the WHO European region has demonstrated that health in all policies truly means all policies.

Olivia Wigzell, Director General, National Board for Health and Welfare, Sweden

Decreasing maternal and child mortality

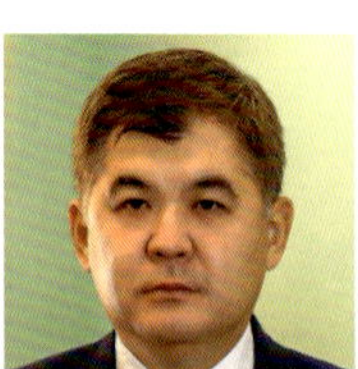

One of the critical improvements we have made over the last five years has been in the area of maternal and child health. With the help of WHO we redesigned the way we assess and treat patients and as a result, our medical statistics improved. These changes have led to a decrease in our country's maternal mortality and child mortality by more than two and half times during the last five years. The quality of our data on maternal and child mortality is now recognized by WHO and global society.

Yelzhan Birtanov, Minister of Healthcare, Kazakhstan

Another area of child health and welfare is the care and support for children with disabilities. Here, I feel a strong personal commitment. I am very pleased that the Regional Committee adopted the *Investing in children: the European child maltreatment prevention action plan 2015–2020. (73)*. This was based on a 2013 European report on preventing child maltreatment, as well as on the 2011 declaration *Better health, better lives: children and young people with intellectual disabilities and their families (140)*. In 2014, the Region also adopted: *Investing in children: the European child and adolescent health strategy 2015–2020 (72)*.

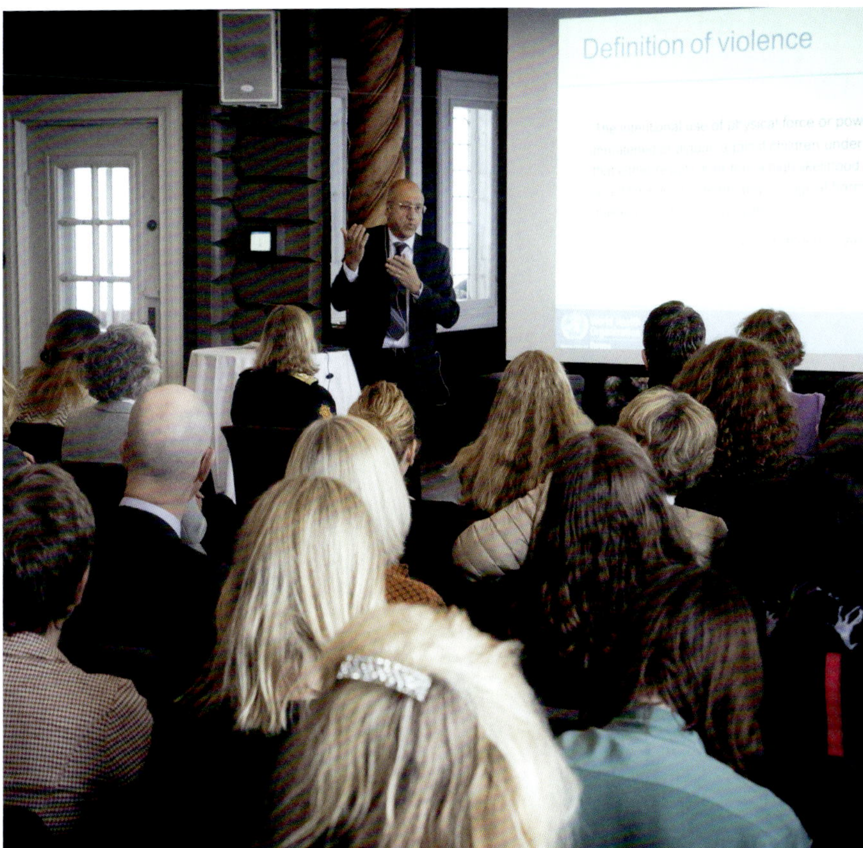

High-level meeting to stop violence against children, Oslo, Norway, 24 April 2017. © WHO

9.3.1.2 Ageing

Ageing has been another relatively neglected area, yet of increasing importance and prominence as our societies age. In 2011, we introduced a new cross-cutting programme on ageing, working with all technical units within the Regional Office on the innovative activities introduced in the *Strategy and action plan for healthy ageing in Europe, 2012–2020, (71)*. Here the Office worked closely with DG Employment, Social Affairs and Inclusion of the European Commission.

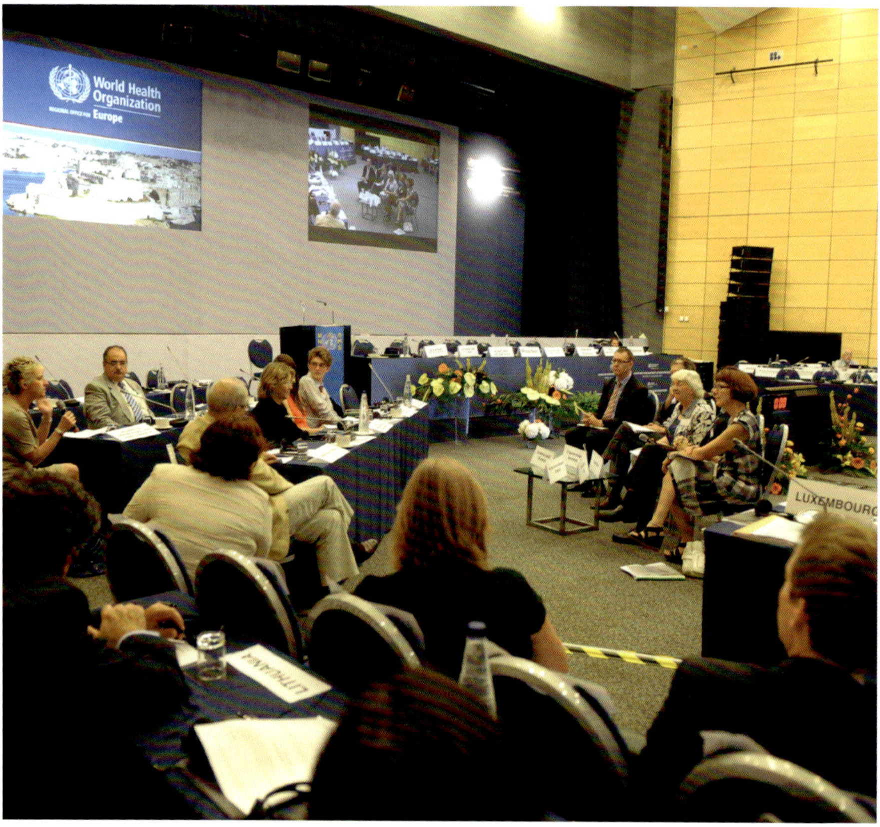

Experts discuss 'Strategy and action plan for healthy ageing in Europe 2012–2020' and challenges to health systems related to health promotion and prevention of age-related chronic diseases at the 62nd session of the Regional Committee for Europe, Malta, 10–13 September, 2012. © Martin Attard

The Office has made real progress. A mid-term review of the Global Strategy and Action Plan on Ageing and Health conducted in 2018 has confirmed that more than 30 countries in the European Region already have national aging and health strategies, policies or plans available *(141)*.

A practical example of progress is the publication of the Age-Friendly Environments in Europe Handbook and policy tool which has served as de facto standard for local policy-makers around the globe *(142)*. Working with the Healthy Ageing Task Force of the European Healthy Cities Network was crucial to this achievement, along with support from the WHO Global Network for Age-friendly Cities and Communities (GNAFCC) that now involves more than 20 countries in Europe and around 280 cities *(143)*.

Healthy Ageing Task Force

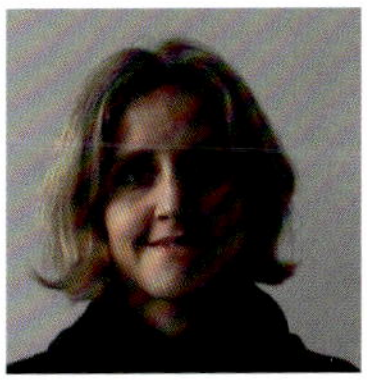

The WHO Healthy Cities Healthy Ageing Task Force was really very useful to us in setting priorities for our city. They helped us start our programmes by doing a profile on healthy ageing in Udine in 2008. This profile was drawn up according to WHO guidance which includes 21 demographic and social indicators, looking at issues ranging from where and how people live to the social determinants of their health *(144)*.

Based on the findings of these profiles we decided on priorities and developed specific programmes. Move Your Minds (MYM), for example, was one of these programmes because dementia is increasing. MYM aims to promote the cognitive process and to counteract loneliness and isolation among older people. This programme is carried out in all the districts of the city and in collaboration with many stakeholders in the city; for example, voluntary associations, toy and book libraries, music and theatre associations, among others. It is a strange collaboration because the partners do not actually get paid, except for a very symbolic amount, and they offer whatever they can do, in different fields – music therapy, yoga, anti-ageing games, writing, English, but not so much to learn the language as to play with it, cookery classes; all sorts of different kinds of activities.

Working with WHO helped us in three ways. First, was in the branding of programme. The WHO connection gives the programme brand scientific credibility. Second, the task force provided opportunities of really exchanging and sharing experiences. For example, we compared data from different cities and co-developed an evaluation and advocacy tool about the promotion of health for older people. Third, we got new ideas for programmes from the network. One of the themes was prevention of falls in homes. We discussed this with some experts during meetings of the Task Force and then we developed a programme.

Stefania Pascut, WHO Healthy Cities Network Coordinator, Udine, Italy

9.3.2 Tackling the European Region's major health challenges– NCDs

Premature death from or living long term with a NCD and its related disability has put an increasing strain on health systems, economic development and the well-being of large parts of our populations. Reduced income and early retirement caused by NCDs can lead individuals and households into poverty. At the societal level, in addition to surging health care costs, there are increased demands for social care and welfare support, as well as the burden of absenteeism from school or work, decreased productivity and increased employee turnover.

In September 2011, heads of state and government, assembled at the United Nations in New York, committed to address the global burden and threat of NCDs with the adoption of a wide-ranging political declaration on the prevention and control of NCDs at the opening of the General Assembly's first United Nations High-level Meeting on the Prevention and Control of NCDs *(153)*.

In July 2014, during the second United Nations High-level Meeting on NCDs, ministers and representatives of states and government and heads of delegations committed to the following four immediate domestic actions (also called the time-bound commitments): setting national NCD targets, developing multisectoral policies and plans, accelerating the reduction of risk factors, and strengthening health systems *(146)*. A third high-level meeting took place in September 2018 and reviewed the global and national progress achieved.

Discussions at the second and third high-level meetings built on guidance set out in the *Global action plan for the prevention and control of noncommunicable diseases 2013-2020 (130)* endorsed during the 66th WHO World Health Assembly in 2013.

The Political Declarations that came out of the high-level meetings highlighted the need for whole-of-government and a whole-of-society responses. At the level of the WHO European Region, these global commitments were followed by the adoption of the *Action plan for the prevention and control of NCDs in the WHO European Region 2016–2025* during the 66th session of the WHO Regional Committee for Europe in 2016 *(12)*.

The goal of the Action plan is to avoid premature death and avoidable mortality, and significantly reduce the disease burden from NCDs, by taking integrated action, improving the quality of life and making healthy life expectancy more equitable within and between Member States. It is fully aligned with Health 2020. It sets out the aspirational vision of a health-promoting European Region free of preventable NCDs, and builds on the relevant strategies and action plans for the underlying determinants.

Importantly while the risk factors for NCDs imply personal behaviours, national public policies in sectors such as trade, taxation, education, agriculture, urban development and food and pharmaceutical production have a major bearing on risk factors for NCDs at the population level. The broader social, economic and environmental determinants of health associated with globalization and urbanization, alongside population ageing, are the underlying drivers of the behavioural risk factors.

This Regional approach has been working. There are three important global targets for reductions in premature mortality and the European Region is likely to be the only WHO Region in which these targets will be met, or even exceeded *(145)*. Because of the rapid decline in premature deaths related to NCDs, the Region is likely to achieve SDG target 3.4, to reduce premature mortality from NCDs by one third earlier than the target date of 2030 and will probably exceed the 33.3% reduction significantly.

How have we succeeded in achieving this? We have intensified our efforts on moving 'upstream' towards health promotion and disease prevention. We have new initiatives on health literacy *(223)*. We have improved governance and have been strengthening comprehensive, integrated and people-centred health systems which are competent to prevent and manage NCDs. One of our highest priority has been addressing behavioural risk factors, particularly tobacco, alcohol, physical activity, nutrition including salt and sugar, as well as the social and environmental determinants. We have also aimed to reduce deaths and illnesses from environmental exposures such as air pollution, chemicals and climate change.

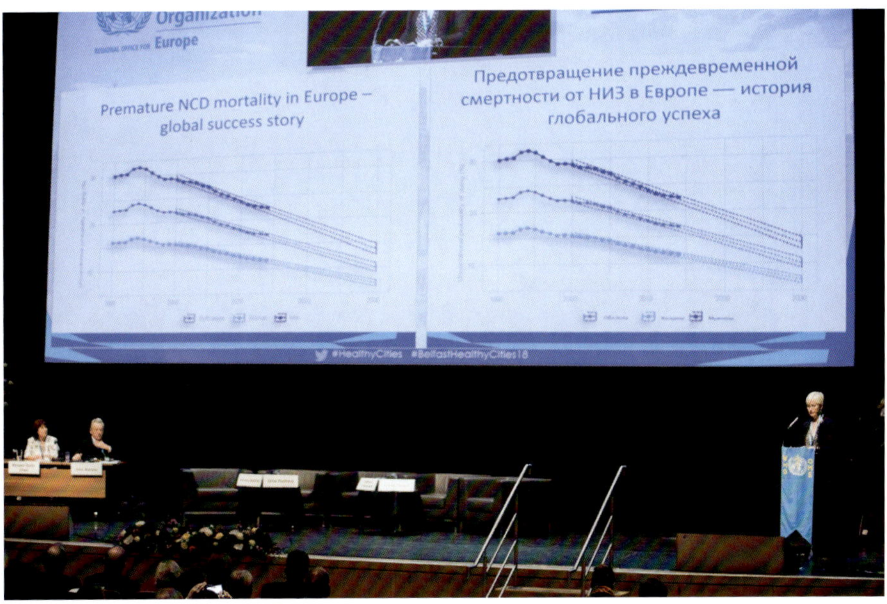

Bente Mikkelsen, Director, Division of Noncommunicable Diseases and Promoting Health through the Life-course, WHO Regional Office for Europe delivers her keynote presentation titled 'Time to deliver: How can WHO Healthy Cities be a vehicle to implement action to prevent and manage noncommunicable diseases and injuries over the life course' at the WHO International Healthy Cities Conference, 1–4 October 2018, Belfast, United Kingdom. © WHO

However, not all is good news. In the European Region tobacco use and alcohol consumption are declining too slowly, and the prevalence of overweight and obesity is rising rapidly. The targets in those areas are unlikely to be achieved. Unfortunately, robust assessment of progress with other important targets – such as salt reduction, physical activity and access to essential medicines and technologies – is currently not possible owing to limited comparable data.

Significant inequalities in premature mortality levels remain between and within countries and reveal strong gender inequity. Most premature deaths occur among men and are caused by cardiovascular diseases. Gender sensitive approaches and hypertension management in primary health care are two important areas of action to further accelerate the decline in premature mortality. Analyses indicate that eliminating excess male cardiovascular disease mortality would reduce absolute inequalities between countries by approximately 50% and contribute substantially to Health 2020 and SDG targets *(206)*. It is vital that governments act resolutely and implement the 'best buys' that have a rapid effect on mortality, such as controlling the price, availability and marketing of tobacco and alcohol *(146)*.

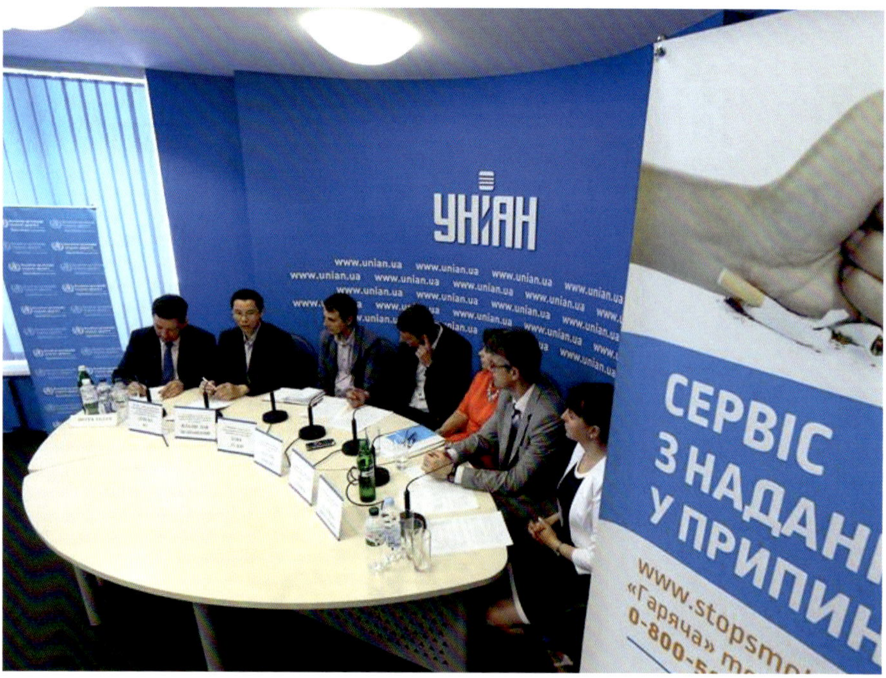

On 20 June 2017 WHO and partners presented a professional smoking cessation service aimed to support Ukrainians who suffer from tobacco dependence. © WHO

NCDs – policy dialogues

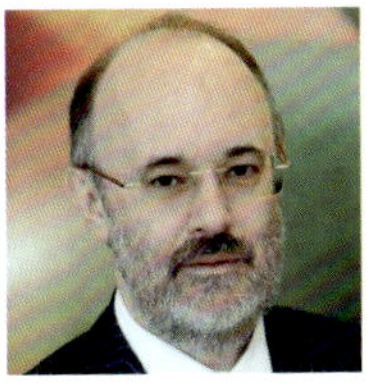

We invited WHO and the Observatory to facilitate our national internal discussions on NCDs. What the international discussions brought to this topic is that the health sector per se is much too small to solve the problem. They introduced the concept of Health in All Policies. Of course, that's very helpful, but if you think of the silos of the national government, it is very, very difficult to overcome the organizational structure of public services. We do not even talk in Regional Committees anymore about Health in All Policies because it is already such a standard, but if you come to my real world it is not a standard.

For those of us in the Ministry of Health, it is always good to have WHO as an ally – because they have the authority to say something that cannot be easily dismissed. We still respect multilateral organizations, and when they say something, we listen. Whether any action ever come of it is another question.

For our policy dialogues on NCDs, and with Health in All Policies, there are a lot of people you need to get into the room. It is complicated. You have to have the officials, the respected bureaucracies, the legal entities, the legal representatives of certain branches, and civil society. You have to bring them all, otherwise you are lost. You need good strong moderators to guide that process to get results. It makes the discussion easier if you have good moderators from outside who are not directly involved or do not have a particular vested interest.

We have good researchers, we have a good public health institute, but the prophet from one's own country is not always listened to. So, what do we do? We do not just invite experts to come in; we prepare the process very carefully. We tell all the experts provided by WHO very precisely what we want to achieve, so they can tailor the information they give. Otherwise they may come up with ideas that do not fit the Austrian reality for example. You have to invest time and effort; but it is time and effort worth spending. The dialogue, for example, helped us draft a strong Primary Health Care bill.

Clemens Martin Auer, Special Envoy for Health, Austria

Whilst our main policy for controlling and reducing the burden of death and ill-health from NCDs must be health promotion and disease prevention, and the effective integration of these approaches into primary care, we need also to give a high priority to the management of existing NCDs, for example by providing adequate population-based management of hypertension and diabetes in primary care, including strengthening health literacy.

We have been working with countries in a systematic way to both assess and strengthen health systems to achieve better NCD outcomes, since 2012. One of our key findings show that cost effective NCD interventions, on both individual and population levels, are not implemented in many Member States. In 2018 we took up this challenge at a High-level regional meeting – Health Systems Respond to

Experience in the European Region –16–18 April in Sitges, Spain. Here the aim was to strengthen health systems to accelerate progress in reducing premature mortality from NCDs, in order to achieve UHC and better NCD outcomes. We drew on the solid evidence accrued over many years working with Member States to articulate and demonstrate what a comprehensive and aligned health systems response to NCDs looks like (see Section 9.3.4.7 and Developmental reflection 8).

The Region has also been advocating for the WHO global STEP-wise approach to Surveillance (STEPS) *(147)*. This is a simple, standardized method for collecting, analyzing and disseminating data in WHO member countries. By using the same standardized questions and protocols, all countries can use STEPS information not only for monitoring within-country trends, but also for making comparisons across countries. The approach encourages the collection of small amounts of useful information on a regular and continuing basis.

Recognizing that strong leadership and urgent action are required at the global, regional and national levels, the WHO European Office for the Prevention and Control of NCDs was launched in Moscow in 2014, funded by a voluntary contribution from the Ministry of Health of the Russian Federation. This NCD Office has catalysed the ability of European and other countries to combat NCDs.

Russian global leadership in combating NCDs

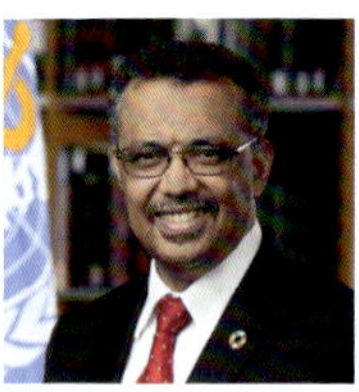

The first global ministerial conference on healthy lifestyles and NCDs control was held in Moscow in 2011 in preparation for the United Nations High-level meeting in New York. The conference had an incredible advocacy impact on Member States. Following this success the Russian Federation has continued its commitment to the fight against NCDs, as one of the countries most affected by premature mortality from NCDs, and has strengthened its engagement with WHO as a donor, at both global and regional levels, with the creation of the GDO on NCDs in Moscow serving all of the European Member States and other Regions.

Tedros Adhanom Ghebreyesus, WHO Director-General

The availability and affordability of essential medicines is also central to UHC and the implementation of the Global action plan for the prevention and control of NCDs 2013–2020. This set a target of ensuring "an 80% availability of the affordable … essential medicines … required to treat major noncommunicable diseases" *(130)*. However, it remains a sad reality that for the most vulnerable segments of the population, life-saving essential medicines may be impossible to afford.

For example, for several countries in the eastern part of the European Region, a one-month course of simple hypertension treatment can cost up to 35 days of wages, most of which is paid out of pocket. Here importantly the countries of the CIS strengthened their collaboration towards affordable medicines by agreeing to a development plan for the Pharmaceutical Pricing and Reimbursement Information (PPRI) network for the CIS *(148)*.

9.3.2.1 Tobacco

Smoking is the second leading risk factor for early death and disability worldwide. The cost to societies is enormous: in 2017 the US National Cancer Institute and WHO jointly estimated that tobacco use globally causes more than US$ 1.4 trillion annually in health care costs and lost productivity *(149)*.

Among WHO regions, Europe has the highest prevalence of tobacco smoking amongst adults, at 28%, and some of the highest prevalence of tobacco use by adolescents. WHO estimates that tobacco use is currently responsible for 16% of all deaths of adults over 30 in the Region *(150)*.

Examples are instructive concerning what works in tobacco control. Firstly, nearly all Member States of the European Region have become a party to the Framework Convention on Tobacco Control (FCTC). They are supported by the six MPOWER measures, which are aligned with the treaty and help countries reduce the demand for tobacco *(211)*. The MPOWER measures are high impact, yet also practical and low cost. Secondly the movement for plain packaging of tobacco products has taken a major boost globally through the leadership of European Member States, seven of whom now (at the time of writing) have legislation to this effect. Thirdly, some Member States are now moving towards becoming tobacco-free, with a smoking prevalence of 5% or less *(151,152)*.

Overall therefore, the European Region has seen positive progress. For example several Member States are moving towards becoming "tobacco free", with a smoking prevalence of 5% or less. If these advances continue and are replicated elsewhere, the Regional trend towards reduction in consumption of tobacco products could accelerate impressively *(150)*.

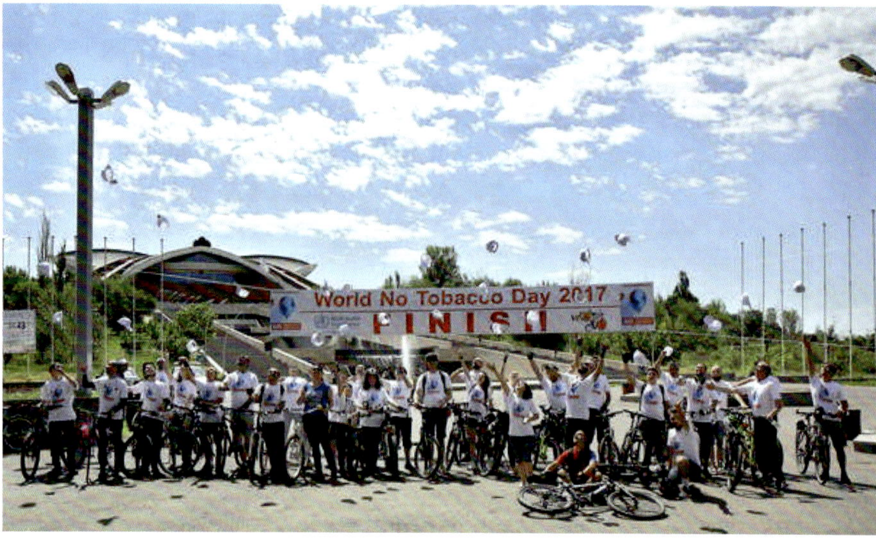

The WHO Country Office in Armenia organized a "Say NO Tobacco" cycling tour in Yerevan to show support for World No Tobacco Day, 31 May 2017. © WHO

Unfortunately, despite our successes tobacco usage in the Region is not reducing as quickly as it should in order to meet the globally agreed targets. Tobacco products are still far too affordable in many countries. Increasing taxation on tobacco products to raise retail prices is the most effective and efficient method to reduce tobacco use as well as a primary engine for the whole Health 2020 and sustainable development agendas.

Regretfully there exists a large body of evidence that lack of progress in implementing tobacco control is associated with interference by the tobacco industry. Tobacco companies use a range of tactics to interfere and reduce the impact of tobacco control measures, including political lobbying and campaign contributions, financing of negative research, challenging the course of policy and regulatory efforts, and engaging in social corporate responsibility initiatives as part of public relations campaigns. That progress that has been made in implementing tobacco control measures, despite this opposition from the tobacco industry, may offer lessons for other areas of public health concern that face opposition to policy initiatives from powerful corporate interests in relation to other behavioural determinants of health, for example alcohol, fat, salt and sugar.

European Tobacco Products Directive

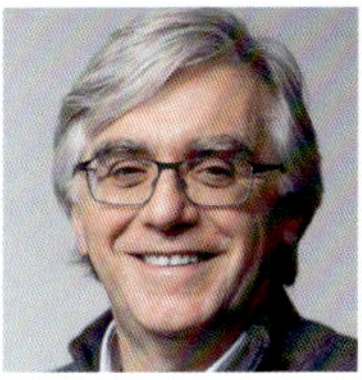

During the EU negotiations on their tobacco control directive, the tobacco industry employed more than 125 lobbyists in Brussels, with an investment of millions of euros to influence the 700 European Parliamentarians. Each lobbyist had a subset of MEPs assigned to them with contact on almost a daily basis to make sure that their 'messages' were heard.

WHO was one of the few voices which were going against these industry voices. Apart from a few NGOs which work on the ground, the legislators are rarely presented with other points of view on issues such as smoking or nutrition. So, our dialogue with the Parliament and the MEPs was key. We successfully managed in several occasions to make sure that the WHO and the public health point of view was part of the conversation.

After long fights and negotiations, eventually the European Commission and the European Parliament, as well as the European Council approved a new tobacco directive: it was somehow weaker than initially planned, but still, provided countries with updated tools to combat the tobacco addiction epidemics.

This was one of the clearest examples on the role WHO can play at the international policy development level to contrast the weight of powerful vested interests in public health policy.

Roberto Bertollini, Former WHO Representative to the EU in Brussels and Former Chief Scientist of the WHO Regional Office for Europe

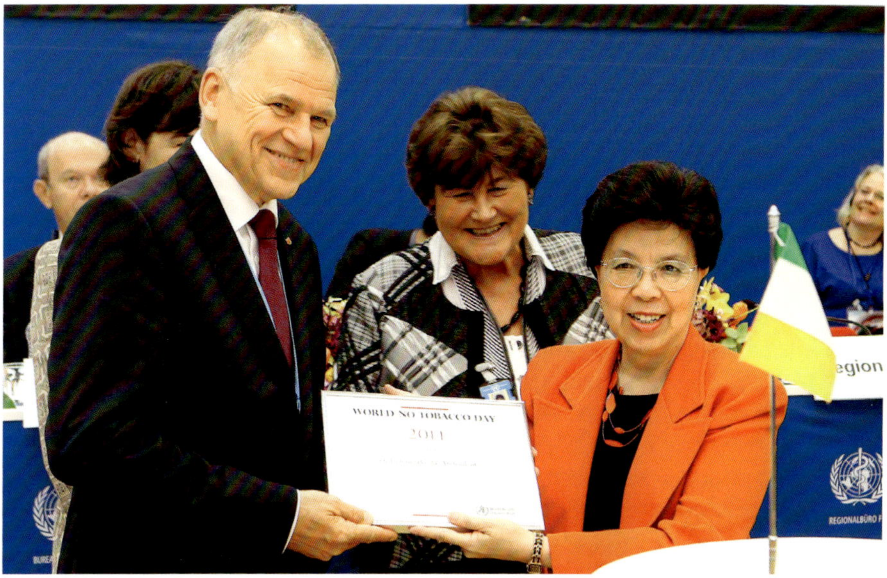

Vytenis Andriukaitis, former Minister of Health of Lithuania and EU Commissioner for Health and Food Safety receives the WHO World No Tobacco Day award from Zsuzsanna Jakab and Margaret Chan, 2014. © Franz Henriksen

WHO FCTC critiques – moving politicians in a healthier direction

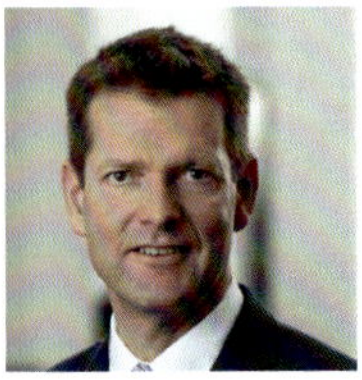

Where we are not achieving well enough is in tobacco regulation. It is a political issue as in most countries. We are not doing yet what some of our neighbouring countries are doing – plain packaging, raising taxes on tobacco etc.

Last year we had the FCTC Regional Office capacity assessment on tobacco regulation. It was critical of several areas of Danish politics, but in a way helpful for us from a public health perspective…

As a civil servant, I have to respect the current political context in my country. But at the same time, as a public health person, I am thankful that the policies of my own country are scrutinized, just as all other countries policies should be. It is nice to have a thing like the FCTC or WHO to help me push democratically elected politicians in healthier directions… It is nice to know we have the WHO never being weak on tobacco regulation.

Søren Brostrøm, Director General, Danish Health Authority, Denmark

Making the case for raising tobacco taxes – WHO's added value

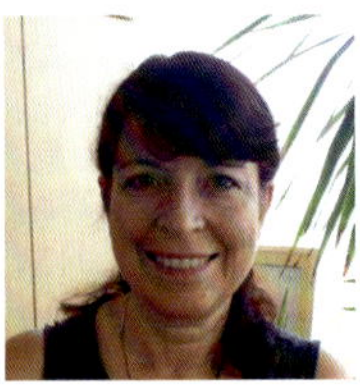

It had been agreed at the Ministry of Health that tobacco prices should be increased to lower consumption, in particular among young people. We had to admit, however, that our capacities in tobacco economics were too limited to enter effective discussions with the Ministry of Finance.

We are a small country of 2 million, and for us it is often crucial to use international expertise. The way to get international expertise without a country having to pay huge amounts to some private agencies is often through WHO.

We all invest in the organization, but in Slovenia we can claim that we also get a lot back. In the case of tobacco prices for example, we were offered the support of an economic expert who had also worked for the World Bank in her previous career and understood the language of finance. This person, sent from WHO, helped us to calculate what it would actually mean if we were to raise taxes, and she explained to our Minister of Finance … about the elasticity of price etc…

They were not very happy because they were also lobbied by the tobacco industry which was providing their own evidence. Nevertheless, the price was raised, maybe not as much as we were expecting, but they could not deny anymore that there is substantial evidence, generated and promoted by international organizations such as WHO, that shows that raising taxes/prices will reduce smoking levels but not reduce revenues significantly. This 'healthy development' was a direct result of support that was organized for Slovenia through WHO.

Vesna-Kerstin Petrič, Head, Division for Health Promotion and Prevention of Noncommunicable Diseases, Ministry of Health, Slovenia

9.3.2.2 Alcohol

Harmful use of alcohol is a serious public health risk, associated with premature death and avoidable disease. Unfortunately, alcohol intake in the WHO European Region is the highest in the world. Alcohol is also a major avoidable risk factor for neuropsychiatric disorders, cardiovascular diseases, cirrhosis of the liver and cancer. It is associated with several infectious diseases, such as HIV/AIDS and tuberculosis, and contributes significantly to unintentional and intentional injuries, including those due to road traffic accidents and suicide. Further, excessive alcohol use during a woman's pregnancy can lead to severe mental handicap of her child.

Beyond avoidable mortality, lives, families, careers, and communities may be devastated by the harmful use of alcohol. WHO estimates that currently this is responsible for around 3.3 million deaths worldwide each year *(207)*. The Political Declaration of the High-level Meeting on the Prevention and Control of NCDs of the General Assembly in 2011 established a global monitoring framework, including a voluntary target of at least a 10% relative reduction in the harmful use of alcohol by 2025, against a baseline of 2010 *(153)*. Now the Region is struggling to reach this voluntary target.

Harmful use has many dimensions. Any effort to protect populations requires wide-ranging support from fiscal policies, trade policies, the judicial system, law enforcement, and a variety of government ministries. WHO supports Member States in improving public health in line with the aims of the Framework for alcohol policy in the WHO European Region *(154)*. Actions include adequate health promotion, disease prevention, disease management research, and evaluation and surveillance activities on alcohol consumption and harm.

WHO also assists countries wishing to strengthen alcohol policies through the *Global strategy to reduce the harmful use of alcohol*, approved by the World Health Assembly in 2010 *(155)*. The Strategy sets out a range of policy options organized around ten areas for targeted action.

As with tobacco, increasing the price of alcoholic beverages is one of the most effective prevention strategies. Having fewer outlets for the purchase of alcohol reduces rates of child maltreatment and drink driving. Restrictions on the hours when alcohol is available for purchase also reduces violent assault.

Since the adoption of the *European action plan to reduce the harmful use of alcohol: 2012–2020 (215)*, 22 Member States have either updated or adopted a national policy on alcohol, and this implementation work will continue. Such national policies are effective, yet also feared and fought by the alcohol industry.

Tobacco and alcohol (and sugar and salt) have come to be understood as examples of the commercial determinants of health, because of the power and influence of the trans-national corporations producing and marketing these unhealthy products and lifestyles. How to respond to these commercial determinants is a major current issue in public and global health. In relation to alcohol in 2013 the then WHO Director-General Margaret Chan made a public statement after the identification of an industry-sponsored group to shape alcohol policies in four countries. She said that the industry cannot have a seat at the table when WHO defines standards and preventive strategies, and the industry cannot supplant governments' role in formulating policies for alcohol control.

Commercial determinants of health

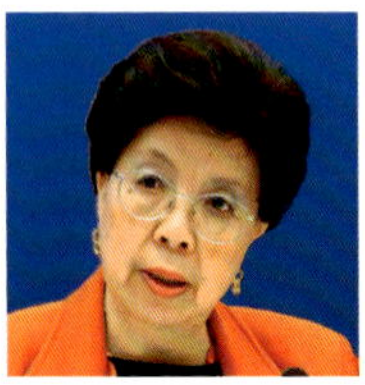

I have been very pleased to see the strong emphasis that Zsuzsanna and the WHO Regional Office for Europe has placed, in Health 2020, on the social, economic and commercial determinants of health.

These were issues I have felt strongly about and was a central theme of an important speech I delivered at the 8th Global Conference on Health Promotion, in Helsinki, Finland, in 2013. In that speech I reminded people how commercial forces were contributing to some of the underlying conditions favouring the rise of NCDs and how the formulation of health policies must be protected from distortion by commercial or vested interests.

Health 2020 provides concrete action options on how countries can address some of these determinants. It is very encouraging to see that many countries are now building their national policies on this framework and its evidence.

Margaret Chan, WHO Director-General, 2006–2017

Not appropriate for industry to be involved

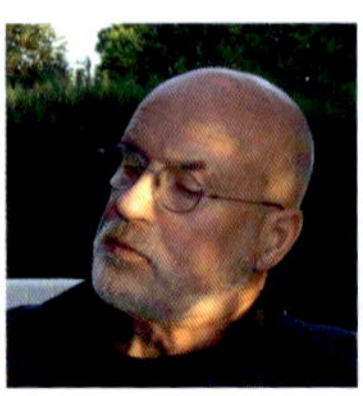

The Global Burden of Disease Studies carried out over the last 25 years have shown very significant and growing public health problems associated with alcohol consumption across the world. There is abundant evidence that a variety of policies and strategies can effectively reduce the harm associated with alcohol consumption.

While there are perhaps some strategies which can reduce alcohol related harm without influencing the amount of alcohol consumed, generally speaking, the less alcohol is drunk in a population the less harm will occur. For public health advocates, therefore, when it comes to alcohol: less is better. The alcohol industry, with a 'bottom-line' interest in advancing its commercial interests has an obvious opposite overall goal. For them more is better. To this end they want to be involved in alcohol policy-making; and in fact, in many countries and in international agencies, the industry currently does play an active role in the policy-making process.

Our European Alcohol Policy Network (APN) is a large group working in governmental and in nongovernmental agencies with an interest in developing and promoting alcohol policies and strategies that serve public health and social welfare. We support and are encouraged by WHO's stand on industry engagement with policies. APN's guidance regarding the role of the industry in alcohol policy-making is that if such a policy is meant to serve public health and social welfare, it is not appropriate for the industry to be involved in the design of the policy. Where the industry is nonetheless involved it is very important that conflicts of interests are transparently managed.

Cees Goos, former WHO acting Director, Chair European Alcohol Policy Network (APN)

9.3.2.3 Diet, overweight and obesity

While we have achieved progress in relation to tobacco and alcohol, we have growing concerns about diet, overweight and obesity in our Region. The increases in overweight among children and adolescents alone risk slowing or reversing the gains made in premature mortality. The increased consumption of highly processed, energy-dense foods high in saturated fats and free sugars, as well as sugar-sweetened beverages, underlie these trends. At the same time to compound the problem the European Region has observed a decrease in levels of physical activity. Poor maternal nutrition, inadequate breastfeeding practices and inappropriate complementary feeding also play a role.

We are taking action, and we need to do much more. In 2010, the World Health Assembly approved a set of recommendations on the marketing of foods and beverages high in sugar, salt and fats to children. In 2014, the then WHO Director-General established the WHO Commission on Ending Childhood Obesity. One of the strongest recommendations in 2016 was for governments to act and implement an effective tax on sugar-sweetened beverages. In 2015, WHO issued new guidelines for free sugars, recommending that these account for less than 10% of total energy intake, and recommended a further reduction to less than 5% to bring additional health benefits *(139, 208)*.

Health 2020 set the tone for the 2013 Vienna Declaration on Nutrition and Noncommunicable Diseases in the Context of Health 2020 and prompted Member States to adopt tools to address the complexity of obesity, notably the European Food and Nutrition Action Plan 2015–2020 *(70, 157)*.

In response governments from across the Region have demonstrated a commitment to tackling obesity. For example, Estonia has unveiled plans to tackle obesity by reducing sugar consumption, starting with a tax on sugar-sweetened beverages that is set to come into force in 2018 *(144)*. The initiative is expected to raise 24 million euros in revenue each year, which is predicted to lead to lower intakes of free sugar and energy and in turn contribute to improvements in obesity and dental health. A catalyst for this innovative step was an Evidence Brief for Policy (EBP), a compelling body of global and local evidence prepared by Estonian policy-makers, public health experts and academic researchers and supported by the WHO Regional Office for Europe. It asserts that the consumption of sugar-sweetened beverages is more associated with increased energy intake, weight gain, overweight and obesity than any other food or beverage, as well as with the development of several NCDs and poor oral health.

In 2018 a WHO progress assessment showed that substantial improvements have been made in areas such as school food, food product reformulation, fiscal approaches and surveillance of childhood obesity *(156)*. However, areas in which implementation is lagging, and which therefore require more attention, include front-of-package labelling and comprehensive marketing restrictions for foods high in fats, sugar and salt. In addition, the assessment report identified scope for reinvigorated or extended action to support breastfeeding and good complementary feeding practices.

An important data–collecting initiative has been the Health Behaviours of School-Aged Children (HBSC) WHO collaborative cross-national study *(158)*. HBSC collects data every four years on 11-, 13- and 15-year-old boys' and girls' health and well-being, social environments and health behaviours. HBSC now includes 49 countries and regions across Europe and North America. The collaboration brings in individuals with a wide range of expertise in areas such as clinical medicine, epidemiology, human biology, paediatrics, pedagogy, psychology, public health, public policy, and sociology. The reports cover a variety of topics, including obesity.

9.3.2.4 Physical inactivity

Physical inactivity is the fourth major risk factor for adult disease. Regular and adequate levels of physical activity reduce the risk of hypertension, coronary heart diseases, stroke, diabetes, and some cancers, including breast and colon cancer. Physical activity also reduces the risk of falls, and hip and vertebral fractures. Evidence also indicates that physical activity can reduce depression and help maintain functional abilities in ageing populations.

Despite these benefits, overall levels of physical activity have declined in almost all countries. Globally, one third of adults do not achieve the recommended levels of physical activity. In Europe, estimates indicate that more than one third of adults are insufficiently active. In response to this, the 65th session of the Regional Committee in 2015 adopted a *Physical activity strategy for the WHO European Region 2016–2025 (159)*.

Urban planning and active mobility – Russian healthy cities

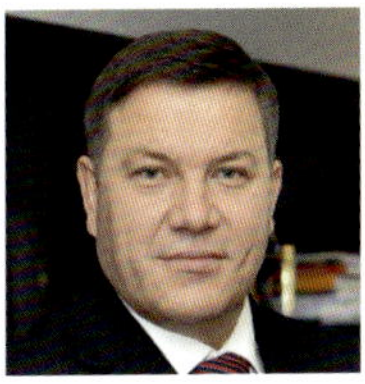

Cities are our future. 70% of the population are living in cities right now, and in the future this number will increase. And the quality of life of the population right now is determined by big cities. Our mission therefore has been and is to develop our Healthy City capacities in the shortest time possible. This has been made possible because we learned early on that we didn't have to create something new – we used the experience of WHO and its European Healthy Cities Network to help build our own programmes.

For example, one area common to many cities in our network has been addressing the challenges of physical inactivity and its many ill-health consequences. The infrastructure of our cities was made for working but not for healthy style of life, so we have been involved in making our urban planning healthier.

Building on models developed in different European Healthy Cities, we implemented projects for renovation of territories, parks, different places for walking and so on. And we changed the exercise facilities available in our city social buildings. They now all have swimming pools, and exercise rooms with equipment. We increased the number of physical education lessons in schools and universities. All these have already helped us to increase the number of people involved in active healthy style of life, from 15% to 30% within the recent ten years.

A key obstacle to this process has been the current Russian mentality that makes people feel they need to consume everything – good cars, good parking places, convenient parking places, bus stops close to each other, etc.

We are working on the ways of changing their mentality. And we are trying to persuade people to change from private to public transport. We created a new system of public transport that helps to change the system of private transport.

With city urban planning, we started to enlarge the space between bus stops and take parking places away from blocks of flats. We are taking these new 'empty spaces' and changing them to parks, to walking places, and activity places. And the population is supporting us.

Other changes are helping this process, as well. It is not a secret that in the former USSR, now Russia, decisions have generally been made without taking account of public opinion. But the situation has changed, and public opinion has become the most important when taking political decisions. People have become more active in public society.

We need to listen to the opinion of the public. Whatever we do right now, whether building parks, spaces for activity, or other places, we will listen to public opinion in special public sessions. This helps us to avoid mistakes by listening to the public, and taking their opinions into account.

We understand that we are on the way to making health a global country idea. Our target is to unite our cities in this endeavour and help us all reach our Sustainable Development Goals. There is so much to be done.

Oleg Kuvshinnikov, Governor of the Vologda Region, Russian Federation, Chairman of the Russian Association of Healthy Cities, Districts and Villages

9.3.2.5 Mental health

In 2013 the Regional Committee endorsed the *European Mental Health Action Plan 2013–2020 (160)*. The Regional Office has assisted countries and areas to develop mental health strategies; suicide prevention strategies; and community-based mental health services that empower people using these services. In some cases, the standards of accommodation and treatment in institutions for adults with intellectual and psychosocial disabilities are grossly inadequate, even appalling. This is a situation about which I feel very strongly, and I was determined that the Regional Office would work to assess quality standards and the protection of human rights in these institutions, working in a collaborative partnership with national authorities and stakeholders.

As a result, WHO has helped train assessment teams in countries and areas, and has evaluated the performance of 75 institutions in 24 Member States and in Kosovo *[1]*. This has led to reports that highlight critical areas which need improvement, and on which we are now working with the authorities.

[1] All references to Kosovo in this document should be understood to be in the context of United Nations Security Council resolution 1244 (1999).

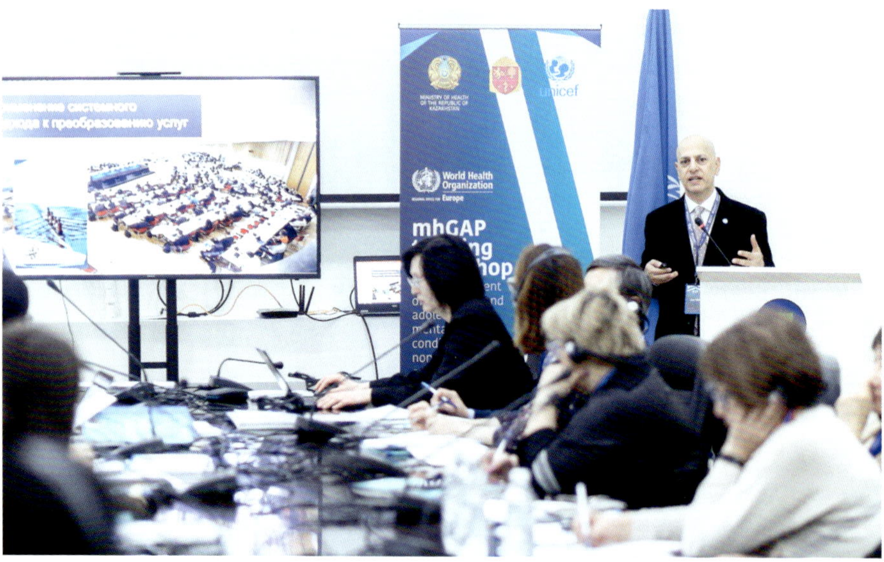

Countries in central Asia, including Kazakhstan, Kyrgyzstan, Turkmenistan and Uzbekistan are embarking on fundamental mental health system reforms to improve the treatment of mental health conditions for their population. Workshop in Kazakhstan in January 2019. © WHO/Jerome Flayosc

Regional Health Development Center on Mental Health in South-eastern Europe

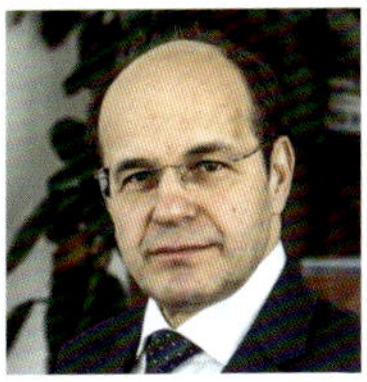

As one of the outcomes of cooperation with countries from the South-eastern European Health Network, the Ministry of Civil Affairs of Bosnia and Herzegovina, in cooperation with counterpart ministries and health authorities, established the Regional Health Development Center on Mental Health in South-eastern Europe.

The activities of this Center aim to strengthen cooperation in South-eastern Europe in the field of mental health and policy development through continuous promotion, prevention, advocacy, publishing and research.

Adil Osmanovic, Minister of Civil Affairs, Bosnia and Herzegovina

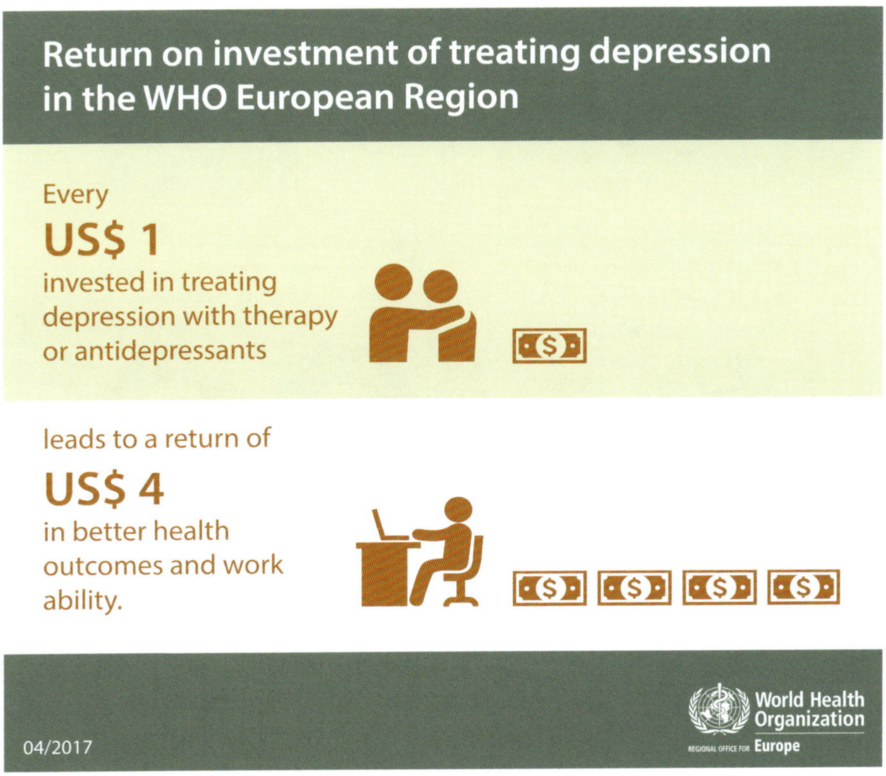

Fig. 12. Example of WHO Regional Office for Europe infographic used to convey health messages to the public through visuals. This message was used for the World Health Day campaign on depression in 2017.

Source: Infographic: Return on investment of treating depression *(212)*.

9.3.2.6 Injuries and violence

There has been a significant fall in deaths from injuries in people aged 5–49 years in the European Region over the last decade.

Road deaths have also fallen over the same period. A global status report on road safety was published in 2009 and 2013. Reducing road traffic fatalities by 50% by 2020 is a key SDG target *(61)*.

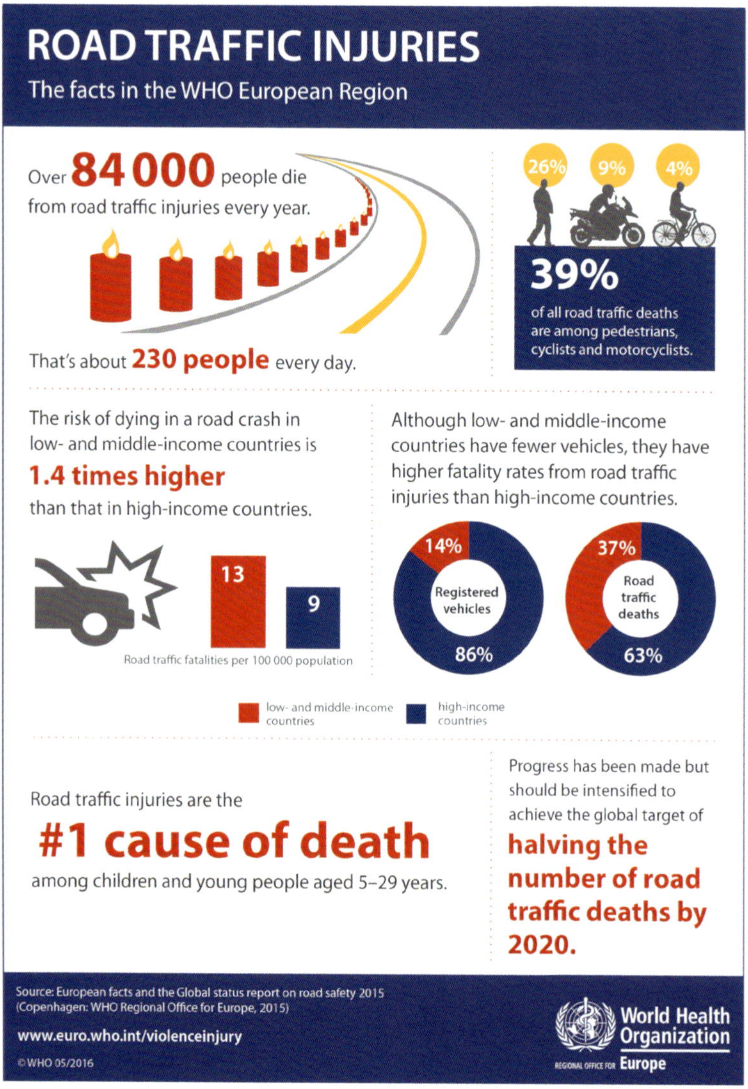

Fig. 13. Example of WHO Regional Office for Europe infographic used to convey health messages to the public through visuals, 2015.
Source: Infographic: Road traffic injuries available at www.euro.who.int

Childhood maltreatment causes both immediate damage to children's health and well-being and long-term harm to their development, resulting in dysfunction throughout life. The Regional Office has continued to support Member States in implementing the *European child maltreatment prevention action plan* adopted by the Regional Committee in 2014, helping Member States measure the problem and develop appropriate policy responses *(73)*.

9.3.3 Tackling the European Region's major health challenges – communicable diseases

The Region has made major progress in the control of communicable diseases, by strengthening health systems and focusing on high-risk populations and vulnerable groups. Regional actions plans have been brought forward in disease areas which place a substantial burden on health in Europe and continue to be of concern: tuberculosis (TB), HIV/AIDS, hepatitis and AMR, vaccine preventable diseases, sustaining polio eradication, malaria, vector borne disease and influenza.

9.3.3.1 Tuberculosis

For tuberculosis the Regional Office has been working with partners such as the Global Fund, United States Agency for International Development (USAID) and others. The Tuberculosis action plan for the WHO European Region 2016–2020 was endorsed in 2017 *(162)*. The good news is that from 2013 to 2016 TB incidence and mortality rates decreased from 36 to 30 new cases and from 4.1 to 2.6 deaths every 100 000 people respectively. This very positive decline is the fastest in all WHO Regions. Also as a result of health system strengthening work with Member States to render services more people-centered, the hospitalization rate has decreased by a quarter from 75 % to 56 % over the period, while the average length of stay in hospitals has also decreased significantly.

The Region has also seen major progress in the fight against multidrug resistant tuberculosis (MDR-TB), is seeing better case detection (increased from 43% to 62%), and treatment success (increased from 49% to 57%). Treatment coverage for MDR-TB patients reached 92% in 2017.This has been due to the rapid scale up of molecular diagnostic tests and strengthening of the health system response with the implementation of people-centred and ambulatory models of care. Yet, despite this progress, the European Region still has the highest rate of MDR-TB in the world, with one out of five people with MDR-TB globally living in our Region *(209)*.

The goal of ending TB in our Region by 2030 is threatened also by an increase of HIV co-infection among TB patients. During the last decade, the HIV prevalence for TB patients quadrupled (from 3 % to 12 %), with now every eighth TB patient being co-infected with HIV (12%).

TB in Romania

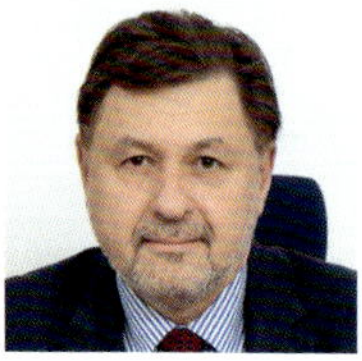

Romania has the most cases of tuberculosis in the European Union, around 12 000 cases each year. We requested technical assistance from WHO Europe to deal with this problem and what came out of this collaboration, I have to say, was one of the most successful partnerships I have ever experienced.

As a result of the technical assistance we got from WHO Europe, we succeeded in designing a national strategy which received approved. This strategy is very comprehensive is more than just medical: it also has some very strong social inputs.

Alexandru Rafila, Ministerial Adviser, Romania

The high rate of multidrug resistant tuberculosis (MDR-TB) in the European Region is in large part due to the inefficiency of health systems to treat the disease effectively and to the ongoing transmission of resistant strains in communities. The Regional action plan has ambitious targets of detecting more than 85% of estimated MDR-TB patients and treating at least 75% of them successfully to curb the epidemic.

Health 2020 identifies a variety of approaches to make further progress in TB control: including, addressing health system barriers and determinants, working with partners, strengthening mechanisms for country support and coordination, and boosting and enabling research. I strongly believe Europe can lead the global efforts in this regard, however national ownership of this work is crucial not only for preparation and launch, but especially for driving sustainable follow-up and ensuring that no groups are left behind.

Roma health mediator – TB action plan Slovakia

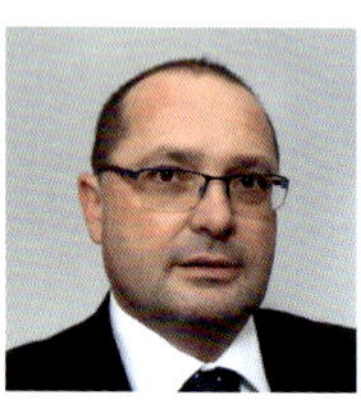

Building on the TB Action Plan 2016 – 2020 of the Regional Office and the Moscow Declaration to end TB 2017, a WHO collaborating centre for work with vulnerable groups was opened at the TB Institute in Vyšné Hágy, Slovakia in April 2018.

In 2017 the total incidence of tuberculosis in persons of Roma ethnicity (estimated at 10% of population) was 37% of the total tuberculosis cases. More alarmingly, children under the age of 14 from the Roma ethnic group accounted for 95% of the total number of tuberculosis in children (44 cases). National studies show that the Roma ethnic group has a high rate of unemployment, poor socioeconomic conditions, multigenerational coexistence in settlements without basic hygienic standard, and a history of poor treatment compliance and high levels of illiteracy.

Active search for patients is hampered by migration and illiteracy. Surveys of health care workers reveal a lack of information about the community, lack of experience, lack of communication skills, language barriers, community bias, and inability to adapt the level of interpretation to the target group.

To address these problems, the Institute of Tuberculosis and Respiratory Diseases in Vyšné Hágy has implemented an educational programme for health education assistants (health mediators) from Roma communities. This is a joint project of the Ministry of Health, our Institute, the WHO Country Office in Slovakia and other actors – e.g. communitiy-based NGOs.

The aim of this activity is to prepare field workers from marginalized groups of the population. These fieldworkers provide cooperative contact tracing for basic examinations as well as follow-up on the continued treatment of patients with tuberculosis under outpatient conditions.

Ivan Solovic, Director WHO TB Collaborating Centre, Slovakia

We are also taking action globally. On 26 September of 2018, the first ever UN General Assembly high-level meeting on TB took place in New York *(161)*. With all its recent experience the Regional Office was able to work with national experts and diplomatic missions to prepare and provide European perspectives to inform the multisectoral accountability framework and the draft declaration.

High priority has been given to supporting countries in implementing effective and efficient TB service delivery systems, shifting towards more outpatient-oriented and integrated models of care, with sustainable financing and well aligned payment mechanisms. This approach is aligned with the United Nations Sustainable Development Goal 3, which includes targets to move towards UHC and end the TB epidemic.

These activities have been implemented through a Tuberculosis Regional Eastern Europe and Central Asia Project (TB-REP) on strengthening national health systems for effective TB and drug-resistant TB prevention and care *(202)*. The project has been funded through a grant from the Global Fund to Fight AIDS, TB and Malaria. It was implemented over three years from 2016 to 2018 by the Center for Health Policies and Studies (PAS Center) as the principal recipient, with the Regional Office as the technical lead agency.

The grant covered activities in 11 eastern European and central Asian Member States (Armenia, Azerbaijan, Belarus, Georgia, Kazakhstan, Kyrgyzstan, Republic of Moldova, Tajikistan, Turkmenistan, Ukraine and Uzbekistan). Project countries have shown their political commitment and nominated high-level focal points who are responsible for national implementation of the TB-REP project and for the development of country specific roadmaps.

Global Fund – The WHO Regional Office for Europe partnership – health systems focus

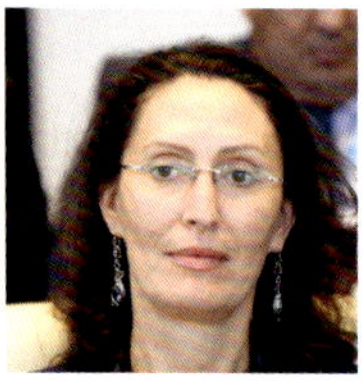

Over the years, we have witnessed a more focused approach to health systems strengthening for both the Regional Office and the Global Fund.

Strong systems for health are the primary line of defence against HIV, TB and malaria, while also enabling prevention, detection and response to new and existing threats to global security. Here in the European Region we are talking about health sector reforms. The countries in the Region are not starting from scratch; they are facing the challenges of bringing systemic changes in the ways HIV and TB services are delivered, financed or integrated.

Health system reforms are generally painful and difficult – it is a challenging area of work, but much needed because without it there would be no effective response to HIV and TB. So our work together, more and more, requires applying an integrated approach for HIV and TB service delivery and financing. Moving forward, our partnership is intensifying support in a wide variety of areas including improving procurement and supply chain systems, strengthening data systems and data use, training qualified health care workers, and building strong community responses. For instance, in the European Region we are working together on revisions of models of care, task shifting, cross-programmatic efficiency such as identifying entry points for integration of TB and HIV services, and other services such as hepatitis C testing, treatment and care. We understand the acute need to support the health care reforms and specifically reform the provider payment mechanisms.

In this regard I must mention the WHO Barcelona Office which has been a very good resource for stakeholders in the region on health financing and health system reforms.

Maria Kirova, Department Head, Asia, Europe, Latin America and the Caribbean, The Global Fund to Fight AIDS, Tuberculosis and Malaria

The Office has designed a blueprint of a people-centred model on improving TB care, including human resource development, health financing and provider payment mechanisms. The Regional Office has also provided a training programme on health systems strengthening for improved TB prevention and care in Barcelona, Spain. The Global Fund has financed this programme through the PAS Center and has been targeting the 11 high-burden countries participating in implementation of the TB-REP *(202)*. The training programme supports transformation in the financing and delivering of TB services in the European Region, identifies problems and generates solutions based on good examples from the Region.

This capacity-building programme has been attended by several stakeholders, including, decision-makers, senior officials and high-level health system administrators from ministries of health and finance, and managers of national TB programmes, health insurance funds and service delivery organizations. In addition to delegates from countries, experts from international organizations supporting TB-REP countries also attended the training programme.

9.3.3.2 The HIV epidemic

The Region has made progress in increasing the number of people receiving treatment for HIV/AIDS and eliminating mother-to-child transmission. There is good progress in several countries, with updated testing policies embracing a treat-all approach. Yet, still one fifth of all people living with HIV in our WHO European Region do not know their HIV status.

We know that the prevention of HIV transmissions among key populations is very important, particularly among people who inject drugs, and their sexual partners, vulnerable young people, men who have sex with men, sex workers and prisoners.

Our gains in HIV treatment are unevenly distributed and as a result overall the Region is not on track to meet HIV targets. While there are great achievements in responding to HIV in the west and in the centre, the challenges are still substantial in eastern Europe and central Asia. In the east of the Region, late diagnosis, low coverage with antiretroviral therapy (ART) and failures to implement evidence-based policy has meant that the numbers of AIDS cases have increased and AIDS-related deaths have plateaued while in the west of the Region, where ART coverage is high, the numbers of AIDS cases and deaths have decreased. Only 50% of all people with HIV in the east of the Region are receiving antiretroviral therapy, compared with 88% in the west and 76% in centre of the Region. The Region has seen increasing rates of new HIV diagnoses. In 2017, of all new HIV diagnoses reported throughout Europe, 82% were from the east *(210)*.

Teenergizer

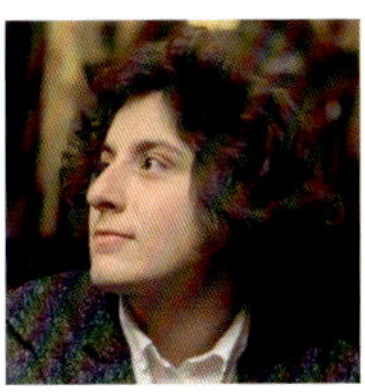

My name is Yana. I am from Ukraine and I am 21. I was born with HIV. I speak openly about this. At the age of 16 I started an organization called Teenergizer *(163)*. It is a movement that unites the HIV positive and HIV negative teenagers of Ukraine, Georgia, Russia and the whole region of Eastern Europe and Central Asia. Our aim is to create a world where every teenager can realize her or his potential; a world free from discrimination in all areas, including HIV; a world where the rights of teenagers and youth do not have to be defended because they are fully respected.

We provide a lot of information about living with HIV; testing, rights, sexual health and sexuality. We have a strong presence on social media and the web and provide a lot of interactive maps helping people find testing facilities and other services. We work with a variety of UN agencies, the Global Fund and other donors. We do a lot of advocacy work. Teenergizer is unique because projects for teenagers are created and embodied by teenagers themselves. Who else would know better what exactly we need!

Yana Panfilova, Founder and Head of the Board of Teenergizer, Ukraine

In July 2018, I invited ministers of health of eastern Europe and central Asia countries to a policy dialogue and we exchanged good practices and agreed on ways to scale up and sustain evidence-informed interventions, in order to make UHC a reality and to end the AIDS epidemic by 2030. Each country is now committed to review the situation, identify the gaps, and make an effort to fill these gaps through a national roadmap coupled with political commitment.

9.3.3.3 Viral hepatitis

Viral hepatitis is a public health threat that affects millions of people *(80)* in the WHO European Region, more than two thirds of whom live in eastern Europe and central Asia. Every day, thousands of people still become infected, due to exposure through unsafe injection practices and insufficient information and tools for prevention. People who inject drugs are particularly vulnerable to hepatitis and co-infection with both viral hepatitis and HIV is common.

Of the 5 main hepatitis viruses that cause acute and/or chronic infection, referred to as types A, B, C, D and E, chronic hepatitis B and C are responsible for approximately 98% of all deaths due to viral hepatitis in the European Region. Hepatitis B and C prevalence ranges from less than 0.5% in western, northern and central Europe to 3–8% in eastern Europe and central Asia *(80)*. An estimated 170 000 people die from viral hepatitis-related causes each year.

The spread of hepatitis can be prevented if countries adopt measures promoted by WHO, including universal new-born immunization against hepatitis B and vaccination against hepatitis A in high-risk groups; prevention of mother-to-child transmission of hepatitis B; promotion of safer sexual behaviour to reduce the risk of infection; reduction of harm related to injecting drug use; the provision of a safe blood supply; and prevention of transmission in health care settings. In addition, access to diagnosis and timely treatment reduces both symptoms of viral hepatitis and complications, including liver failure and primary liver cancer. This improves quality of life and reduces mortality.

Recognizing the tremendous burden caused by viral hepatitis, the World Health Assembly adopted resolution WHA63.18 in 2010, calling for a comprehensive approach to the prevention and control of viral hepatitis.

In 2017, Member States in the European Region adopted the first ever *Action plan for the health sector response to viral hepatitis in the WHO European Region (80)*. They also committed to the global goal of eliminating viral hepatitis as a public health threat by 2030, in line with the United Nations 2030 Agenda for Sustainable Development.

Since then, many countries have demonstrated increasing commitment in scaling up the response to viral hepatitis and setting national elimination goals. The WHO Regional Office for Europe is working closely with several Member States to develop national action plans. The Regional Office is also supporting countries to raise awareness, strengthen surveillance and laboratory capacity, and update national treatment and care guidelines.

9.3.3.4 Antimicrobial resistance (AMR)

AMR is a complex public health concern necessitating the involvement of diverse stakeholders across sectors and levels of organization and governance. National, regional and global policies should address the complex factors driving AMR and be based on public health principles such as surveillance, prevention, containment and research.

Since 1998, WHO has highlighted the need for joint global action on AMR. When I took office in 2010, I made AMR a priority in the Region, and in 2011 the Regional Committee adopted a *European strategic action plan on antibiotic resistance (76)*. This regional action contributed to AMR becoming a global priority, and the Global action plan on antimicrobial resistance was endorsed at the Sixty-eighth World Health Assembly in May 2015 *(165)*.

Supportive and comprehensive regulatory and legislative changes are needed in Member States. The Regional Office has supported the development of national action plans on AMR which are aligned with the objectives of the Global action plan to be in place by 2017. To facilitate intersectoral coordination in line with national plans and policies countries have appointed national AMR focal points. The Region has provided technical guidance to selected countries in the Region on developing and setting up these national action plans. As of March 2019, 39 Member States had finalized national plans of action on AMR.

Surveillance provides a basis for taking action to control AMR. The main surveillance mechanisms gathering and presenting AMR data from countries in the Region are the European Antimicrobial Resistance Surveillance Network (EARS-Net) hosted by ECDC and the Central Asian and Eastern European Surveillance of Antimicrobial Resistance (CAESAR) network, which has enrolled Member States since its inception in 2011. In combination, these two networks provide AMR surveillance data for Member States in the WHO European Region *(164, 191)*.

To further strengthen the evidence base through enhanced and standardized global surveillance and research, in 2015 WHO developed the Global Antimicrobial Resistance Surveillance System (GLASS), which currently collects and reports data on AMR rates aggregated at the national level *(213)*. GLASS also collects data on the implementation status of national surveillance systems.

In line with Objectives 1 and 2 of the Global Action Plan on AMR, the Regional Office supports the establishment of effective antimicrobial stewardship programmes. To that end a massive open online course (MOOC) entitled: 'Antimicrobial stewardship: A competency-based approach' has been developed in collaboration with the University of Stanford (USA). In January 2018 the course was launched on OpenWHO *(192)*, and one year later the course has reached over 22 000 persons from more than 170 countries representing all WHO regions.

Tackling AMR requires multisectoral coordination including involvement of human and animal health sectors (the 'One Health' approach). In this context, the Food and Agriculture Organization of the United Nations (FAO), the World Organisation for Animal Health (OIE), and the World Health Organization (WHO) have come together to support governments, health care workers, veterinary and plant professionals, and other stakeholders, to promote the responsible use of antimicrobials in humans, animals, and plants. The Regional Office supports such a strong tripartite approach through joint meetings and AMR missions in Member States. Whilst this is particularly true for AMR, it also applies to food safety, influenza and other emerging infections.

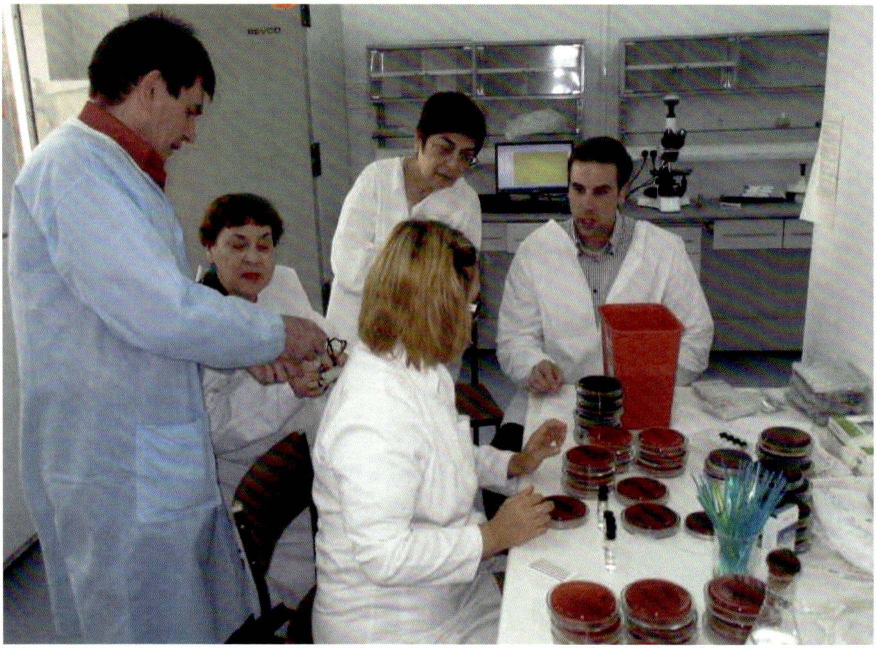

Training in laboratory techniques for combating foodborne diseases and related antimicrobial resistance was held for representatives of the Uzbekistan ministries of health and agriculture, 27 February 2015. © WHO/Uzbekistan

The Regional Office supports the implementation of the revised core components for Infection, Prevention and Control (IPC) in European Member States as one of the key activities. The 'Save Lives: Clean Your Hands Campaign' on 5 May 2017 focused on antibiotic resistance through the slogan 'Fight antibiotic resistance – it's in your hands'.

On the communication and advocacy side, the Regional Office has championed the UN General Assembly's call for immediate action against AMR and has been urging all countries in the European Region to take part in World Antibiotic Awareness Week (WAAW). WAAW continues to gain global momentum and builds on the success of the European Antibiotic Awareness Day, a European initiative that the Regional Office for Europe joined in 2012 and extended to non-European Union countries.

The work of the Regional Office to support Member States to prevent and control AMR is carried out in collaboration with many partners among which are the National Institute for Public Health and the Environment (RIVM) of the Netherlands and the European Society of Clinical Microbiology and Infectious Diseases (ESCMID), founding partners of the CAESAR network and with support of WHO Collaborating Centres and many other financial and technical partners.

9.3.3.5. Vaccine preventable diseases

Vaccine preventable diseases remain a priority as our great achievement of the past few decades in reducing the incidence of measles and rubella and our current polio-free status do not mean that all our challenges have been overcome. Universal immunization is a vital component of UHC. Its success contributes not only to achieving strong and sustainable health systems, but also to equity, protection of human rights and child survival.

However, the current situation is not satisfactory. Since the beginning of 2017 a serious outbreak of measles has affected the Region, with an increasing number of countries affected. In the period 1 January 2018 – 30 May 2019, 49 of the 53 countries in the Region have together reported over 160 000 measles cases and over 100 measles-related deaths *(193)*.

It is vital to raise political and public awareness of the problem and its devastating consequences, respond to vaccine hesitancy, and help strengthen European health systems in the longer term to avoid future outbreaks. This includes strengthening disease surveillance systems to ensure early detection and response; improving vaccine procurement and immunization programmes to ensure that vaccines reach those who need these; and identifying the extent and causes of vaccine hesitancy to ensure that all parents are empowered to choose vaccination for their children.

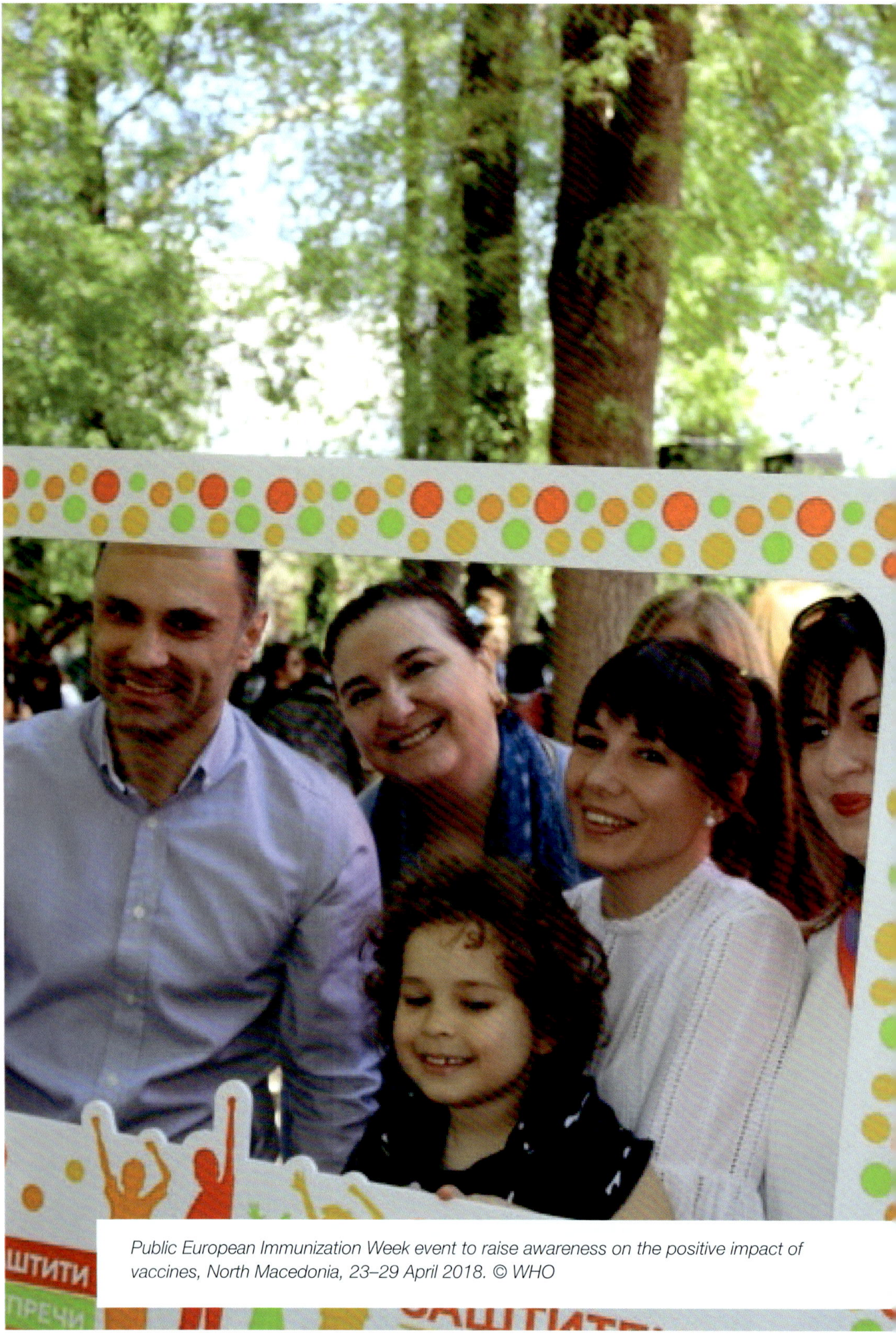

Public European Immunization Week event to raise awareness on the positive impact of vaccines, North Macedonia, 23–29 April 2018. © WHO

Measles in Romania

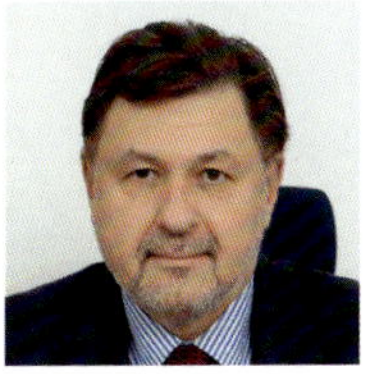

Our Romanian measles outbreak started in 2016 due to the decreasing coverage in MMR vaccination in children at national level. We started in 2008 with 95% coverage, as WHO recommends, and little by little the coverage decreased and by 2016 was 85% for the first dose of MMR and around 75% for the second dose. Over the period 1 January 2017 – 30 May 2019 14 000 cases have been documented with 35 deaths. WHO has been supporting us with technical people from the European Regional Verification Commission for Measles and Rubella Elimination and one year ago with some common joint exercises regarding a communication strategy. These were focused on improving trust of parents and perceptions of the mass media regarding vaccination in general, and the measles vaccination in particular. We are also developing, with WHO assistance, a redesign of our communication strategy in vaccination and adopting a more intense 'closer' approach to the population regarding vaccination with a door-to-door campaign of information, and vaccination especially in the rural areas and with poorly reached populations. This later strategy acknowledges and addresses the fact that the main epidemics are concentrated in pockets around the country where children are not vaccinated or where the coverage is not very high.

Alexandru Rafila, Ministerial Adviser, Romania

It is the responsibility of Member States to ensure equitable access to affordable, safe and effective vaccines. WHO however can play a vital role. The European Vaccine Action Plan 2015–2020 (EVAP), which was unanimously adopted by all Member States in 2014 contributes directly to achievement of Sustainable Development Goal 3, by acknowledging the right of every person to be protected from vaccine-preventable diseases, as an integral part of our global pledge within the SDGs to 'leave no one behind'.

The WHO European Region, with WHO HQ support, has made substantial progress towards attaining the EVAP goals. By the end of 2017, 32 Member States had achieved the routine immunization coverage target of third dose of DTP containing vaccine *(194)*, and 43 had interrupted endemic measles transmission. An increasing number of Member States are taking advantage of the significant health gains offered by the new and underutilized vaccines.

One area where the focus on vaccination is of importance is migration, and it is vital to ensure culturally appropriate immunization services for migrants and refugees.

Our Region is privileged to have the support of HRH Crown Princess Mary, Patron of WHO/Regional Office for Europe, for this key part of our work. Throughout the past decade she has spoken on the occasion of European Immunization Week and other opportunities to underline the contribution vaccines make to our health and well-being.

Investing in children

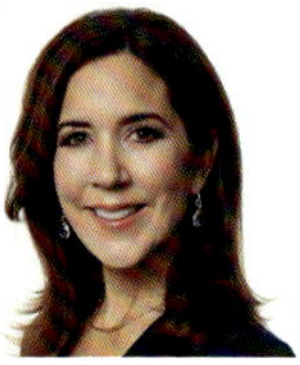

© Daniel Stjerne

We cannot – and must not – forget the importance of investing in children and adolescents. They are our future. From the earliest stages in life, children need protection and vaccination programmes are the foundation of any strong health system. We must ensure that the next generation is afforded the opportunity to achieve their full potential without the threat of illness or death due to vaccine-preventable diseases.

The young generation's ability and possibility to fulfil their full potential will be a testament to the actions we take today. If we fail them, their chance of success is questionable but, if we provide for them, then they will be more likely to succeed.

HRH Crown Princess Mary, Patron of WHO/Regional Office for Europe

Joining the campaign in Romania in 2018, I was pleased to see the engagement of high-level leaders, national health authorities, media, civil society and the public in European Immunization Week. Their participation clearly demonstrates that immunization is a cross-cutting issue that affects everyone.

Awakening policy-makers

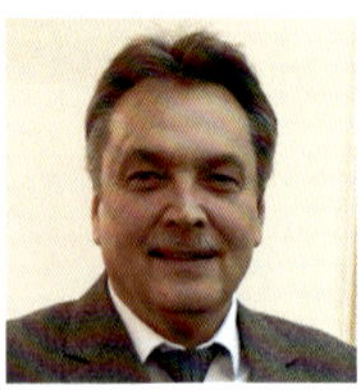

If you are look at the public debates in Romania, health problems have just not been a very high priority in the last 10–15 years. Therefore, it is a huge help when WHO 'awakens' our politicians to their roles and obligations to take action and put into practice the Regional goals of the declarations and resolutions they signed.

We have a very good in example in the law of vaccination. In 2005 we adopted a new health law in Romania without much debate in parliament. Since 2005, we have made 1400 changes to that law. We have articles which were changed six times in the same year! It is not an organic or foundational law but one which you can change easily with amendments. That is why we have been proposing new vaccination laws first in 2012, and then in 2016.

We want to make a foundational law that you cannot change so easily. A law that has very clear goals, and is in line with the rest of the world and European policies and strategies to which Romania is a part. That's why we are very privileged to have a relationship with WHO. We have all kinds of technical support from WHO, from policy development to communication, data systems and reporting, to vaccine procurement and quality control etc. Help has even come from the Regional Director. When, for example, we had a problem with measles in 2012, Zsuzsanna Jakab came to Bucharest and made presentations and suggestions at the highest political level on ways to address identified problems and improve our situation with vaccination in Romania.

László Attila, Parliamentarian, Romania

9.3.3.6 Vaccine hesitancy

Most parents continue to demand vaccination as the surest and safest way to protect their children. However, the delay or refusal of vaccination by some parents, despite the availability of immunization services, known as 'vaccine hesitancy' appears to have contributed to a decline in vaccine uptake in some areas.

Predictive analytics

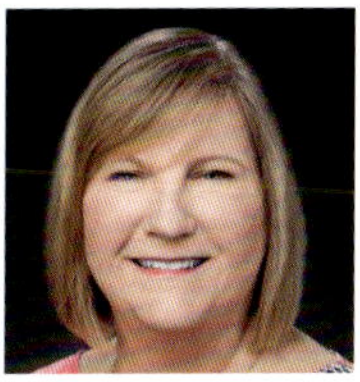

The US Centers for Disease Control and Prevention (CDC) is a domestic agency, but we have been working globally for more than 60 years. Since the 1990s, we have collaborated technically with WHO around many different outbreaks. More recently, we do a lot of trilateral work with the WHO Regional Office for Europe and ECDC in setting up surveillance systems and ensuring strong, quality-assured laboratories.

In the last few years, we have been seeing opportunities for predictive analytics to understand more about the risk of where disease burden may occur or where the gaps are, so we are able to think more about the preventative piece, building core capacities, rather than just responding to outbreaks. An example of such preventative measures are immunisation programmes; to understand why communities may lack access or why somebody is refusing vaccines and to understand what needs to be done with health care providers, with parents or guardians, as well as with government, to improve coverage. When I was detached to the WHO Regional Office for Europe from 2008–2011, we helped develop the Tailoring Immunization Programmes (TIP) tool that countries could use to identify what were the causes of low coverage and what could be done to improve efforts and save lives *(167)*.

We invest in the European Region because we see the benefit to everybody of protecting populations around the world. The US government is very much about stopping diseases where they start, before they cross national borders, before they reach our shores, to minimize loss of life and economic impact. Today, all WHO regions are experiencing measles outbreaks, which has led to importations from Europe to the US. We can trace those through the genetics and the typing of the viruses themselves, so our partnership and efforts in Europe to protect our borders and at-risk populations around the world and to prevent the spread of disease, is as vital today as ever.

Rebecca Martin, Director, Center for Global Health at the US Centers for Disease Control and Prevention (CDC), USA

Our studies have shown that vaccine hesitancy is a complex and context specific phenomenon, varying over time, place and individual vaccines *(166)*. It includes factors such as complacency, convenience and confidence. To equip Member States to better identify the factors influencing vaccination intentions, decisions and behaviours, the Office has developed the *Guide to Tailoring Immunization Programmes (TIP) (167)*. This consists of proven methods and tools to:

- identify populations susceptible to vaccine-preventable disease;
- diagnose supply and demand side barriers and enablers to vaccination; and,
- recommend evidence-informed responses to build and sustain vaccination uptake.

Among the range of efforts needed to sustain high immunization coverage, we must all effectively communicate the facts about immunization, through European Immunization Week and other means, to ensure our communities remain resilient to misinformation and that parents can make informed, responsible choices.

9.3.3.7 Polio, malaria, vector borne, parasitic diseases and influenza

Happily, despite a major polio outbreak in 2010 (see Developmental reflection 6), the Region has kept its polio-free status through effective outbreak response. Our most recent assessment by the European Regional Commission for the Certification of Poliomyelitis Eradication in May 2019, concluded that there was no poliovirus transmission in the Region in 2018 and that any importation or circulation of a poliovirus would have been detected promptly by existing health/surveillance systems.

Developmental reflection 6

Polio outbreak and response in Tajikistan and neighbouring countries

"It is not over till it is over"

Our Region has been polio-free since 2002, a status that we are all determined to maintain by all means. In 2009–2010, we therefore responded rapidly to the polio outbreak in Tajikistan, which also affected four other countries – Kazakhstan, the Russian Federation, Turkmenistan and Uzbekistan – that required preventive responses by other neighbouring countries. Along with the UNICEF and other partners we acted swiftly and effectively to support the Government in implementation of supplementary immunization campaigns targeting 2.7 million children aged less than 15 years.

By 4 July 2010, no new acute flaccid paralysis cases had been detected. I visited the country myself, as soon as the first polio cases were reported, to work out a joint response strategy with the then Minister of Health, Mr Salimov, and to launch the first round of the immunization campaign. I met with President Emomali Rahmon and many government officials of Tajikistan. I was very pleased to see that their leadership took immediate open, transparent and appropriate action in close collaboration with WHO and that they used active communication to reach out to every family and child in the country.

I also visited Uzbekistan, with the Deputy Regional Director of UNICEF, to launch the second round of their immunization campaign with the Minister of Health, Dr Ikramov. In Uzbekistan, 2.85 million children aged less than 5 years were targeted with 3 rounds of supplementary immunization activities.

Thanks to effective surveillance systems in all countries, imported polio cases were detected outside Tajikistan, including 3 cases in Turkmenistan and some cases in the Russian Federation, for which control measures were rapidly put in place.

The Government of the Russian Federation gave strong support to WHO and the affected countries throughout this outbreak through the quick and efficient work of the regional polio laboratory, to which all the samples were sent for analysis.

This polio outbreak in Tajikistan and the cases detected in neighbouring countries – causing paralysis in 475 people and 30 deaths – reminded us of the Region's vulnerability, and it was a clear signal to us that we have an unfinished agenda which needs full commitment and determination. It reinforced for us the Region's needs for strong public health functions and capacities, strong surveillance, high immunization coverage and full transparency, and compliance with the IHR (2005) to avoid similar outbreaks.

All of these priorities are addressed in our Health 2020 framework. And our staff, throughout the Region, continue to develop tools and interventions to support Member States to strengthen the scientific and political leadership needed to maintain the polio-free status which the European Region has enjoyed since 2002!

Our aim at Regional and national levels is to maintain malaria elimination; achieve improved surveillance and control of invasive vectors and re-emerging mosquito-borne diseases; control of leishmaniasis; control and prevent soil-transmitted helminthiases; and promote the use of sustainable vector-control alternatives to persistent insecticides.

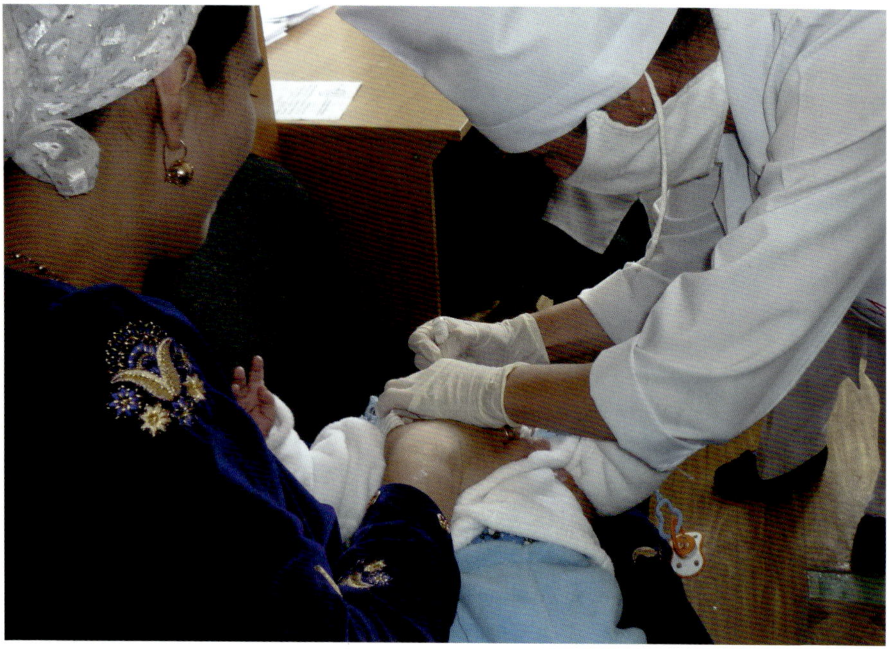

A baby being vaccinated during the fifth round of polio immunization in Tajikistan, October 2010. © WHO/Nukra Sinavbarova

In 2015, for the first time, the WHO European Region reported zero indigenous malaria cases, in line with the goal of the Tashkent Declaration to eliminate malaria from the Region by 2015 *(168)*.

The achievement of zero indigenous malaria cases in the WHO European Region is extraordinary but fragile. The Region is prone to continual importation of cases from endemic regions, with the threat of re-establishment of transmission. Maintaining zero cases in the European Region will require sustained political commitment, resources and constant vigilance, as indicated in the Ashgabat Statement *(195)*. The *Regional framework for prevention of malaria reintroduction and certification of malaria elimination 2014–2020* is available for European countries and should be fully implemented *(169)*.

Implementation of the Regional framework for surveillance and control of invasive mosquito vectors and re-emerging vector-borne diseases, 2014–2020 *(170)* and two Regional frameworks on parasitic diseases *(81, 196)*, has reduced the burden of vector-borne (such as dengue and chikungunya fever) and parasitic diseases, by providing strategic guidance and technical assistance, building capacity, strengthening operational research, promoting cross-border cooperation (involving both the WHO Regional Office for Europe and the WHO Regional Office for the Eastern Mediterranean) and enhancing intersectoral collaboration *(170)*.

This work supports the implementation of World Health Assembly resolutions on the prevention and control of soil-transmitted helminthiases, dengue and leishmaniasis, and the improvement of health through safe management of waste and obsolete chemicals.

We have continued our close collaboration with Member States in the past year in the area of influenza and other high threat pathogens. We conducted a review of high impact outbreaks in the Region during the past decade. We have also carried out combined surveillance with the ECDC resulting in the publication of the joint Flu News Europe bulletin for the third consecutive season.

We have made significant progress in implementing the Pandemic Influenza Preparedness (PIP) Framework, and we have strengthened national systems for influenza surveillance and outbreak response, including the development of guidelines for the treatment of severe respiratory illness in five recipient countries.

The Regional Office has also been very active in the prevention and control of seasonal influenza. It published guidance for managing outbreaks in long-term care facilities and raised awareness for seasonal influenza vaccination by conducting our fourth Flu Awareness Campaign in 11 countries.

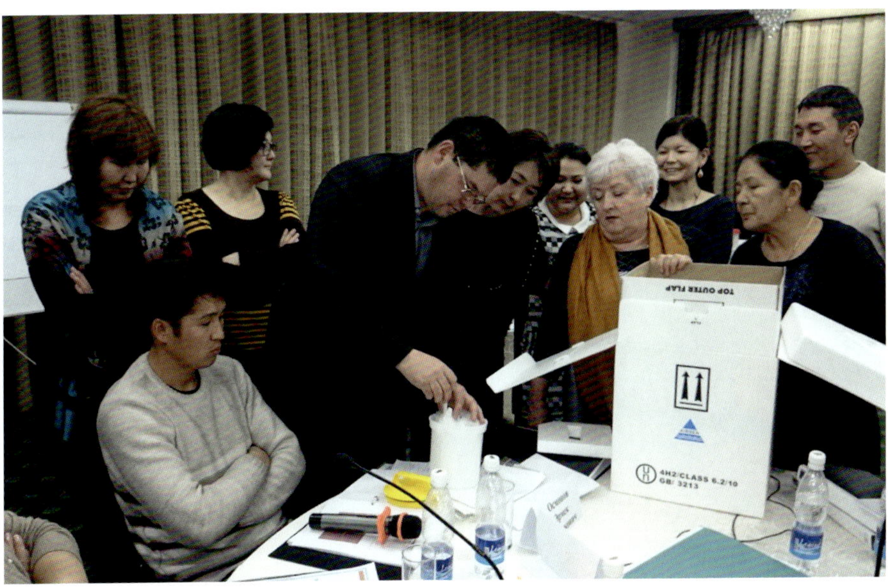

Biorisk management and infectious substances shipping training for specialists in Kyrgyzstan as part of the Pandemic Influenza Preparedness Framework Partnership Contribution Implementation Plan 2013–2016, 1–4 December 2015. © WHO

Fifty Member States, however, have provided data showing a declining use of seasonal influenza vaccine across the Region since 2009. This is worrying not only because of the risk of severe disease and death which may be caused by influenza, but also because of the potential negative impact on pandemic preparedness in the long-term.

The Better Labs for Better Health initiative is building laboratory core capacities: five countries developed national policies and three are implementing operational plans on licensing and accreditation, and sample referral and transport. One country has improved its national curriculum for laboratory managers and eight countries are receiving mentoring in lab quality.

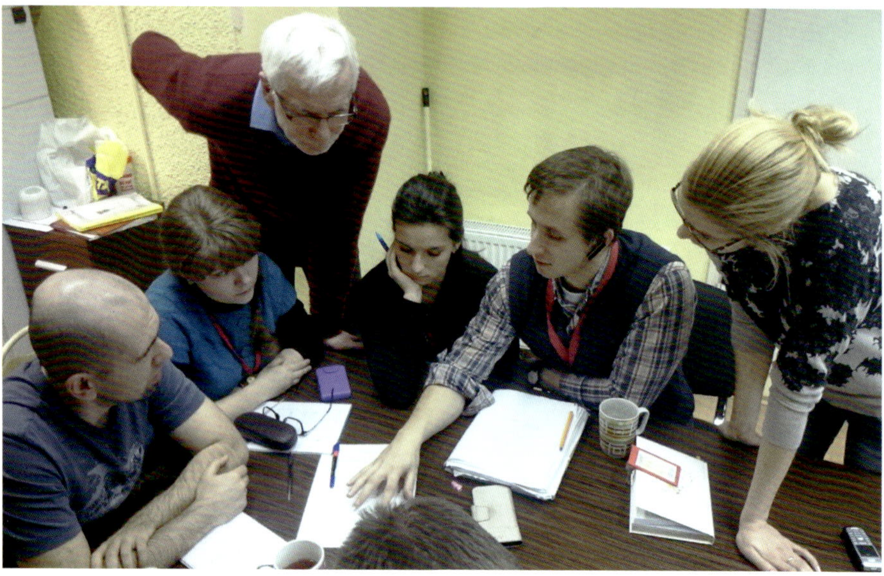

Under the Better Labs for Better Health initiative, staff at the WHO National Influenza Centre of Russia in St Petersburg, Russian Federation, received training in internal laboratory auditing and performed a risk assessment exercise, 29 February–4 March 2016. © WHO

9.3.4 Strengthening people-centred health systems, public health capacity and emergency preparedness, surveillance and response

Consistent with the drive to achieve UHC, the Regional Office has focused on health services as an important determinant of health. We must offer people higher quality, integrated and people centred safe health services that meet their needs and preferences. These services should provide the full range of interventions including health promotion, disease prevention, treatment, rehabilitation and palliative care.

The Regional Office has developed several new tools and areas of work to support countries to lead and manage this transformation.

9.3.4.1 Coordinated and integrated health services delivery

We are committed to the implementation of a new *European Framework for Action towards Coordinated and Integrated Health Service Delivery (CIHSD)* focused on people-centred care and the appropriate use of treatments and medicines *(171)*. This has been developed through an iterative and consultative process with the Member States. The Framework identifies ways to improve coverage of core services and remove barriers that limit access and quality of care for all.

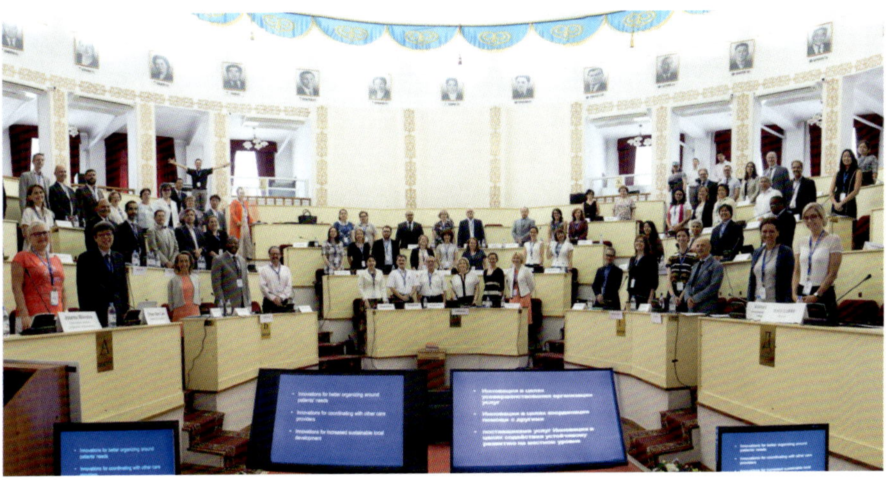

Country delegates from nearly 30 European countries and experts from around the world convened in Almaty, Kazakhstan, 22–23 June 2017, to exchange lessons learned from integrated health services delivery initiatives. © WHO

The Framework aims to create health systems that are sustainable, fit for purpose, people-centred and evidence-informed. This requires prioritizing disease prevention; integrated service delivery; continuity of care; continual quality improvement; support for self-care by patients; and, community care provided as close to home as is safe and cost–effective.

Our vision of primary health care, fully integrated with public health, is at the centre of this work. Every five years we have revisited and celebrated the Alma-Ata Declaration in our Region to keep primary health care high on our agenda. That vision was renewed at a global meeting in Astana, Kazakhstan in October 2018 to mark the 40th anniversary of the Alma-Ata Declaration on primary health care (see Section 9.3.4.6).

Astana meeting outputs

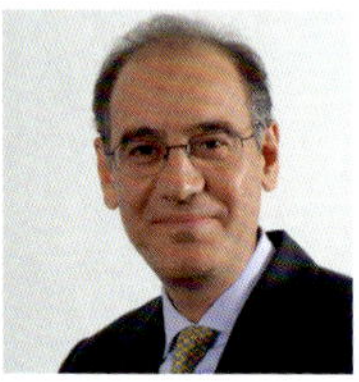

This meeting brought much-needed energy and direction to our global health system development debates. It was indeed timely and important for three reasons.

First of all, it clearly reaffirmed primary health care services as the core of integrated health systems and the critical element for realizing universal health coverage.

Secondly it emphasized the need for more rapid and effective translation of research to practice and implementation. There was a call for national policy-makers to work with academic institutions and others to identify ways to implement globally emerging public health evidence which might be useful in their countries, taking into account contextual differences that exist.

And thirdly the new Astana Declaration provides for a global recommitment to the principles of the Alma-Ata Declaration and should play an important role in shaping the global health agenda going forward.

Rifat Atun, Professor of Global Health Systems, Harvard University, USA

Other important areas of health systems strengthening include: enhancing human resources for health in line with the WHO Global Code of Practice on International Recruitment of Health Personnel; assessing the rational use of medicines and health products and their affordability; and safeguarding quality of services and patient safety. Also important is making full use of modern tools and innovations such as communication technology and social media, and digitalization of health including medical records, telemedicine, and e-health (see Section 9.3.4.8).

9.3.4.2 Support for implementing the Tallinn Charter

Marking the 10–year anniversary of the signing of the Tallinn Charter, the Office held a high-level technical meeting again in Tallinn in June 2018 to review progress, with a focus on 'include, invest and innovate'.

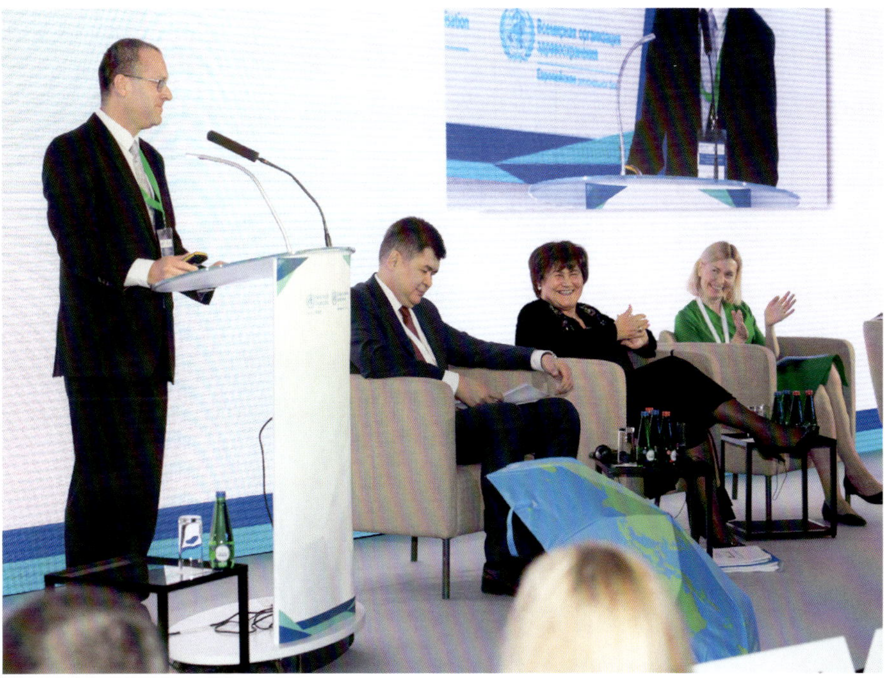

Hans Kluge, Director, Health Systems and Public Health Services speaking at the WHO high-level regional meeting, Health Systems for Prosperity and Solidarity: leaving no one behind. Panel included: Yelzhan Birtanov, Minister of Healthcare, Kazakhstan; Zsuzsanna Jakab, WHO Regional Director for Europe; and, Riina Sikkut, Minister of Health and Labour, Estonia. 13-14 June 2018, Tallinn, Estonia. © WHO/Erik Peinar

PART 2

Not glib statements

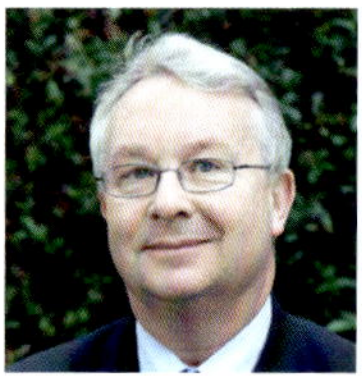

I would say that all three Tallinn conferences have been very heavily based on evidence and have produced really quite original thinking. They have pushed forward the boundaries of how we conceptualize health systems and the ideas of 'include, invest and innovate' at the most recent Tallinn conference on health systems. These are not just glib statements. These are backed up by very solid evidence, and I think we are now seeing that symbiotic relationship where WHO is drawing on high-quality evidence from researchers, but at the same time is helping to set the agenda and ask the policy relevant questions. This two-way process has been the biggest change that I've seen I think in the last ten years.

Martin McKee, Professor of European Public Health, London School of Hygiene and Tropical Medicine (LSHTM), United Kingdom

The objectives were to celebrate the Tallinn Charter and its achievements, reflect on progress in health systems strengthening in the WHO European Region; and outline potential future directions for health systems in Europe.

Health 2020 reaffirms the central principles of the Tallinn Charter by putting forward both a vision and actions for health system strengthening. Health 2020 implementation actions have aimed to improve the performance of health systems through innovative approaches that reinforce core health system functions, while allowing systems to stay resilient to economic downturns.

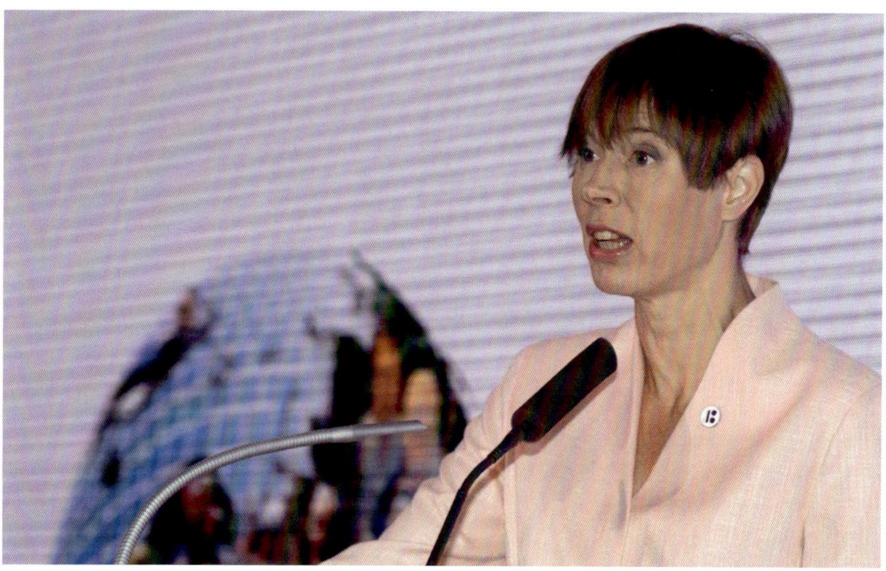

Kersti Kaljulaid, President of Estonia, addresses WHO high-level regional meeting, Health Systems for Prosperity and Solidarity: leaving no one behind, Tallinn, Estonia 13–14 June 2018. © WHO /Erik Peinar

9.3.4.3 Economics, the financial crisis and austerity

The Regional Office has invested substantially in identifying and communicating about the health consequences and impacts of the economic and financial crises and the austerity and economic efficiency measures taken in response in different Member States. This work has been supported by both the European Observatory on Health Systems and Policies and the WHO Barcelona Office for Health Systems Strengthening.

Addressing the financial crisis

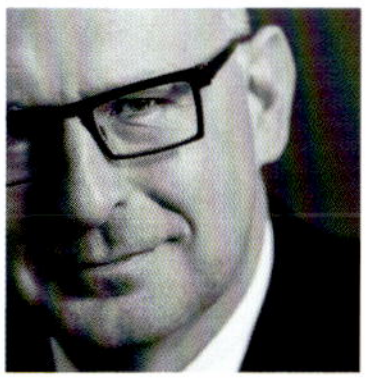

Following the financial crisis, the WHO Regional Office for Europe took significant steps to put health on Europe's political agenda by drawing attention to the impact of the economic crisis and austerity on health and health care. In 2013, the Office organized an important conference on the impact of the crisis on health systems and developed improved methods to evaluate access to health care and its impact on health.

Tom Auwers, Secretary General, Federal Ministry of Health, Food Safety and Environment, Belgium

In 2013 we held a high-level meeting in Oslo to review the impact of the ongoing economic crisis on health and health systems across the Region *(172)*. The Oslo review showed that where there is political will, it is possible for health systems to address inefficiencies such as high drug prices. It has also shown us that coverage reductions can undermine equitable access to needed health services, which causes suffering for many individuals – particularly poorer people but also those who rely on regular access to health care, for example, people with chronic conditions. The clear message is that policies should focus on addressing inefficiencies and avoid damaging access to effective services.

There are, however, limits to how much can be achieved through increased efficiency. Studies show that whilst efficiency gains can absorb some budget reductions, sustained financial pressure may result in policies that damage access to needed services. And ultimately, efficiency gains may not be enough to bridge the gap between revenue and expenditure. Additionally, some of the deeper structural reforms health system need are difficult to make under financial and time pressure because they require additional investment and may not deliver savings immediately.

The Oslo review concluded that countries need to find ways to secure additional revenue for the health system, especially countries in which health spending is already low by European standards. It also highlighted the crucial role of governance – not only in strengthening health systems generally – but in ensuring they are resilient when they come under pressure.

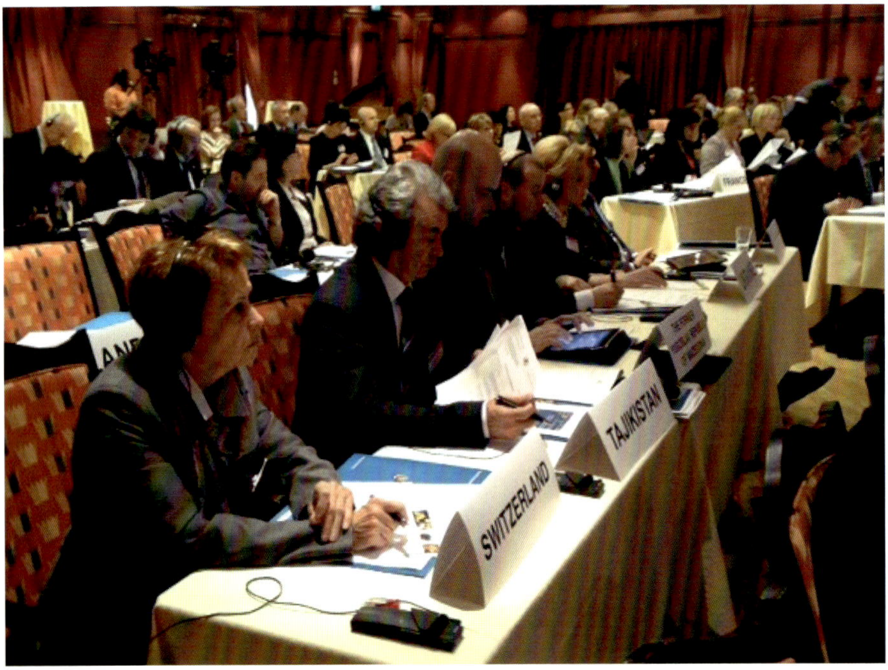

Delegates at the high-level technical meeting on health systems to review the impact of the ongoing economic crisis on health and health systems across the Region, held in Oslo, Norway, on 17–18 April, 2013. © WHO/Mellita Jakab

There is also good evidence that a wide range of preventive approaches are cost-effective in both the short and longer term. These include interventions that address the environmental and social determinants of health, build resilience and promote healthy behaviours, as well as vaccination and screening. In addition, investing in public health generates cost-effective health outcomes and can contribute to wider sustainability, with economic, social and environmental benefits *(173)*.

A key test for good governance is to ensure that policy actions in the short term are consistent with health system goals in the longer term, for example moving towards and sustaining UHC; protecting access; preventing financial hardship; promoting and prioritizing cost–effective services; ensuring people-centred, coordinated service delivery-based on primary and community care; protecting what works well; and addressing inefficiencies rather than damaging access.

And of course, good governance relies on strong information and monitoring systems. Here, the crisis has confirmed what we already knew, namely that our health information systems are not always fit for purpose. Often, we do not have the data we need and, where there is data, it may not be timely. We need to be thinking now of ways to address this issue in the longer term, but we should also be sure we are making full use of the information currently available.

Health 2020 implementation experience has shown that achievement of all these goals will require much political, managerial, professional and public commitment, as well as close collaboration with partners and stakeholders.

Seeking economic solutions

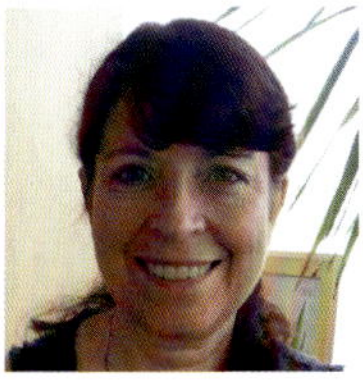

In 2014, after the financial crises, we were looking for solutions to make our health system more resilient and sustainable. Discussions were going on among all key stakeholders and it became evident that too often they were based on perceptions rather than on solid evidence.

It had been identified at the Ministry that an objective analysis of all components of the health system should be made immediately, using figures as well as qualitative information, as a background for the reform proposals.

Based on very good cooperation in the past it was decided that we would do the analysis with WHO Regional Office and European Observatory for Health Systems and Policies. The response of the organizations was immediate and several international experts were mobilized to do the job in 2015.

The process was very inclusive and at least 60 Slovenian experts were included in the focus groups and writing of final papers on financing, purchasing, service delivery and long-term care. In less than one year the analysis was there and was used for the development of our National Health Care Plan 2016–2025, which was adopted by the parliament. This common venture was immensely important to reach consensus among stakeholders on what were the priorities and possible solutions.

Vesna-Kerstin Petrič, Head, Division for Health Promotion and Prevention of Noncommunicable Diseases, Ministry of Health, Slovenia

PART 2

9.3.3.4 Implementing universal health coverage (UHC)

UHC has become a major goal for health reform in many countries and a priority objective of WHO. UHC is defined as ensuring that all people have access to needed health services (including prevention, promotion, treatment, rehabilitation and palliation) of sufficient quality to be effective while also ensuring that the use of these services does not expose the user to financial hardship. Making progress towards UHC will play a major role in reducing health inequities by promoting equity of access and outcomes. As Dr Tedros has said: "No one should get sick and die just because they are poor, or because they cannot access the health services they need."

Health 2020 identified UHC as a core political objective which should guide the strengthening work of health systems. One core component of UHC is financial protection, as out-of-pocket payments can create a financial barrier to access, resulting in unmet need, and lead to financial hardship among people using health services, including medicines. The WHO Regional Office for Europe has worked extensively with Member States to monitor financial protection and find ways of reducing out-of-pocket payments for the people most in need of protection.

Instituting UHC in Georgia – creating a paradigm shift

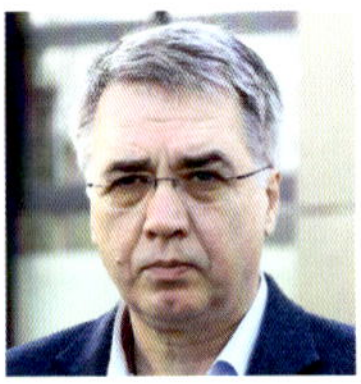

Until recently, UHC was considered a luxury that only rich countries could afford. Low/middle income countries could not even dream about implementation of such general health coverage. In 2012 when our new government came to power we set ourselves the ambitious mission of establishing UHC even though, unfortunately, we belong to low/mid income countries and for us, especially for the Ministry of Health, it was huge challenge as we had an extremely limited budget. We had to look for creative solutions.

Our first thought was to consult WHO and we made contact with the European Office and its Regional Director, Zsuzsanna Jakab. Her reaction was immediate and within an unusually short period of time, two weeks, she arranged for two distinguished experts of global health to come to Georgia to help us.

We worked together as one team for a couple of months, from the end of 2012 to the beginning of 2013. Apart from our own political commitment, this was the main factor that allowed us to tackle the challenge. It was and is extremely important not only for Georgia, but also for global health. This process and engagement, by WHO and ourselves, has created an absolutely new paradigm that we can call 'no one left behind'. Even in low/mid income countries health and health care can no longer be seen as a privilege for the few but a right for everyone. UHC is not a luxury but the most cost–effective approach to tackle the challenges of health care.

To implement this programme requires a variety of elements. A key mandatory factor is a financial budget, but that is not sufficient on its own. An ability to manage the project is essential. How to implement it? How to utilize resources correctly? How to tackle health care needs of the 50% of population who were not covered before?

Almost immediately, within a few months, the number of people who could apply for medical services doubled. Before the implementation of the programme, 50% of Georgians were paying the full cost out of their pockets, so they were only applying for medical services in an emergency, bypassing primary health care, prevention, early detection, etc. Now all Georgians are able to access services for prevention, early detection of diseases and the governmental programme.

We have had to overcome several obstacles to be able to sustain these changes. The first has been the rising costs of health care globally, as technologies develop and become more expensive. Another has been general inflation in Georgian economy. Thirdly, there is the health care paradox, where supply creates demand. In 2013, we went back to WHO for help in developing a single-payer governmental system where one institution supplies the health care needs of the population. This has allowed us to shape our services and keep expenditure within our budget.

In May 2017, new criteria for differentiation of beneficiaries (according to beneficiaries' revenue) have been implemented for provision of more needs orientated services and development of a 'social justice' approach. From July 2017, persons suffering from chronic conditions became eligible for the state programme providing drugs for chronic conditions.

David Sergeenko, Minister of Internally Displaced Persons from the Occupied Territories, Labour, Health and Social Affairs, Georgia

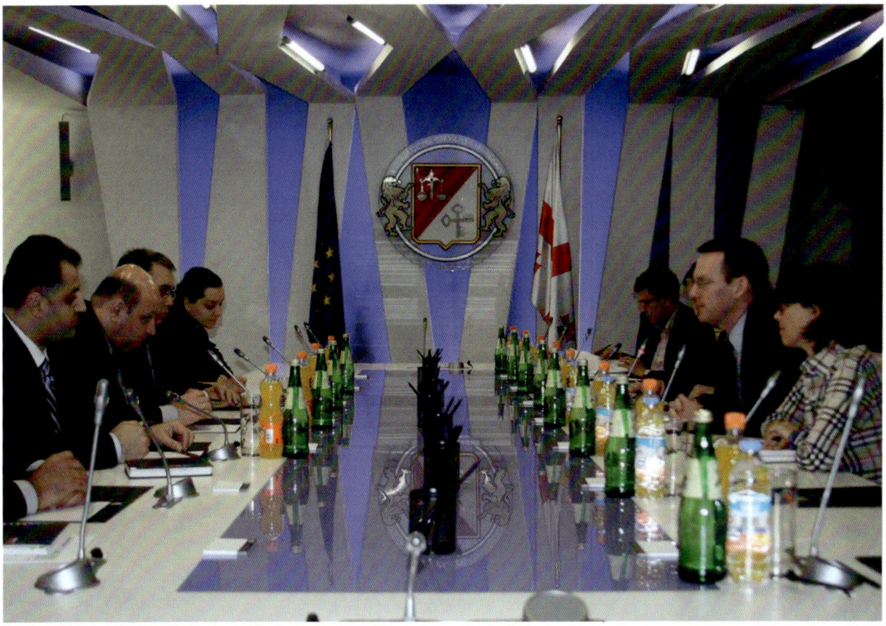

Advisors from WHO Regional Office for Europe, the World Bank and the United States Agency for International Development meeting with the Georgian Government on 4–6 December 2012 to discuss and advise on measures to establish a universal benefit package of health services for the population. © Ministry of Finance of Georgia/ Tea Begiashvili

PART 2

UHC pilot project in Tajikistan

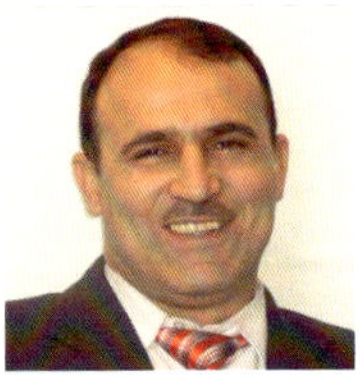

With the support of WHO Regional Office for Europe, the Republic of Tajikistan was selected as a pilot country for the introduction of UHC. The mechanism proposed aimed for achievement of the best results with the least cost, through rational use of resources for coverage of everyone by different kind of services.

WHO Guidelines, proposed in the framework of services coverage, were adapted to consider the specific context of Tajikistan with special attention to health promotion, prevention of diseases and treatment, with indicators linked to those controlled by our Ministry in the framework of our 2010–20 National Health Strategy.

As for the financial aspects of UHC, it was agreed to define indicators based on the WHO Regional Office for Europe methodology developed by the WHO Barcelona Office *(174)*. There are three key types of indicators: catastrophic costs, impoverishment, and unmet needs. These indicators are focused on payments for health care and associated costs at the expense of households.

Salomudin Jabbor Yusufi, Head of the Department of Medical and Pharmaceutical Education, Health Personnel Policy and Science Ministry of Health and Social Protection, Republic of Tajikistan

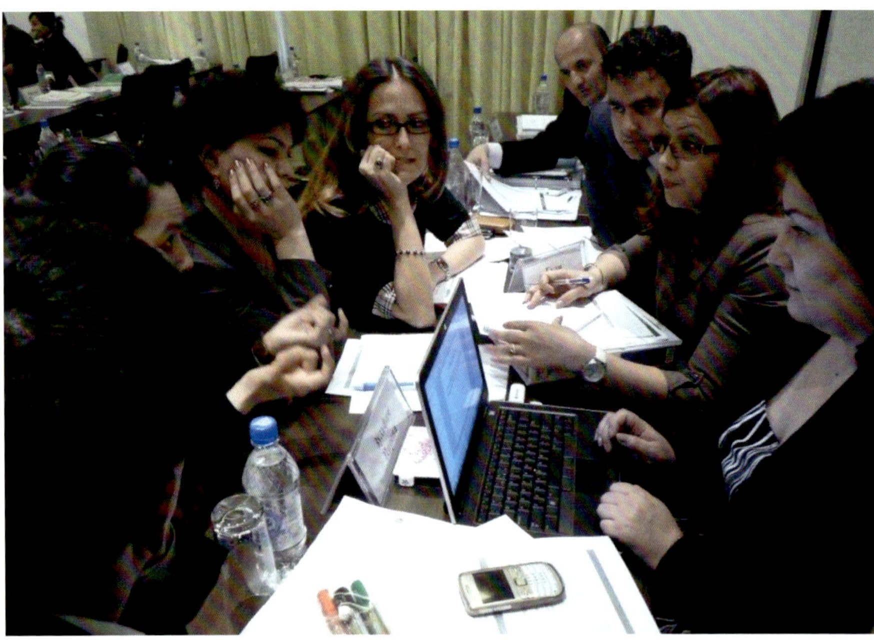

Participants from health sector gathered around a computer discussing ideas at a training course on moving forward towards UHC. Tajikistan, 15 April 2014. © WHO/Tahmina Alimamedova

9.3.4.5 Financing for universal health coverage (UHC)

In 2016 the Regional Office stepped up efforts to generate evidence to support UHC, initiating a new programme of work to monitor coverage, access and financial protection across the Region.

The question of whether people can afford to pay for health care is central to UHC. In the past, however, monitoring of this crucial dimension of health system performance has focused on barriers to access without considering the financial hardship people experience when they use health services and require medicines and health products.

To address this major gap in health system performance assessment, the Regional Office has developed work in three areas:

1. Developing measures of financial hardship that are more suited to high- and middle-income countries and using these to generate actionable evidence in all the Region's Member States. We have developed these refined metrics through wide consultation and discussed them at the International Health Economics Association (IHEA) Conference in Boston in June 2018.
2. Working with national experts in 25 countries to provide context-specific analysis and carefully tailored recommendations for national policy development. This includes concrete guidance on how to reduce out-of-pocket payments, especially for medicines. Several countries benefitted from the policy recommendations based on these country-specific reports and related policy dialogues.
3. Drawing lessons from and for the Region through a regional assessment of coverage, access and financial protection. The Regional Office presented the findings from the regional analysis at the high-level conference to celebrate the 10th anniversary of the Tallinn Charter. While some of the Member States progress well, we still have a long way to go to achieve our target: a Europe free of impoverishing out-of-pocket payments for health. In the countries covered by the study, the share of households impoverished or further impoverished due to out-of-pocket payments ranged between 0.3% and 9%. Overall the study suggests that it is possible to avoid poverty due to ill-health through a combination of higher public spending and pro-poor coverage policies. In 2019, the first-ever regional report on financial protection in Europe was published on World Health Day.

As important has been our Barcelona course on health financing for UHC which has been running since 2011 and has trained more than 600 government officials and experts from across the European Region and beyond (see Developmental reflection 7).

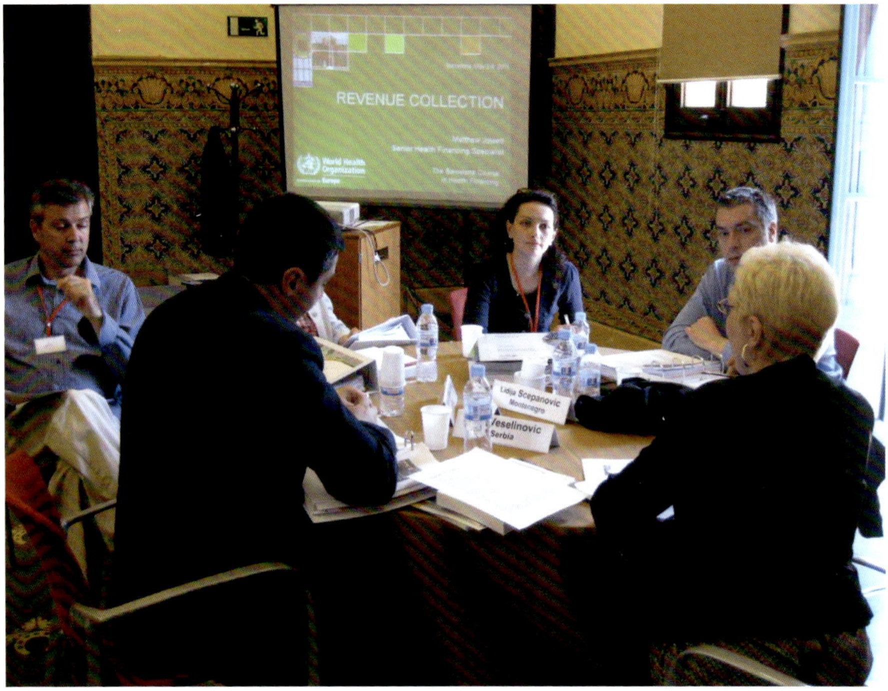

The second WHO Barcelona course on health financing was held 14–18 May 2012, Barcelona, Spain. The course reviewed effective policy instruments to improve health system performance through better health financing policy. A special theme of the course was moving towards and sustaining UHC, with a highlight on how to counter the impact of economic downturns. © WHO

Developmental reflection 7

WHO Barcelona course on health financing for UHC.

The WHO Barcelona course on health financing for universal health coverage is one of the most sought-after products of our Office. It stands out with its high-quality programme and has had excellent feedback from participants and significant policy impact.

We launched this WHO course in 2011 for the first time. It is a one-week course which targets policy-makers and those who support decision-making in ministries of health, finance, other government agencies, and health insurance agencies. We have found this to be a very effective platform, not just for capacity-building, but also to communicate key policy messages related to UHC. It allows us to reach more countries than what we could otherwise advise on a one-to-one country-specific basis. In addition to the materials, participants also enjoy exchanging information and experience with each other.

By focusing on the real daily challenges of developing and implementing health financing systems, it provides a unique learning environment for participants.

We have also run country-specific courses where we get different stakeholders together and seek to create consensus.

The course is based on a systematic framework that participants can use to problem solve when they go back to their countries. In addition, we rely extensively on country case studies and narratives of reform experiences. We also include a pre-course health financing exercise identifying and analysing a problem, which is further developed during the course and then implemented when participants go back to their country.

Combining country work with this regional capacity-building effort over time has allowed us to have more impact at country level because we have a network of people who have taken our courses, 'talk the same language' and have been systematically applying their learning in their own contexts.

Much appreciated by those people who attend, these courses have an overall rating of 4.8/5, both in terms of content and delivery. The demand for our course typically exceeds three times the number of places that we could provide and we are not seeing a drop in demand.

With the prominence of UHC in the agenda of WHO for the years to come, this course and other global and regional variants, will remain a key product for WHO to provide to interested Member States.

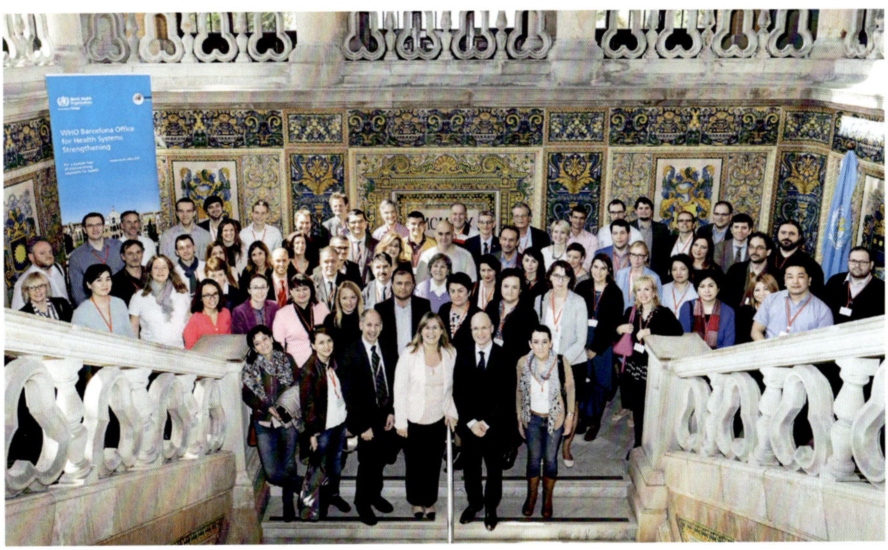

The seventh WHO Barcelona course on health financing for UHC, was held in March 2017 and covered systematic thinking about health systems and health financing with an interactive, practical focus on ways of improving health system performance through better policy analysis, design and implementation. © WHO

9.3.4.6 Developing primary health care models

If we look at the many global health challenges faced by today's societies we can see that traditional approaches based on disease-specific, reactive, fragmented and episodic interventions are no longer appropriate. What we need is a fundamental shift towards a primary health care approach anticipated long ago in Health for All and at the Alma-Ata Conference in 1978 and reaffirmed at the Astana conference in 2018.

This approach promotes health and well-being along the life-course, mitigates risks, and manages the social circumstances of health. Such an approach would empower and engage individuals and communities as partners not as passive recipients. In addition, the health sector alone cannot meet these challenges and needs to be part of a joint effort that includes other sectors including education, social services, transport, etc.

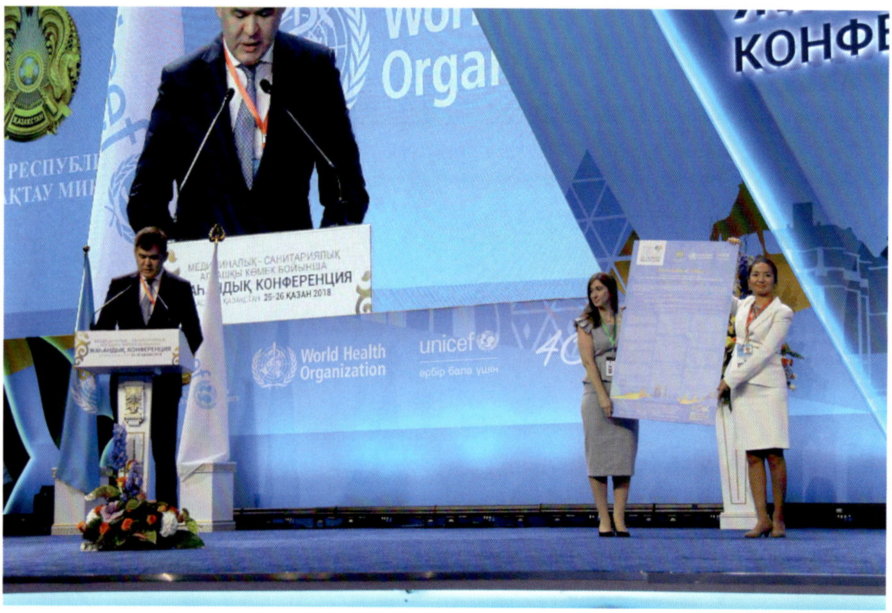

Yelzhan Birtanov, Minister of Healthcare of Kazakhstan, announces the adoption of the Declaration of Astana, at the Global Conference on Primary Health Care, 25–26 October 2018, Kazakhstan. © Ministry of Health, Kazakhstan

From Alma-Ata to Astana

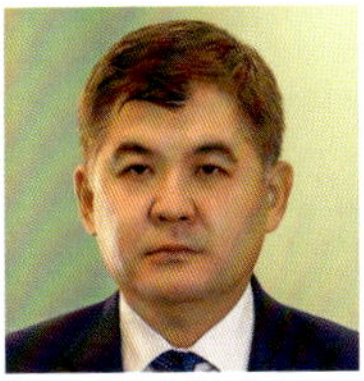

Our partnership with WHO started many years ago with the famous 1978 International conference on primary health care when the Declaration of Alma-Ata was adopted, in which all countries agreed on the essential role primary health care has in health care systems, providing access for the whole population to medical services.

Of course, we are still certain that primary health care should remain as the basis for health care systems to provide universal health care for everyone. But over the last 40 years many global trends have changed health care systems around the world. Therefore, we came back again to Kazakhstan in the new capital, Astana, to talk about the future of primary health care. We adopted the Declaration of Astana on primary health care to illustrate the new directions we should take, including innovations in the areas of biomedical sciences and digital health technologies, to make our primary care more effective.

We are now working intensively on improving our primary health care and making it provide more patient-oriented services. We have also started a new WHO geographically dispersed office on primary health care, which we propose to transform to Global centre for primary health care – this helps us to gather the best ideas and the best experience as to how we can improve primary health care globally, as well as in our country.

Yelzhan Birtanov, Minister of Healthcare, Kazakhstan

The WHO European Centre for Primary Health Care in Almaty (see Developmental reflection 1), is already doing normative global work to develop the global agenda in the implementation of primary health care. One element of work, for example, was to identify key primary health care policy accelerators (see Box 16) prior to the Astana Conference to help develop the new WHO vision on PHC. The Centre also organized an event prior to the conference to review how cities and mayors, together with other 'settings' in which Health for All can be implemented, can contribute to the implementation of primary health care. This global dimension of the work will continue and dependent upon the availability of additional resources it can be further expanded.

BOX 16. Primary health care policy accelerators

1. Realize a population health management approach for integrated public health and primary health care;
2. Adopt a community care model to integrate with social care;
3. Empower communities and engage patients to formulate problems, make decisions and take action;
4. Network providers to ensure responsive and multiprofiled delivery;
5. Invest in the competencies of family doctors and general practitioners and nurses to increase the response capacity of primary health care;
6. Establish learning loops in clinical settings for quality improvement;
7. Ensure the responsible use of medicines;
8. Optimize services with evidence-informed transformations;
9. Upgrade facilities for the optimal use of eHealth and health technologies in primary health care; and,
10. Align accountability and incentives with new models of care *(198)*.

Making the case for investment in primary health care

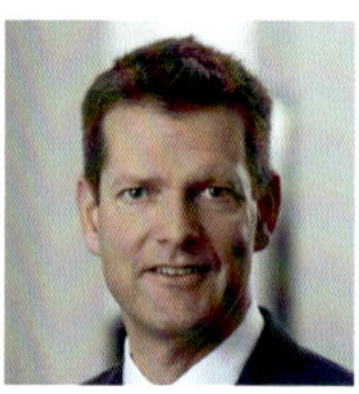

Universal health coverage is a very strong point for us in Denmark, and always has been. We adopted the NHS model from the United Kingdom in the 1970s and converted from insurance-based into the very strong taxpayer-funded equal-access free-of-charge health care system now in place. It has had broad political support from everyone in my country for the last 40–50 years. Whoever is in government, they do not waver from strong support for taxpayer-funded equal-access. But of course, that system has its challenges because it relies on very heavy taxpayer funding, and there is a limit to how much people will pay taxes. That limit has been reached.

So our challenge now is how to continue to provide universal health coverage without increasing taxes. That challenge was increased when we were hit by the financial crisis of 2008. Before that we had net growth of approximately 3% in our health care spending until 2008. And there is even some discussion that our politicians were overspending on health care before the financial crisis hit us. Since then it has gone down to around 1%. On top of that we have a 2% productivity increase annually. But that's not a net growth because we are still challenged by demographic changes; e.g., people live longer and there are more NCDs, that have put more of a burden on health care – so actually we have had negative growth of around 0 or 0.5%. These are our challenges.

In adapting our health care system, I think we have shown that we can adapt under more difficult economic circumstances. We're struggling currently, because the hospital system cannot take any more patients, and we have to reinvent, refocus our primary health care. We are not the only ones facing this big challenge. We can use our collaborations and contributions within the European Region to help tackle these challenges. That is why, when I was contacted by the Regional Office to collaborate on a Task Force for primary health care, I was very happy to agree. It is one of our strong points, even though we do not have any solutions in Denmark, it is something we are thinking about ourselves.

I agreed with the Regional Office that Denmark would be a major contributor to the work of that Task Force which is basically going to make the case for investment in primary health care for a stronger health care system in the future.

Søren Brostrøm, Director General, Danish Health Authority, Denmark

9.3.4.7 Health systems and NCDs

The Regional Office, the European Observatory for Health Systems and Policies and the OECD have undertaken a lot of work in this area, showing that promoting health and preventing chronic diseases through interventions aimed at modifying individual behavioural risk factors is possible, and cost-effective.

During the period 2012–2014 we developed an ambitious multidisciplinary programme – 'Strengthening Health Systems, Supporting NCD Action' – to enable health systems to respond effectively to the growing burden of NCDs. This multidisciplinary and interdivisional work programme was motivated by increasing calls from Member States for a comprehensive health system response to NCDs (see Developmental reflection 8).

The Regional Office completed multidisciplinary country assessments as entry points in 13 countries and focused on sharing a series of good practices and effective instruments with country base teams. Several needs emerged in the countries assessed, including universal access to essential medicines; helping working age men with high NCD burden and yet low to no utilisation of services; responding to the currently low rates of cardiovascular risk assessment and quality management; and inappropriate use of cancer screening.

The Office has also carried out capacity-building in the form of an annual training programme based at the WHO Barcelona Office reaching more than 300 participants.

Developmental reflection 8

NCDs, health systems and change management

Our pioneering work programme on strengthening health system response to NCDs, one of the first major interdivisional and interprogrammatic initiatives of its kind, has shown the way forward. This more comprehensive way of working has now become the new standard in the WHO Regional Office for Europe.

Our Health Systems and NCD divisions have been working together on this programme since 2013. Our aim was to strengthen our capacities to give more practical and pragmatic advice on health system strengthening by looking through the lens of specific health conditions. We also looked for ways to make all our disease-specific work more system-oriented. For the first five years, we carried out country specific missions with multidisciplinary teams with the aim of developing and providing pragmatic and actionable recommendations on health system strengthening for combating NCDs. Our international multidisciplinary teams were mirrored by national multidisciplinary teams. We worked together to make a consensus-based assessment of the main health system barriers and good practices in implementing the NCDs 'best buys'.

What we found when we went to many countries was that they had a lot of disease-specific plans. They had a diabetes plan, a cardiovascular plan, a stroke plan, a hypertension plan, an obesity plan, and they were all trying to do the same thing. The content was, essentially, identical and they all needed to involve the same primary health care and health promotion units to develop the same kind of support services. To get people to stop smoking, for example, was part of every hypertension, stroke etc. plan. The individual disease-based plans were fragmented and did not have much clout. So, our teams started working on an umbrella NCD policy framework which identified the health system support elements that were needed.

In each case we followed it up with a big policy workshop that often brought a lot of attention to these issues, even from parliament. Member States loved it because it was interdisciplinary. They were congratulating us for finally stepping out of our silos: we were congratulating them for stepping out of theirs. We synthesized these experiences into a regional report *Health systems respond to noncommunicable diseases: time for ambition (175)* and a high level regional meeting in Sitges, Spain. Both have been very well received.

Most importantly, we found that people were excited to connect their programmatic work to something larger. They found that they could keep doing their good, programmatic work, for example, on primary care and or on health workforces, but now reframe it as part of a 'larger' comprehensive health system response to NCDs.

We learned from this experience that people wanted to work more widely. We also learned that structural barriers could be overcome with good will. When there were enthusiastic people who were both willing and wanting to put their programmatic budget towards this kind of interdisciplinary type of work it could be done.

This was an important lesson for us as we now start looking at the transformation agenda of the Director-General and GPW13 which is really all about breaking down the programmatic silos that cross the organization and finding new ways to work together.

We learned that two essential components of managing such a change are having very strong top-level management support, and some very enthusiastic people.

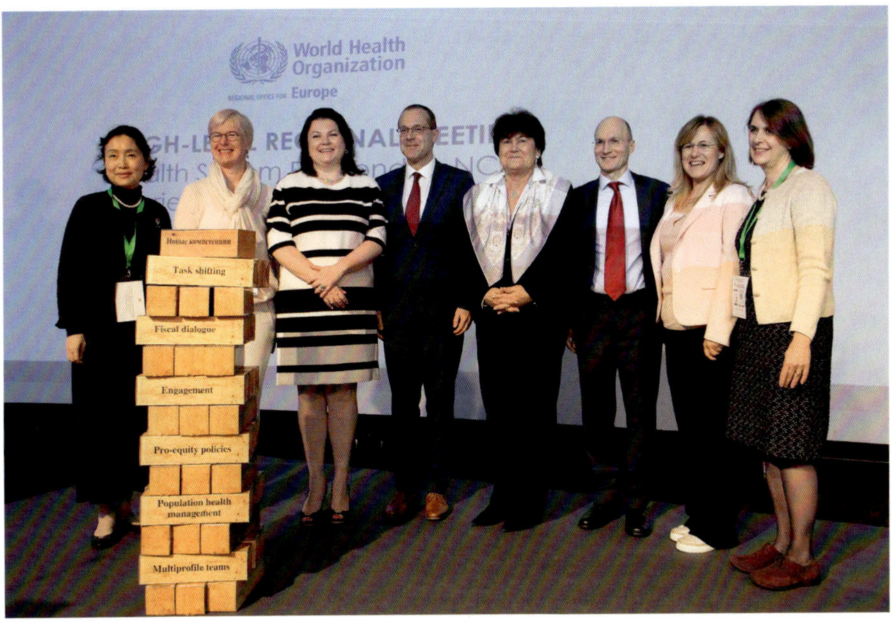

The high-level regional meeting - Health Systems Respond to NCDs - provided policy-makers with a platform to share country experiences of strengthening health systems for better NCD outcomes, celebrate and understand successes, and inspire action for accelerating health systems transformation to reduce premature NCD-related mortality. 16–18 April 2018, Sitges, Spain. © WHO\Joan Valera

9.3.4.8 Digitalization of health systems

I firmly believe that digitalizing health systems is a key component in achieving UHC. Digital health can improve the reach, impact and efficiency of modern health care and the delivery of patient-centred services, and support health professionals and institutions to be more effective and efficient. It can empower communities and individuals to improve their health and well-being in unprecedented ways, in environments that are comfortable and familiar, bringing care closer to home and out of hospitals and at times that are convenient. Smart devices have a developing role in the tracking, management and improvement of health.

However, there are challenges which we need to tackle when extending digital health. They relate to governance: for example, confidentiality; who holds and owns the data; how the data is used and by whom; what policies are followed in this regard; and what are the regulations and the legislation in place governing these issues.

We held a symposium, co-sponsored by the Norwegian Centre for e-Health Research, on the Future of Digital Health Systems in the European Region in Copenhagen, in February 2019 to share country experience and gather input in a process to inform new global initiatives in this are; to develop guidance for our Member States; and to expand collaboration and sharing of good practices across and beyond the region.

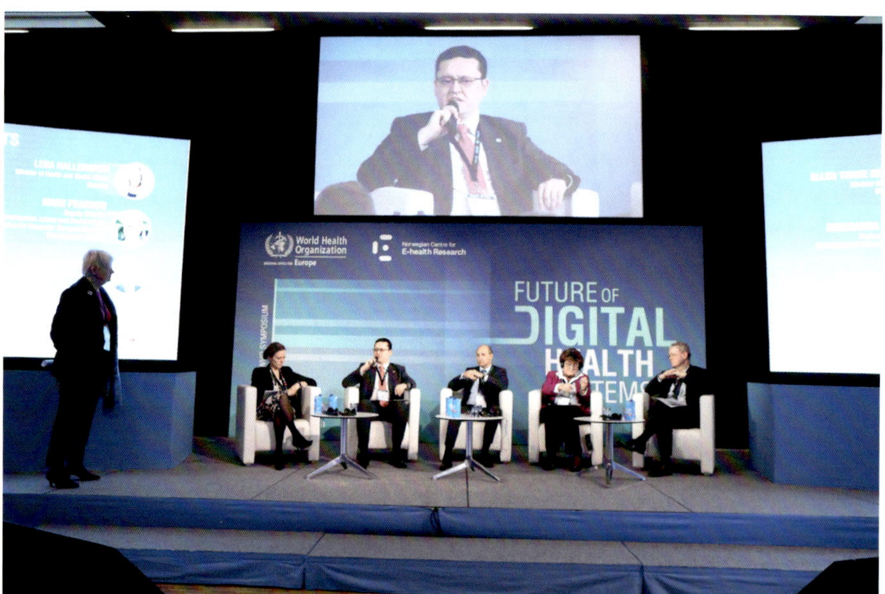

Opening panel on the digitalization of national health systems at the WHO Symposium on the Future of Digital Health Systems in the European Region, Copenhagen, Denmark 6–8 February 2019. © WHO

Visionary and courageous

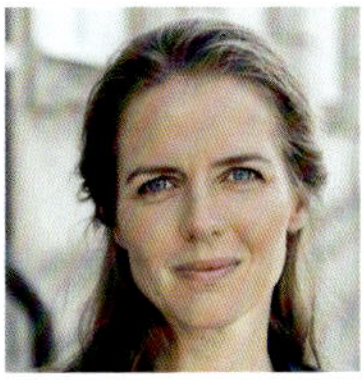

Digitalization has helped us create a wide variety of tools to make our health and health care easier. A very recent example is our nationwide 'My Doctor's App' which facilitates the exchange between patients and family doctors, saves time in the waiting rooms, and can provide the same functions and information as the websites of doctors.

Another example is the app called the Medicine Card [Medicinkortet], where you can just swipe to request a renewal of your medical prescription.

Another example is the web portal sundhed.dk, launched in 2003, which allows patients to access and take control of their health data.

Like many other countries, we are working to release the full potential of digital technologies to support predictive and personal care. We see huge potentials here.

We also understand the need to take political responsibility and show political leadership in this field. We need to be visionary and courageous.

We need to embrace digitalization and the world of opportunities it provides, but also set boundaries where we see that this is not the way that we should go forward.

We need to have a strong political focus on the regulation that is needed. Otherwise, we will not reach the goals we would like to see, where digitalization can provide better health care for all our citizens.

Ellen Trane Nørby, Minister for Health, Denmark

Health systems without digitalization will become obsolete

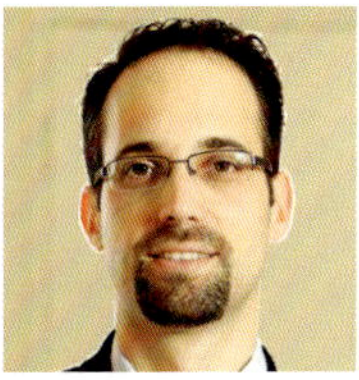

The current functioning structure of most health care systems is unsustainable by design. We do not have enough workforce or funding to sustain the current model of health care provision while maintaining the basic core values that drive us and WHO: solidarity, universal access, and equity.

When we look closely at our health systems, we can see a whole set of futile activities being performed that are wasteful of our scarce resources. There are a lot of opportunities to provide more adequate care being missed. There are far too many mistakes and errors systematically embedded in the way we provide care; most importantly, the continued predominant attention being focused on the therapeutic, reactive approaches rather than the preventive, proactive approaches which are much more sustainable in the longer term in this era of noncommunicable disease multi-morbidity.

The only way to go beyond that and to truly be able to provide universal, equitable access to effective care is by making some profound changes in the way health care is provided and to push forward a new meaningful digital agenda.

Led by RD Zsuzsanna Jakab and her Division Heads, WHO has been active in supporting this strategic thinking from very early on. Our Clalit WHO Collaborating Centre on NCD Research, Prevention and Control is focused on innovative digital ways of looking at the most basic problems of the way health systems deal with NCDs. At the Clalit Research Institute we have about fifty data scientists, epidemiologists, clinicians and mathematicians all working together in ad hoc groups trying to solve key questions and create new digital tools to allow better tackling of noncommunicable disease prevention and control.

Take, for example, chronic kidney disease. The usual way of tackling people already symptomatic with chronic kidney disease taught us that it is too late to make a true impact on the morbidity incidence curves of end-stage renal disease. We knew that to be effective we needed to be preventive in approach and predictive. We needed to identify and intervene early when the patient is still asymptomatic but is already experiencing the first level steps of the cascade that would bring him/her in five years towards renal failure.

We created predictive models based on phenotypic data, usual data from the electronic medical record and lab tests, that allows you to identify those patients. We then tackle them early through several not-costly and not-complex changes: in the medications they are receiving, in the way they handle and balance their other chronic diseases like diabetes and hypertension, and by refraining from risky behaviours and treatments like getting contrast during some of their imaging tests.

Through such changes we are able to redirect them from a course that was taking them downhill towards the inevitable end of chronic renal disease and renal failure. We started implementing this programme in 2011 in our 1500 outpatient clinics serving 4.5 million people across Israel (more than half the Israeli population). We are now already able to measure some of the impact on reducing the rates of new cases of renal failures in Israel.

We have had several obstacles to overcome. When we started this, the concepts of predictive modelling in health care were not yet spoken about; they were completely 'out of the box'. People were not always comfortable with doing these kinds of data-driven health care decision-making processes.

Secondly, physicians do not trust black boxes. They want to understand why some patients are flagged and others are not, and what is the patho-physiological process that leads you to the understanding that a patient is at risk. So we had to re-engineer the models to explain to them why specific patients were at risk. We had to go to educate the physicians about this new tool. And finally, you have to meld these kinds of interventions into the usual care processes, otherwise physicians would not want to add to their already hectic and over-burdened everyday work load. We really had to integrate this process into the usual care patterns, into their electronic medical records, as seamlessly as possible. When you come to a single primary-care physician, then the large numbers of patients at risk suddenly become three. And they can deal with three patients, which when done across our whole system can make a massive impact on the society as a whole.

We have now done this for several other diseases. It is becoming the way we conduct business. We have predictive-modelling-based interventions for the at-risk elderly; preventing patients with pre-diabetes becoming diabetic; identifying patients at risk for colon cancer; prioritizing influenza vaccines to those at flu and pneumonia risk; preventing future cases of stroke and of osteoporotic fractures. The list is growing rapidly. We are also now using our data to allow more personalised care and more personalised data-driven treatment selection according to what the data on millions of patients can teach us which goes way beyond the experience of a single physician.

These types of approaches are now in place and we believe that in a few years they will become the mainstay of health care everywhere.

Having an organization like WHO showcase these kinds of new approaches in a very careful and critical way is very important. The WHO Regional Office for Europe has taken on a global leadership role in this area; especially as it fits well with the basic values of affordable universal care, and provides leapfrogging opportunities for less affluent countries. They understand well its potential, and the need for their active participation in helping to set independent governance standards and ensure that the digitalization changes underway maintain and strengthen our core values.

Ran Balicer, Founding Director, Clalit Research Institute and Director of Health Policy Planning at Clalit Health Services, Israel

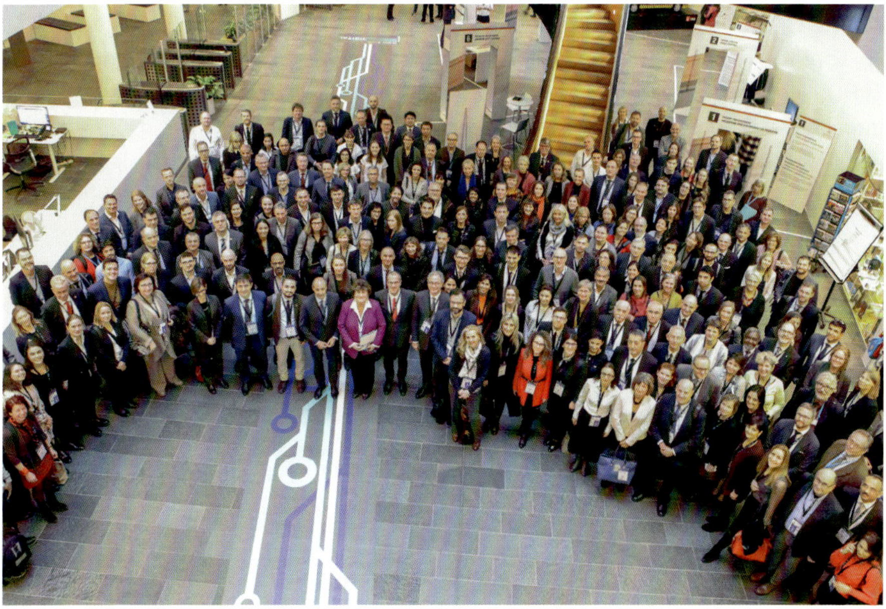

Group photo at the WHO Symposium on the Future of Digital Health Systems in the European Region, Copenhagen, Denmark 6–8 February 2019. © WHO

9.3.4.9 The contribution of public health to Health 2020 and the SDGs

The EPHOs were defined within the European Action Plan for Strengthening Public Health Capacities and Services (EAP-PHS), and subsequently EPHO self-assessment tools were developed. Member States have been using these tools to strengthen public health services in the Region, as a cornerstone of SDG and Health 2020 implementation *(214)*.

The Regional Office has now developed the self-assessment tool in electronic form which has been available since early 2016 *(176)*. It has also been made available in Russian. It allows countries to assess the state of their public health services and capacities, with various stakeholders coming together to look at the provision of public health services in a comprehensive and systematic way. Following this assessment, countries identify the priorities for strengthening public health services, with further technical assistance provided from the Regional Office where appropriate.

Following an evaluation of the EAP-PHS at the Regional Committee, since 2016 countries are increasingly requesting support in strengthening the three 'enabler' EPHOs; assuring governance for health and well-being; assuring a sufficient and competent public health workforce; and assuring sustainable organizational structures and financing. The Regional Office has now started to build a powerful collaboration establishing a Coalition of Partners (CoP) to strengthen these enabler EPHOs in a more coordinated, systematic and proactive way *(177)*. The CoP seeks innovative approaches to public health reform, both in terms of applying expertise and in funding its activities, to support Member States. Importantly the collaboration is directly and continuously informed and driven by Member State needs.

The Coalition of Partners

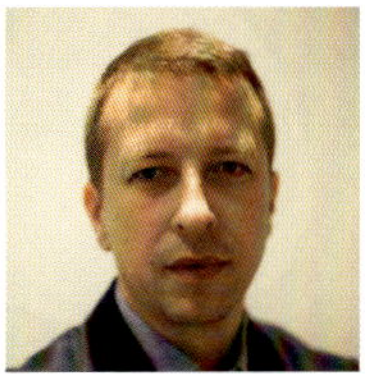

Over the past ten years ASPHER has undergone a veritable 'explosion' of activity (with more than 100% growth) and that's been largely due to our partnership interactions with the WHO policy framework of Health 2020 and the European Action Plan for Strengthening Public Health Capacities and Services. These WHO Regional Office for Europe initiatives and accompanying work have been of great importance and benefit to ASPHER as they really have helped put public health higher on the policy agenda and reposition our European organization globally.

Since the early nineties, with the competency in public health introduced by the Treaty of Maastricht, the EU has made some good efforts and stimulated public health actions around the internal market context and its free movement principles (of people, capital, services and goods). However, it never actually addressed the full extent of public health, nor did it ever provide a clear framework for how all its components should/could operate. This arrived only with the introduction of Health 2020 and the European Action Plan with the EPHOs which have changed everything for us.

Following the mid-term evaluation of Health 2020 and the Action Plan, a new stakeholder platform was created by WHO called the Coalition of Partners for strengthening public health. This is a platform for communicating with different agencies and networks who will then take on further responsibility to become active and involved in implementation. ASPHER continued its focus on EPHO 7, and we worked with partners on the development of a roadmap for public workforce professionalisation and guidelines on how to professionalise the wider workforce context through competency-based education, sound human resource (HR) practices, continuing professional development (CPD) and professional credentials, as well as formalisation and development of codes of professional conduct.

These tools have proved to be of interest to countries and we've now worked several country missions. Some policies have already been implemented and some mechanisms have already been introduced in countries across the WHO European Region.

Another project has been the development of a public health competency framework for the public health workforce to support relevant HR practices. ASPHER has always been involved in the development of competences. Most of this work has been focused on academic settings (our core membership), i.e. schools and programmes of public health. ASPHER's core competences lists have served as guidelines for developing and accrediting curricula and enabling different kinds of exchange and networking between organizations providing training in public health, as well as for individual career and system human capacity planning. However, until now, there has been a lack of knowledge about the standards and competences suitable for work-based HR practices; for recruitment, performance assessment, professional credentialing and CPD. Here I must compliment the Coalition of Partners, which has facilitated access to resources at the country and regional level, as well as mobilized the involvement of relevant networks, such as the International Association of National Public Health Institutes (IANPHI). It has catalysed new opportunities for European Public Health agencies and associations to work together with policy-makers in countries on these issues.

I feel that these initiatives have allowed us, for the first time, to start closing the gap between public health training and practice. For years we have observed the situation in which a large part of the public health workforce lacked any kind of training or education in public health, while on the other hand graduates of public health schools and programmes lacked employment opportunities and clear career paths. Of course, the public health workforce ought to remain multidisciplinary and multi-professional, contributing from across sectors. However, ideally it should allow for a strong sense of identification and belonging, supported by sound professional development. This is now being realized through the work of the Coalition of Partners.

The impact we are making through these programmes has raised the profile of European public health globally. We look forward to sharing our relevant experience with colleagues from around the world at the 2020 European Public Health Conference in Rome, which will serve as a platform for the 16th World Congress on Public Health – the public health meeting of the year 2020!

Robert Otok, Director, Association of Schools of Public Health in the European Region (ASPHER), Belgium

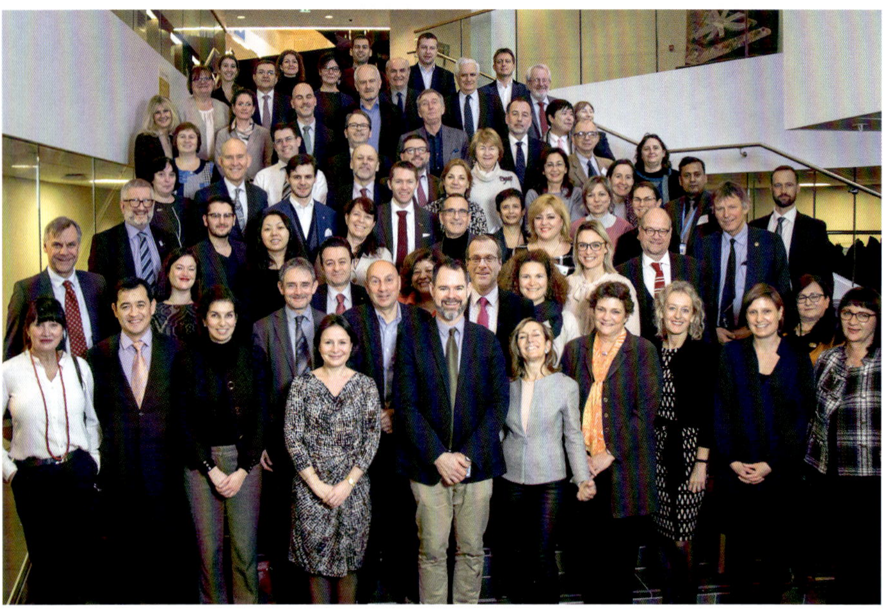

The Coalition of Partners Expert Meeting on Strengthening Public Health Capacities and Services in the European Region at WHO Regional Office for Europe in Copenhagen, Denmark, 2018. © WHO/Lasse Badsberg-Hansen

The CoP and IANPHI

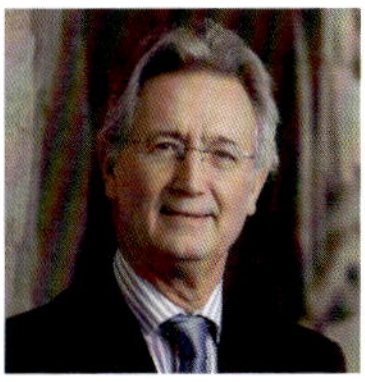

IANPHI is a well identified action partner within the CoP. Together with WHO country offices, for example, IANPHI organized a leadership workshop for the Public Health Center of Ukraine in April 2017, to help support the redesign of its approach and structure.

Our country development work with WHO concentrates on a Staged (peer-to-peer) Development tool. We start by looking at what could be the next step for the public health institute, or what would be best practices that could be used to improve key elements. We focus on assessing and giving help to institutes' movement forward in a staged manner. Most countries appreciate this sort of framing and approach, because we are never judging or saying you are better or worse. We talk colleague to colleague and work to help countries reach the next stage.

I think our partnerships with WHO work well because of our fantastic complementarity. WHO brings normative standards and leadership, the IANPHI brings in experienced national public health institutions and colleagues.

Andre Van der Zande, President of the International Association of National Public health Institutes (IANPHI)

To promote further public health across the Region, I commissioned a new vision for public health in the 21st century, which was adopted by the Regional Committee in 2018 *(51)*. This process helped us rethink the contribution of public health in facing today's complex health problems. Obesity is a good example of such complexity. In tackling such a problem no single intervention will be sufficient on its own. We need coordinated multilevel regulatory and policy interventions at the whole-of-society and whole-of-government level, as well as targeted behavioural interventions at the more individual level. Also, we need to think of interventions across the whole of life-course, and not focus only on adults. To rise to these challenges, we need to enhance the institutional basis for public health practice, as well as promote a public health workforce with new skills of advocacy, negotiation and persuasion.

9.3.4.10 Health emergencies

Every continent is vulnerable to emergencies. Europe is no exception. Every year on average, the WHO Regional Office for Europe receives more than 20 000 warnings of potential health threats, out of which 2 000 require the Organization to conduct formal assessments and about 50, or one every week, need a response.

During the 21st century, Europe's emergencies have become more complex and demanding due to growing global trends. These hit the Region with a wide range of hazards, like measles epidemics; outbreaks of vector-borne diseases; outbreaks of food-borne diseases and growing AMR; floods, heatwaves, forest fires and other extreme events due to climate change; earthquakes and other natural disasters– possibly combined with chemical or nuclear contamination; conflicts and terrorist attacks.

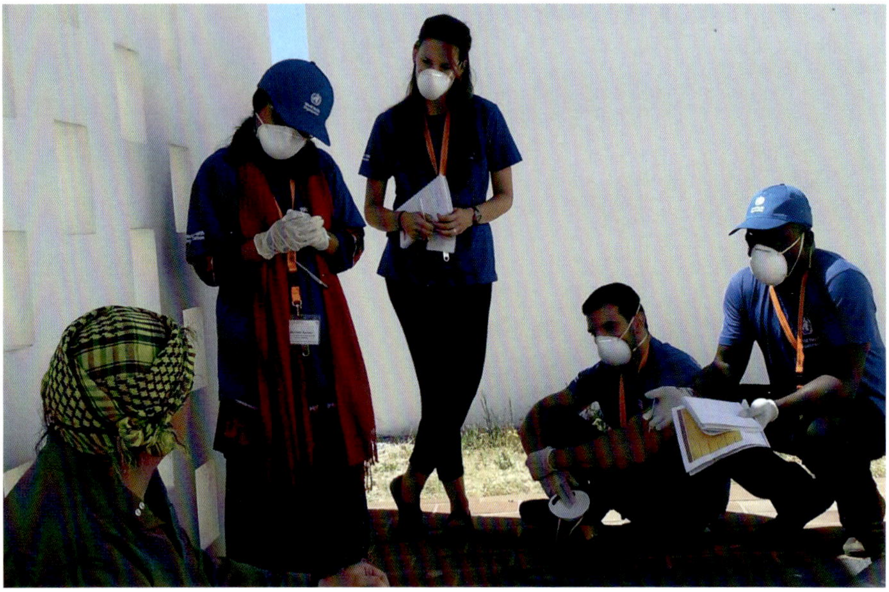

Outbreak investigation team collecting information from a survivor of an unknown disease during a simulation exercise at a training in effective field response to outbreaks and health emergencies, Lisbon, 9–15 July 2017. The training was provided by WHO Regional Office for Europe and the Global Outbreak Alert and Response Network (GOARN).
© WHO/Alex Ruswelt

As the European Region is part of a highly interconnected world, an emergency in one country often impacts many others globally. Striking examples of emergencies in other parts of the world with repercussions in Europe are outbreaks of Ebola and Zika viruses, and the Syrian humanitarian crisis.

All disasters and emergencies have common features. They threaten people's health, disrupt communities and impose high economic costs. Their impact can also be greatly reduced by investing in preparedness. That is why WHO is working with countries in its European Region to strengthen their capacities to prevent, prepare for, respond to and recover from all types of health emergencies.

The WHO Health Emergencies Programme (WHE), established in 2016, provides the Organization's response to more and more demanding crises. Mainstreamed across all levels of WHO, it is geared to better protect people from health emergencies by establishing people-centred health systems which can detect, assess, communicate and respond to crises in a matter of hours.

As WHO Director-General Dr Tedros has said: "Universal health coverage and health emergencies are two sides of the same coin". In fact, "all roads lead to universal health coverage". These are ultimately political choices and require political commitment.

This is why I am proud that European countries have adopted a 5-year *Action plan to improve public health preparedness and response in the WHO European Region 2018–2023 (216)*. This Action plan is tailored to the European context and needs. It is meant to bond countries with comparable levels of capacity and capability to avert or respond to emergencies. The approach of linking emergency preparedness with health systems strengthening and essential public health functions represents a real breakthrough on the way to UHC and United Nations 2030 Agenda for Sustainable Development.

9.3.4.10.1 Emergency preparedness

Countries that are well prepared see fewer deaths and suffer less disruption when an emergency happens. Investment in preparedness pays a dividend in terms of lives saved and illnesses avoided. It also pays a dividend in terms of a timely, more efficient emergency response. This leads to swifter recovery, less economic impact and a lower overall cost for the health system.

GPW13 makes a clear case for investment in prevention, preparedness for, response to and recovery from health emergencies. Total global investment required over the coming five years is estimated at US$ 28.9 billion. Success will be measured against WHO's goal of better protecting at least 1 billion more people from health emergencies and providing life-saving health services to 100 million vulnerable people. It will save between 1.5 million lives and provide estimated economic gains of US$ 240 billion. The return on investment is US$ 8.30 for every US$ 1 provided – a more than eightfold return.

At the core of the WHE programme, the scaling up of the IHR (2005) core capacities is central to our health emergency work in the European Region. Entered into force more than 10 years ago, it has made a difference in guiding countries towards achieving common approaches and capacities to detect, assess and respond to health threats. Strengthened IHR core capacities and resilient health systems are foundations for attaining the relevant SDGs and have contributed greatly to the implementation of Health 2020.

WHO has identified countries and territories in the European Region where support for strengthening IHR core capacities should be a particular priority. Each of them faces significant hazards, and each has vulnerabilities in their health system that hinder their ability to respond to those hazards. This means health emergencies can have a high impact in these countries and territories. It also means they are the places in the Region where investment in IHR core capacities can produce the greatest return on investment.

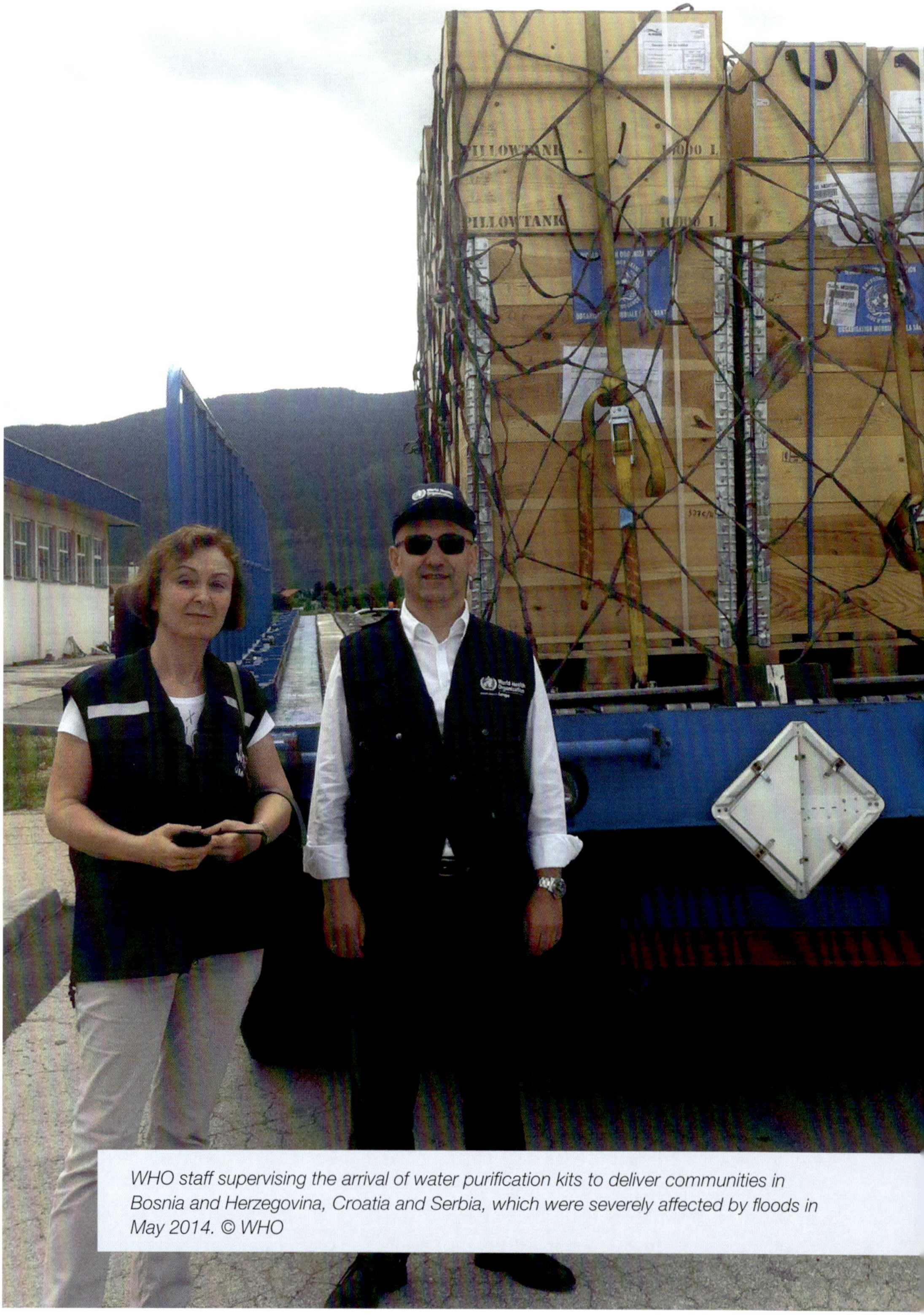

WHO staff supervising the arrival of water purification kits to deliver communities in Bosnia and Herzegovina, Croatia and Serbia, which were severely affected by floods in May 2014. © WHO

As each country is unique, the WHE Programme tailors its support to country's specific situation. This means looking at the key hazards the country faces, its vulnerability to emergencies and its health system's capacities and capabilities to prevent, prepare and respond to emergencies. The findings of the monitoring and evaluation tools identify capacity-building activities to address the specific gaps and needs of Member States.

In addition to the obligatory State Party self-assessment annual reporting (SPAR), the WHE programme offers three voluntary assessment opportunities of core capacities; namely, simulation exercises, after-action reviews and external evaluations.

We place specific emphasis on the development of national evidence-based action plans, tailored to strengthen the needed capacities. These include, for example, improving hospital safety and functionality and mass casualty management, establishing a laboratory network of excellence, setting up systems for disease surveillance, and engaging communities to communicate risks. For this, the IHR implementation and preparedness activities follow a cyclical approach, with tailored all-hazards National Action Plans developed, costed and funded *(178)*.

Partnerships with EU and its agencies has strengthened and can further strengthen preparedness and response capacities in the Region.

Health emergencies – collaboration between WHO and EU

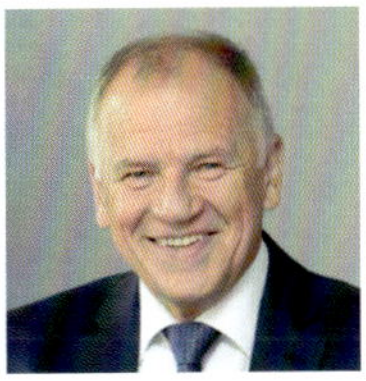

Ensuring the highest possible level of health security is a major priority for both the Commission and WHO. Major joint efforts are invested to implement the WHO International Health Regulations and support countries in building core capacities to prepare for and respond effectively to dangerous infectious diseases and other health threats. The close cooperation between the Commission departments of Health, Development Cooperation, Humanitarian Aid and Research, the European Centre for Disease Prevention and Control, and WHO in the past and current outbreaks such as Ebola, Zika, Polio and Measles has contributed to effective responses and crisis management in Europe and beyond. Furthermore, preparedness cooperation was intensified through targeted collaboration, thus contributing to stronger response capacities in our region.

Vytenis P. Andriukaitis, EU Commissioner for Health and Food Safety

9.3.4.10.2 Emergency response

Through its fully functional WHE programme *(179)*, the Regional Office provides direct support to Member States in response to public health emergencies of any type including life-saving interventions and aid, contributes to anticipate potential risks, and offers its support to crises in other WHO Regions.

The all hazards approach is used for the whole emergency cycle, from prevention, to preparedness and from response to recovery. What is more, linkages and synergies made with other health programmes and health system strengthening initiatives have had positive impacts on the health of the people beyond the emergency response. Importantly, we link operations with recovery and development, working with countries to make sure that their health systems become fully capable of coping with health emergencies.

A Flood emergency in Republika Srpska, Bosnia and Herzegovina

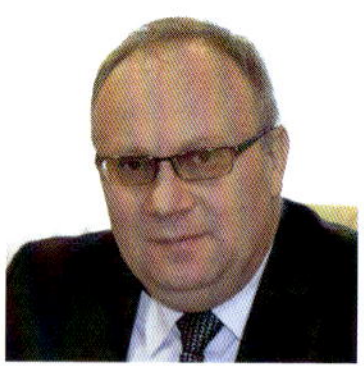

Heavy rainfall which started on 14 May 2014, caused flooding of 24 municipalities/cities in Republika Srpska, Bosnia and Herzegovina. Floods caused death, injuries and suffering of people and animals and substantial damage to the affected areas. Thousands of people lost their homes. Mudslides, landslides, provision of clean water, sanitation, protection from outbreaks and waste management became the main concerns. Key infrastructure as roads, bridges, health and educational facilities were severely damaged too.

As a part of Republika Srpska, Bosnia and Herzegovina risk assessment and management activities, the Ministry of Health and Social Welfare responded by activating our Crisis Communication Plan in Public Health, developed with input from the WHO Regional Office for Europe. An operational team consisting of leading experts in the health area among others, was formed, in line with the challenges that we faced. Their role was to communicate daily, estimating possible scenarios and offer solutions and suggestions. An Action Plan for Flood Disaster Management was prepared and activated, emphasizing roles and responsibilities, as well as organization and functioning of all relevant stakeholders from health sector. The plan was monitored weekly and regularly updated, and covered the need for adequate health care, risk mitigation, coordination and communication.

The Ministry of Health and Social Welfare and the Republika Srpska, Bosnia and Herzegovina Public Health Institute worked together with other ministries, institutions, and health-related facilities. Support came from member countries of SEEHN including Croatia, Serbia, Slovenia, and Montenegro: for example, patient treatment was provided in a hospital in Slavonski Brod in Croatia; and exemptions were made to border procedures among countries affected by floods.

Support from international organizations was significant. Coordination of all activities in the field of health was accomplished by WHO. Daily communication through the IHR (2005) platform provided appropriate involvement in the international mechanism for emergency preparedness and response. The emergency mission of WHO experts further confirmed that our plans and activities were appropriate and effective.

Dragan Bogdanic, Former Minister of Health and Social Welfare, Republika Srpska, Bosnia and Herzegovina

IHR National Focal Points and their networks are critical to ensure early detection and identification of outbreaks and other emergencies. Supported by WHO Emergency teams they work to prevent and control the international spread of diseases and other hazards potentially impacting human health, in line with SDG Target 3.d.

The WHO Regional Contact Point in the Regional Office is in daily contact with IHR NFPs to detect, verify, assess and respond to potential public health emergencies of international concern. This function is watching 24 hours a day, seven days a week, for any outbreak or emergency that puts people's lives or health at risk, by screening more than 20 000 signals per year.

New standard operating procedures (SOPs) are now in place. An updated Emergency Response Framework (ERF) is already being implemented, defining roles, responsibilities, accountabilities, timelines and partnerships. It provides coordination and leadership functions in responding to emergencies using Incident Management Systems (IMS), which allows for information to be shared better across the Organization and for clearer coordination and planning mechanisms.

The Contingency Fund for Emergencies can provide an initial tranche of funds within 24 hours of a request, allowing WHO to deploy experts and supplies more quickly than before. Coordination within the three levels of WHO is now stronger as a result of the establishment of one WHO-wide emergency programme. Staff of the WHO Regional Office for Europe, for example, have recently been deployed to the Eastern Mediterranean Region and the African Region to support response.

Our experience tells us that no single organization can protect people in health emergencies, but jointly we can. Therefore, we are working with countries and partners to pre-position health professionals and other experts for rapid deployment.

The concept of the Global Health Emergency Workforce, comprising national responders and international responders from networks and partnerships, is central to improved coordination. These partnerships have been strengthened (including the Global Outbreak Alert and Response Network (GOARN), the Global Health Cluster, Emergency Medical Teams (EMTs), standby partners and other members of the Inter-Agency Standing Committee (IASC), resulting in faster, more predictable response capacities and actions.

It has been a priority to enhance and expand the GOARN, a system of more than 200 multidisciplinary technical partners, who work together to monitor, assess and respond to communicable disease outbreaks of concern. In the European Region we have been supporting the Network's oversight, policies and secretariat functions, and engaging new partners. Since the beginning of 2016, Network partners have been more involved in alert, risk assessment, preparedness and response activities. They have also supported early joint assessment of developing outbreaks and strengthened coordination and planning of international response and country support.

There are 49 Health Cluster partners at the global level and more than 300 partners in countries, a collective force led and coordinated by WHO, guaranteeing that the response to health emergencies becomes more timely, effective and predictable. These partners include international organizations, UN agencies, nongovernmental organizations, national authorities, specialized agencies, affected communities, academic and training institutes and donor agencies.

The number of WHO EMTs is increasing, and the WHO Secretariat manages the training, capacity-building, standard-setting and quality assurance processes for this global initiative. More EMTs are now ready to support their national and other nations' capacities to respond to emergencies with health consequences, consistent with the principles of the IHR (2005). Approximately one third of the EMTs that have so far requested global classification by WHO are from the European Region.

9.3.4.10.3 Emergency operations

The Regional Office continues to lead and coordinate the work in two protracted emergencies in the Region with partners and through field offices in Turkey and Ukraine (see Developmental reflections 9 and 10).

More recently, the Regional Office has assessed the measles outbreaks affecting the Region a 'grade 2' emergency on a scale of 1 to 3 under the internal Emergency Response Framework (ERF). This was based on the growing number of children and adults affected by and dying from the disease, the persistence of pockets of non-immunized or under-immunized individuals in many countries, and the conclusion that more support is needed from WHO to accelerate action to control the outbreaks *(200)*.

Developmental reflection 9

Health services for northern Syria

Millions of refugees have fled Syria over the past 8 years of conflict. Many are seeking to build new lives elsewhere, including in neighbouring countries such as Turkey – now host to almost 4 million Syrian refugees. WHO's Refugee Health Programme in Turkey, established in 2016, supports Turkey's Ministry of Health in ensuring that Syrian refugees have access to culturally sensitive health services with the same standard as those offered to other residents and citizens[9]. This is achieved by training and integrating Syrian health workers into the national health system, giving them a new opportunity for a career and a life. These efforts align directly with two WHO's strategic priorities, outlined in the GPW13 to ensure that 1 billion more people are protected from health emergencies, and 1 billion more people benefit from universal health coverage, as well as the SDGs.

In line with the UN's 'whole-of-Syria' approach, WHO brings together and coordinates health care groups providing life-saving interventions to people in need, across lines and borders. The WHO field office in Gaziantep, a Turkish city near the Syrian border, has served as operational hub since 2013. As health cluster lead agency, WHO has a key role in the coordination of all health-related cross-border activities, overall priority-setting, contingency planning and provision of health information in order to support an effective humanitarian response. This includes delivering medicines and other supplies and providing primary health care; vaccinating hundreds of thousands of Syrian children against polio, measles, diphtheria and other diseases; treating burns and severe injuries; caring for patients with NCDs and mental health; and training health care workers *(199)*.

PART 2

[9] The Refugee Health programme operates from the WHO Country Office in Ankara. Its activities are defined within the scope of a Regional Refugee and Resilience Plan (3RP), a broad partnership platform that has brought together more than 270 development and humanitarian partners to provide coordinated support in countries bordering Syria that are heavily impacted by the influx of refugees. WHO's activities are complementary to the SIHHAT Health and Well-being project, a joint initiative by the European Union and Ministry of Health of Turkey aimed at improving health care services for Syrian refugees in the country.

Mainstreaming refugee – migrant health services: there is no other way

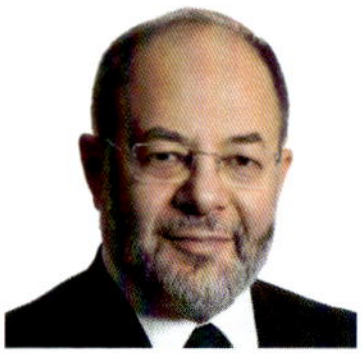

We have almost four million refugee–migrants in our country – almost three and a half million Syrians and 500 000 from Afghanistan and other countries. You can imagine that it is a huge burden to deal with. But hopefully we can overcome all the problems, especially health issues. I have national data. All the migrants in our country can take all the health services that we can give to our children. Primary health care services, prevention services, emergency transport and hospital services, they are all free of charge. No matter what they need, they can access health services. There is no restriction. There is no difference between the Syrians, or other migrants, and our citizens in terms of receiving health services. WHO's guidance on migrant health has been very helpful in this sense.

Why and how can we do this? It is a moral issue! If you accept it as a humanitarian issue in your mind, you can do it! It is not very difficult. This is built on our morals, our cultural values, our religious values, all of them. These values tell us that we can deal with this problem sincerely. Because they are our brothers and sisters, our neighbours, we should do our best for them. There is no other way... You can find the necessary resources.

That's why we have achieved this in our country. It is not a big problem for us! Our minds and hearts are ready for it. Yes, there is some debate in our country, especially from the opposition parties who ask why we have to keep these people in our country. But the majority of the public think that it can be done. So, we do it.

Recep Akdag, Former Deputy Prime Minister,
Former Minister of Health, Turkey

Developmental reflection 10

Ukraine conflict and health transformation

The story of Ukraine is illustrative. A country already suffering health system weaknesses and low life expectancy since its independence, was further burdened by a conflict started in 2014 which had a direct impact on the health of more than 3.7 million people – counting 580 000 children – living in the affected areas including those internally displaced. More than 2.7 million people are living in nongovernment-controlled areas with limited freedom of movement and limited access to social and humanitarian assistance. An estimated 800 000 people are living in difficult and dangerous conditions on both sides of the contact line, faced with ongoing hostilities. It was estimated that 77 out of 350 and 26 out of 250 health care facilities have been damaged or destroyed in the Donetsk and Luhansk regions, respectively.

To address this situation, WHO – through its main Office in Kyiv and four field offices – has continued to procure medicines, medical supplies and medical equipment for selected health care facilities; and train health care specialists to improve the quality of the health care services. Its priorities are improving access to health services; increasing availability of equipment, supplies and medicines; rehabilitating damaged health facilities; and integrating comprehensive mental health care at the primary health care level.

Of particular concern were the very low rates of immunization coverage, which dropped from full compliance in the 1990s to 70% in the 2000s and less than 50% in 2014 *(181)*. From the start of the crisis in 2014, polio became an imminent threat for Ukraine as the already stretched health system was overloaded with other priorities, and routine health services, already suboptimal, were jeopardized *(180)*. An outbreak of circulating vaccine-derived polio in 2015 triggered WHO, UNICEF and UNDP advice to hand over the procurement of vaccines to a consortium of three agencies (UNDP, UNICEF and Crown Agents) supported and guided by WHO.

The humanitarian crisis was the opportunity for the Ministry of Health, WHO and the Health Cluster partners to design joint gap-filling operations that would become the model and the forerunners of the health transformation process in Ukraine. This model was based on Health 2020 and supported by the WHO European Action Plan for the Strengthening of Public Health Capacities and Services. Strengthening primary and emergency care, and improving public health functions became the immediate objective, together with the need to communicate these changes effectively to health workers, patients and the general public.

A network of Mobile Emergency Primary Health Care Units (MEPUs) was established with the technical support from all WHO Health Programmes at all levels. Physician and nurse organizations defined a package of quality essential primary and emergency health services. The package was shared with health workers using a hand-held, real-time, web-based health information tool, which included the newly developed standard operating procedures (SOPs), algorithms and patient management decision-making trees, linked to the WHO Essential Medicines concept.

WHO and the UN Humanitarian Teams successfully advised the government about revising its legal framework to allow for rapid importation of WHO, UNICEF and International Committee of Red Cross (ICRC) medical supplies. In November 2014 a Tripartite Agreement between the Ministry of Health, the Ukrainian Red Cross Society (URCS) and WHO authorized the URCS and the Hippocrates Greek Medical Foundation (HGMF) health workers to provide the comprehensive package of services through the MEPUs. The health workers were fully trained, for example, on clinical pathways and the use of the hand-held devices. The reporting system was established and included on-line and weekly updates to the Ministry of Health and the WHO Country Office.

The MEPUs' model inspired the upgrade of primary health care services in Ukraine and represented a critical step towards improved access to and utilization of quality essential primary care services (also called the Health Protection Package).

Since then, the Ministry of Health, supported by partners, has been reforming many aspects of the health system functions, including the prevention of NCDs. A health policy dialogue platform has supported the Ministry in designing a concrete health reform strategy and action plan, aiming to improve national health services with a health financing mechanism in an effort to attain UHC.

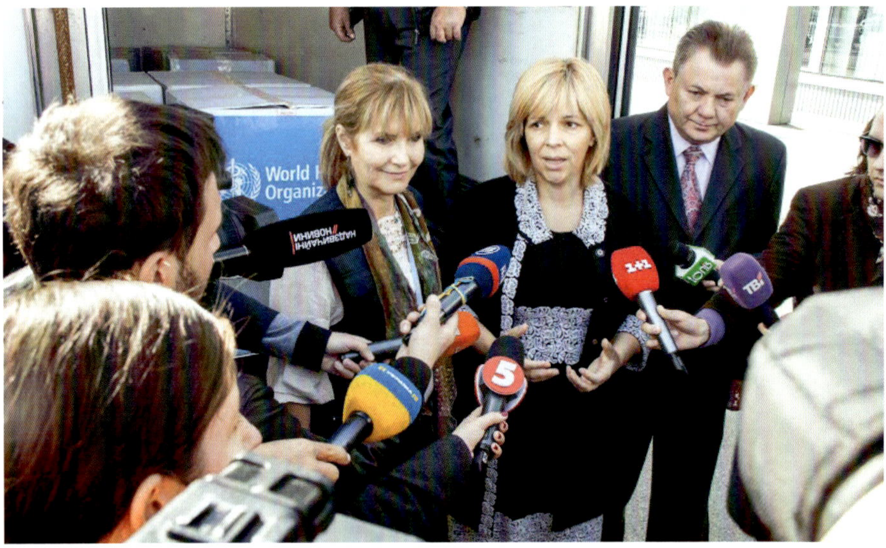

Dorit Nitzan, WHO Representative to Ukraine, Olga Bogomolets, Advisor to the President and Vasyl Lasoryshynets, Deputy Minister of Health of Ukraine, explaining to the media the importance of a shipment of tetanus toxoid vaccine. © WHO

9.3.5 Creating resilient communities and supportive environments

Health and health inequalities are substantially socially determined *(182)*. Accordingly, creating resilient communities and supportive environments for health was one of the key priority areas of Health 2020. Communities are one locus for governance for equitable health and well-being. Building community resilience is a main factor in protecting and promoting health and well-being at both the individual and community levels. Resilient communities respond proactively to new or adverse situations; prepare for economic, social and environmental change; and deal more competently with crisis and hardship.

Enhancing resilience– Health 2020 to SDGs

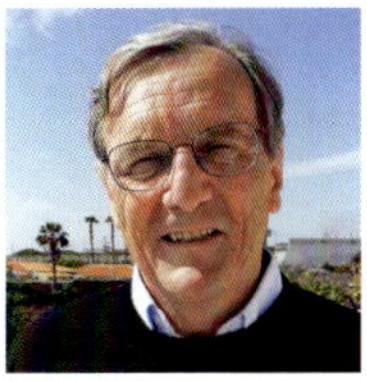

After I retired from WHO, I was very pleased when Zsuzsanna asked me to consult and help coordinate the Regional Office's work on resilience as part of the Health 2020 development process. Health 2020 identifies resilience as 'a key factor in protecting and promoting health and well-being at both the individual and community levels'. I knew that this was going to help catalyse awareness raising, knowledge generation and most importantly public health action to enhance resilience on all levels.

Resilience is connected to processes and skills that result in good individual and community health outcomes in spite of negative events, serious threats and hazards. Basically, it is the capability of individuals, communities (families, groups) and systems to cope successfully in the face of significant adversity, hazards and stress.

The key merit of the Health 2020 approach is that it views resilience as a developmental process rather than a genetically determined personal gift or an unmodifiable characteristic. Resilience is seen as a capability that can be strengthened over time and circumstances; and importantly, as an individual, community and system level competence that public health and health systems can greatly influence.

The central task for those of us working on this issue was to gather practical evidence that could inform country policies and interventions aimed at strengthening resilience on all levels. Countries wanted to know not just what they should do but how they could take effective action in this area. We worked closely with academic institutions, WHO collaborating centres and most importantly Member States and networks like the Small country initiative in gathering scientific evidence which linked the strengthening of resilience to health outcomes.

To date we have been able to produce several compendia which summarize current research and also present narratives and well analysed examples of how resilience can be strengthened in practice at individual, community and system level *(47, 183–185)*.

Nowadays, research on resilience has become a domain encompassing many different variables including personal and community characteristics, coping processes, a sense of coherence in the lives of individuals and other protective factors. Such factors stem from the social and cultural environment where people are born, grow and age. They include resources amenable to policy action, such as parental support, community organizations, self-help, mutual support and other community resources available to individuals and groups including high-quality health services and public health programmes.

More particularly, regaining a sense of 'being in control' contributes to both individual and community resilience. The level of control (or lack of it) that communities and individuals have over their life has been shown to be a key factor in the social determination of health and health inequities. The Regional Office experience points to the need for action that aims at building resilience to address the power dynamics underlying people's vulnerability and health inequities.

It is worth noting that resilience has a very prominent role basically in all the SDGs. Thus, lessons European Member States are learning in addressing resilience within the context of Health 2020 can now help us all to more easily find ways to address both the political and scientific requirements needed to position population health within the development agenda advocated by the SDGs.

Erio Ziglio, Former Head, WHO European Office for Investment for Health and Development, Venice, Italy

An example of an approach to building resilience is our WHO 7-country initiative *(47)*. The 7-country initiative covers four different geographical and climatic zones: arid and semi-arid water-stressed areas (Kazakhstan and Uzbekistan); high mountainous areas (Kyrgyzstan and Tajikistan); Mediterranean countries (Albania and North Macedonia); and a sub-Arctic region in the northern Russian Federation (Arkhangelsk Oblast and Nenets Autonomous Okrug).

A number of countries have experienced climate-related exposure, including extreme events such as water scarcity, glacier melting and permafrost thawing. By drawing upon the experiences of countries already affected by climate emergencies, this initiative offers a firm foundation for future action by providing examples of the priorities, challenges, and emerging solutions utilized by the seven participating countries. The overall aim is to protect population health from climate emergencies by building capacity for assessing vulnerability, impact and adaptivity, thereby strengthening the health systems of the countries.

The initiative has enabled the development of national health-adaptation strategies or action plans to counter the impact of climate emergencies. It has also facilitated awareness-raising activities and the sharing of knowledge and experiences in this complex field. Institutional capacity to adapt and to prevent the negative impact of these events on health is linked to the creation of supportive environments that strengthen resilience at individual, community and societal levels.

Building city sustainability and resilience – Health 2020 and SDGs

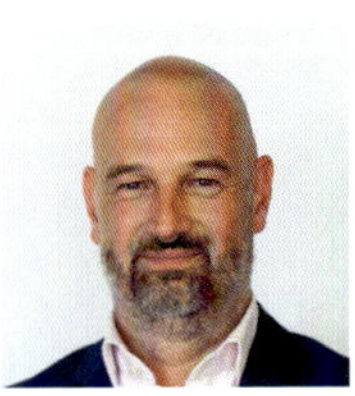

© Desiree Meulemans

We know that good urban development strategies can make our citizens happier, our environment healthier, and our economy more sustainable. We are convinced that for any such strategy, health should be a part of our policy-making. This has led us to giving health and well-being priority in all of our policies, consistent with the healthy urban living for everybody outlined in Health 2020 and the Sustainable Development Goals.

How do we do this? Our 'Healthy City Future' is a long-term commitment and not only by the current political board, but the joined-up actions of many, including, divisions of government, private sectors, research institutes and, most importantly the residents themselves. We are redesigning our city to be a healthy city for everybody which protects and promotes health in environment and spatial planning.

We want more space for pedestrians and cyclists and thus get cars out of our public space. We have begun to use electric boats in the city canals for distributing goods in the inner city. All diesel cars are banned from the city centre through our low emissions zone. We are creating electric car-sharing schemes. This initiative is supported by private industry, specializing in batteries which are charged by solar energy. They are not only capable of moving cars, but also capable of absorbing the peak problems, that mark the distribution of sustainable energy. All this also involves the reduction of noise exposure.

We have found bright investors to help build new parts of the city. Their advertising line is 'Please come here to live and it will add five years in good health to your life.' This is a big break-through: private money working for public good. Health and happiness will be measured and will be key indicators in the tenant procedures and the use of the community buildings and facilities.

We also understand that this transformation to a more inclusive, sustainable and resilient society requires a shared responsibility at international, national and local level. We can learn a lot from each other and that is one reason we cherish our partnership with the WHO European Healthy Cities Network. We are looking forward to mutual inspiration for a healthy and happy future.

Victor Everhardt, Deputy Mayor for Health, Utrecht, Netherlands

9.3.5.1 Environment and health

The environment is a major determinant of health, estimated to account for almost 1.4 million deaths a year in the WHO European Region. Air quality, poor water and sanitation, chemicals in the environment, housing conditions, occupational exposures and the impact of climate -related emergencies all significantly affect human health.

One year of life expectancy is lost for every person in the WHO European Region due to the air-borne exposure to particulate matter (PM), mainly because of the increased risk of cardiovascular and respiratory diseases and lung cancer. Such factors interact with the social determinants of health. For example, while deaths from ambient air pollution occur in all European countries regardless of their income, those from indoor air pollution are more than five times greater in low and middle-income countries than in wealthier ones. Expanding interdisciplinary and intersectoral collaboration between human, environmental and animal health enhances public health effectiveness.

Health 2020 considered the health co-benefits of environmental policies in the context of 'Rio+20', the United Nations Conference on Sustainable Development held in 2012 *(186)*. Today the ECEH in Bonn, generously supported by the Ministry of Environment of Germany, is at the heart of the Region's technical achievement in environment and health. For example, the Centre has coordinated several projects to support the comprehensive revision of EU air quality, drinking water quality and climate change related policies and regulations by providing evidence-based advice on health aspects of these determinants. The Centre plays also an important normative role, notably with respect to the update of the WHO Air Quality Guidelines *(89)*, and the launch, in October 2018, of the Environmental Noise Guidelines for the European Region *(197)*.

Collaboration between WHO and the European Environment Agency (EEA)

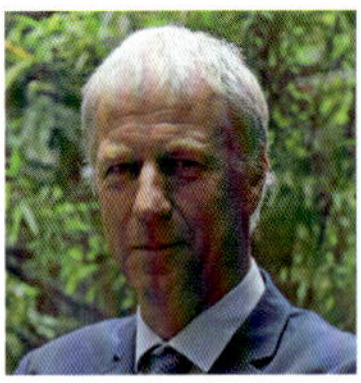

Our key collaborative work is on air pollution and noise. What we get from WHO are the guidelines and the methodologies to make estimates on the impact of exposure to different levels of air pollution and noise. Since we do not do the fundamental research that sets these standards, we rely on WHO's authority to benchmark European policies against the standards they are setting.

If you look at discussions at the European level on air quality, it is obvious that we need to base our arguments on solid air quality measurements and science. People have a lot of questions and concerns about these findings and that is why WHO standards on air quality are so important.

By making the WHO standards very explicit in our reporting, you could say that indirectly these standards are driving the type of knowledge that is supporting stronger environmental policies. This has also a big communication impact. When we come with our annual air quality report, with the estimates of premature deaths in Europe based on WHO methodology, it gets a lot of media coverage, which helps keep the issue on the political agenda.

Similarly, we are doing these assessments for noise. Noise has been a bit of a forgotten issue at the European level and we know that we have quite a bit of terrain to cover to have solid measurements on noise exposure. However, here again, the WHO guidelines for noise exposure have been very helpful.

Hans Bruyninckx, Executive Director, European Environment Agency (EEA)

We believe that health systems should take a lead in responding to environmental pollution. Here the Region has focused on identifying and articulating the impact of environmental pollution from health care. An expert meeting in 2013 identified the main challenges, including the emissions from health systems. Proper management of waste, medicines consumption, chemical and water pollution were amongst the issues identified.

City 'Air Ambassadors' tackle pollution

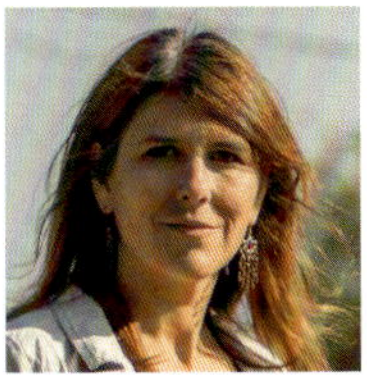

© Camille Desmot

In 2014 when I got elected as the chair of the WHO Healthy Cities Network in France we began to focus our advocacy on environmental issues challenging our cities. We now have more than 90 cities in the Network. Because of our strong and visible advocacy at the city level, I got nominated to the national air council and was invited to join several big national environmental events and initiatives.

Coincidentally, this national and European recognition gave us more power locally, so we could push bolder actions and stronger policies in our city. Air quality was a particular important issue in our city because we were one of the cities with very high and contentious levels of pollution by European Union standards. Contentious because some people thought we were exaggerating and saying that there is no such air pollution problem. Others were saying "there is even more air pollution than you are admitting and we are all dying and you are minimizing the problem".

So, we had a big problem of confidence. And a big problem of: what do we do as a city? How can we address this dilemma? In keeping with our city commitment to doing things in an 'equitable participatory way', we decided to engage our population in measuring our own air quality. We went for a national call for action to find an independent NGO to coordinate workshops to help people learn about air quality, and train community people in ways to use sensors to measure pollution in priority neighbourhoods, especially in poorer areas where air quality was generally worse.

And the people actually invented new ways of measuring: e.g., multiple level measurements – one on the ground floor and one on the seventh floor. And some became neighbourhood 'ambassadors for air'. They even had – actually, still have – 'ambassador business cards' so that they really felt empowered to talk about the air quality in the city and take steps to change things. They, for example, campaigned to shift public policies to support more cycling and public transportation issues. And when they learned that many in their neighbourhoods didn't know how to ride bicycles, the ambassadors started developing bike riding training classes and creating free bike sharing schemes to address inequities in this area.

These programmes gave us national visibility with the press, and when I went back to the national meetings everything changed. When I was first there the people on the cabinet criticized us for questioning 'official measures'. Now, everybody wants to do something like we did.

Our relationship with WHO Region Office helped enable us. It helped make us more legitimate in the eyes of other policy-makers and the public. Every time we tweeted from a WHO conference, for example the Ministerial Conference in Ostrava, people could see that we were being acknowledged as positive innovators in major European arenas. We also have found WHO tools, like the HEAT tool very useful in our advocacy work *(187)*. Our cities love it. It allows our mayors, for example, to quantify the impact of their policies and say, for example, that "S/he can save 600 lives in the next five years" with this biking initiative. That's a really good tool.

Charlotte Marchandise, Deputy Mayor for Health, Rennes, France

PART 2

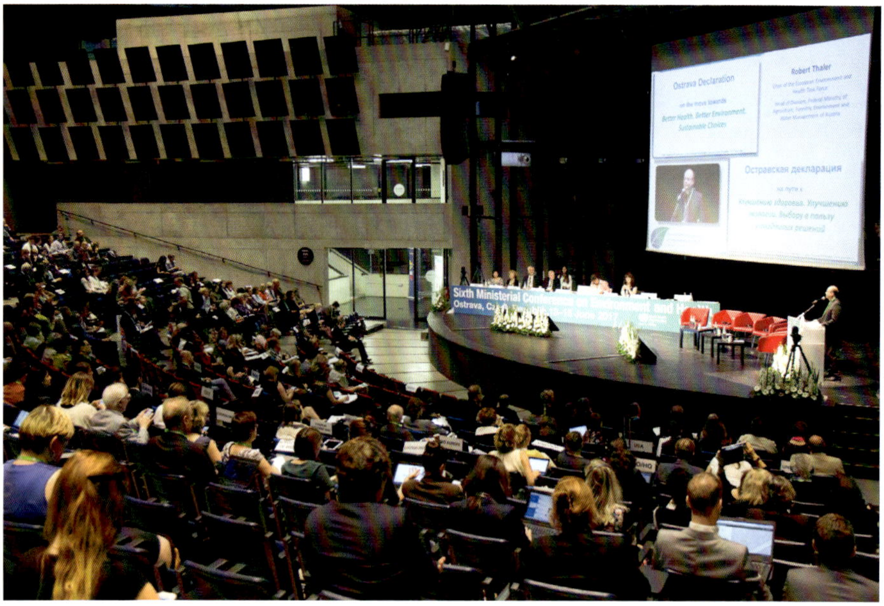

The Ostrava Declaration is presented to the plenary prior to the official signing at the Sixth Ministerial Conference on Environment and Health, Ostrava, Czechia, 13–15 June 2017.
© WHO/David Barrett

Protecting and improving public health by providing access to safe water and sanitation is supported by the Protocol on Water and Health *(217)*. At the policy level there is a significant momentum building to scale up adoption of the WHO-recommended Water safety plan manual (WSP manual) *(188)*.

The ministerial conferences of the European Environment and Health Process provide a unique intersectoral policy platform bringing together relevant sectors and partners to shape policies and actions on environment and health (see Section 2.6 and Box 11).

The Fifth Ministerial Conference on Environment and Health, organized by the WHO European Regional Office for Europe, and hosted by the Government of Italy in Parma, 10–12 March 2010, focused on protecting children's health in a changing environment. The Parma Declaration was the first time-bound outcome of the environment and health process. Member States set clear targets to reduce the harm to health from environmental threats over the succeeding decade *(189)*.

The Sixth Ministerial Conference, hosted by the Government of Czechia, the Moravian-Silesian Region and the City of Ostrava, was held in Ostrava, Czechia on 13-15 June 2017. It was organized by the Regional Office in close partnership with the United Nations Economic Commission for Europe and the United Nations Environment Programme. It was generously hosted by the Government of Czechia, the Moravian-Silesian Region and the City of Ostrava.

The Conference focused on the creation of supportive environments and resilient communities, aiming to position the European Environment and Health Process as a platform for implementing selected and relevant environment and health goals and targets from the United Nations 2030 Agenda for Sustainable Development.

The Sixth Conference also considered the urgent need to continue and strengthen efforts to address the leading environmental determinants of ill health, including air pollution, inadequate water and sanitation services, hazardous chemicals, waste and contaminated sites, climate change, as well as new responses to these multiple challenges, including through a new emphasis on the importance of action at the sub-national and local, and by highlighting opportunities from developing environmentally sustainable health systems.

At the Conference, Member States adopted a declaration, which included a commitment to develop national portfolios for action on environment and health by 2018, a compendium of possible actions for its implementation and an agreement on revised institutional arrangements for the European Environment and Health Process.

Ostrava Declaration – taking action in line with UN 2030 Agenda for Sustainable Development

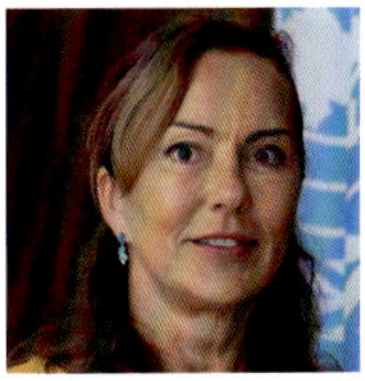

Through our cooperation with WHO Regional Office for Europe we have had the pleasure to contribute to the European environment and health process.

I really want to highlight the consistent and continuous commitment of Zsuzsanna Jakab, to this process. After the adoption of the Ostrava Declaration in 2017 at the Sixth Ministerial Conference on environment and health, she personally promoted the development of a compendium of possible actions to advance its implementation. This outlined a broad range of actions that both our organizations could take in support of Member States.

The interlinked and interconnected way UNECE works with WHO in these areas in very much in line with approaches being promoted by UN 2030 Agenda for Sustainable Development and the SDGs.

Olga Algayerova, Executive Secretary, United Nations Economic Commission for Europe (UNECE)

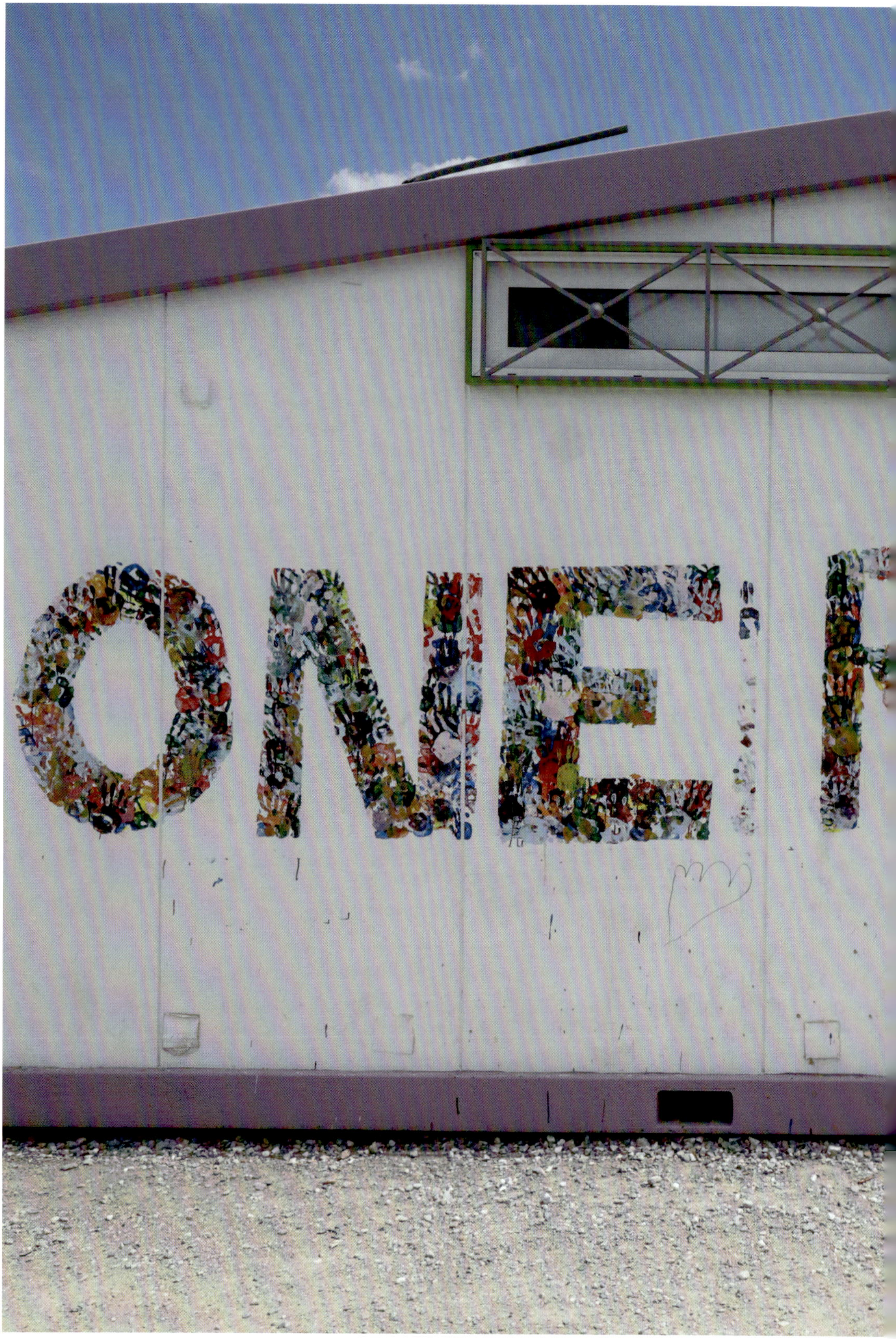
ONE

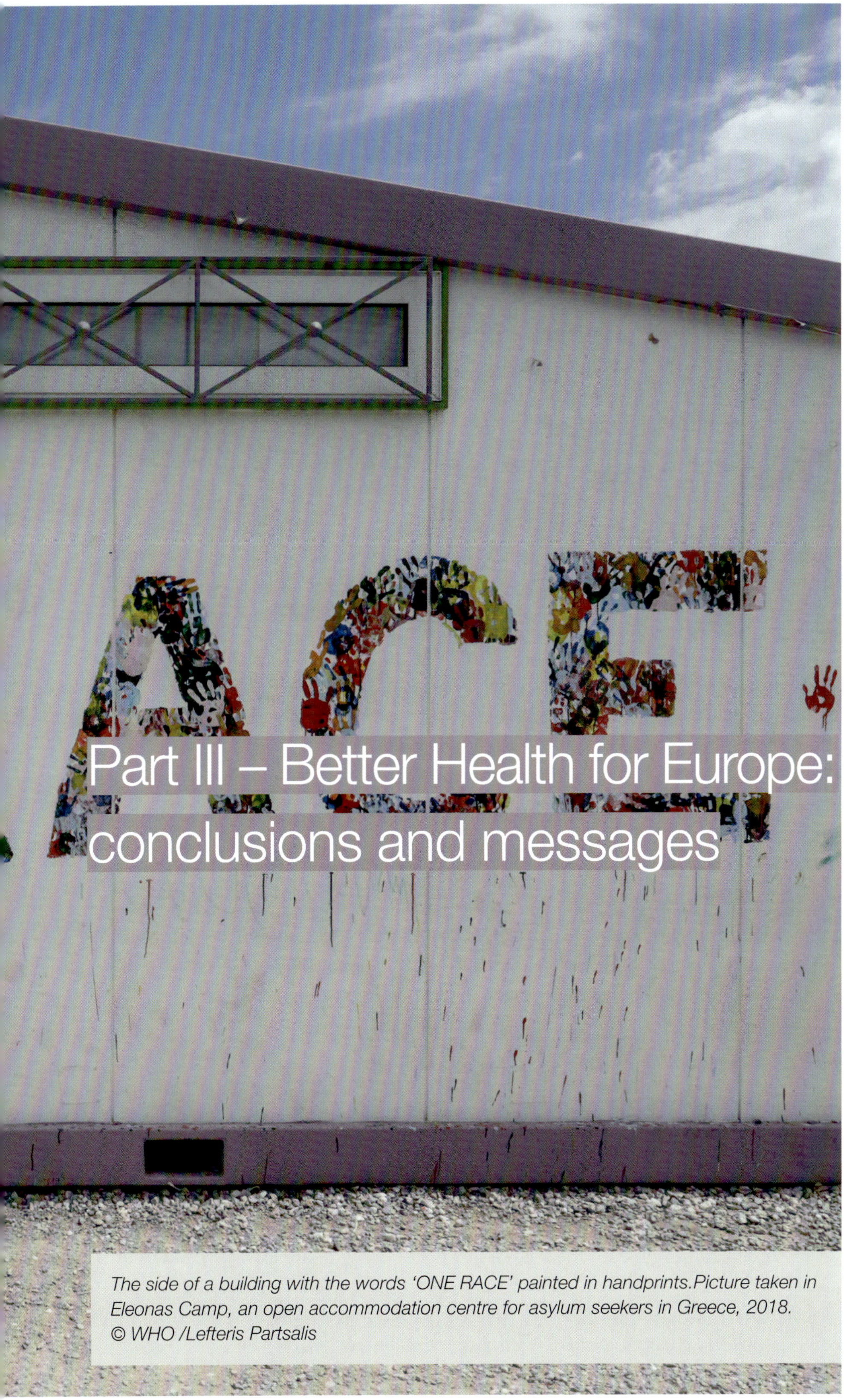

Part III – Better Health for Europe: conclusions and messages

The side of a building with the words 'ONE RACE' painted in handprints.Picture taken in Eleonas Camp, an open accommodation centre for asylum seekers in Greece, 2018.

These last 10 years have been transformative for public policies and health in the WHO European Region and beyond. New and significant challenges to health and health equity continue to arise, yet two key developments have changed everything.

The first key development is our changing developmental narrative. The neo-liberal economic models that have dominated and determined disease investment and development thinking since the 1990s focused on competition, privatization and efficiency. Models have now shifted to focus more on the human development goals, which are explicit in the United Nations 2030 Agenda for Sustainable Development and the Sustainable Development Goals (SDGs), which include a wider set of development outcomes than solely economic gain.

Health 2020 presented an early example of this thinking. It is fully consistent with the 2030 Agenda for Sustainable Development and the SDGs, reflecting a world in which health is considered much more seriously on national and global agendas. Health is seen as a public good, as a human right, and as a matter of social justice. It is a vital issue for economy, trade and security; an investment sector for human, economic and social development; and a major economic sector in its own right. Today, health really matters.

Health is so important that it must be for everyone. Universal health coverage is one of the most compelling concepts of our time, promoting the goal that all people should have access to the quality care they need without suffering financial hardship in accessing it. UHC is central to ensuring healthy populations and well-functioning, well-governed health systems. WHO's goal today is to see another billion people in the world enjoying UHC by 2030. The WHO European Region must play a full part in making sure that this goal is achieved by making health the political choice.

Importantly, health impact has emerged as a key metric, driver, lens and barometer of this new development narrative and agenda. Health is a precondition, outcome and indicator of sustainable development. Health is being effectively repositioned in the centre of local, national, regional and global political debates.

Over the last 10 years, the focus of the work of the Regional Office and the central thread running through Health 2020 has been to catalyse these changes and support the capacities of Member States and public health communities to deliver on this agenda.

The second key development relates to transformative change in people and public health leadership. Our collaborative work and collective experience in developing and implementing Health 2020 related polices at regional, national and local levels has strengthened the voice and work of existing public health leaders in all 53 Member States and beyond, and has created new public health leaders for the 21st century. Public health advocates have been empowered with new tools, skills and competencies to champion the new developmental narrative.

We now have a strong cohort of public health leaders who understand the importance of value-based, evidence-informed action on public health. They can adapt effectively and efficiently to rapidly changing environments and take full advantage of the collective wisdom, experience and know-how of our vast and diverse Region. They can take health into other sectors of government and make health a joined-up governmental responsibility, where every minister is a minister of health in his or her area. They can help their communities of practice address common, yet complex, challenges.

We have gained much more understanding about the role and importance of public health and the need to respond to health inequities. We know so much more about the range of determinants of disease, particularly the social determinants and social circumstances, and about their interactions over the life course. This has created new opportunities for improving health and well-being on an equitable basis. We also have more evidence-based information about what works and what does not.

The notion of good health is evolving, shifting towards a world in which we create and maintain good health and well-being, rather than merely treating disease and illness. Powerful new scientific understanding and technologies are changing health and health care, and offering so many more opportunities to intervene across the spectrum of health promotion, disease prevention, treatment, rehabilitation and palliation.

The global context has become much more complex. The number of players has increased and there is a growing diversity in the institutional landscape, characterized by more partnerships, foundations, financial instruments, bilateral and multilateral agencies, and civil society engagement. Today, no country or agency can resolve all of the challenges to health and well-being on its own, nor can it harness the potential of innovation without extensive cooperation. Reasonable solutions to the most complex problems require well-managed intergovernmental and interagency negotiations to reach a fair deal for all.

Today, we also have a much better understanding of the relationship between health and wealth. We know that health systems contribute to societal well-being in three main ways. Firstly, health systems contribute to health both as a direct component of well-being and through impact on wealth creation. Secondly, health systems have a direct impact on wealth as a significant component of the economy, which again has an impact on well-being. And thirdly, health systems contribute directly to well-being because societies and the people within them draw satisfaction from the existence of health services and the ability to access the services they provide. This triangular relationship is context specific, and in any country reflects the particular social, economic, cultural and political environment.

The 2030 Agenda for Sustainable Development will continue to underpin all that WHO and the Regional Office will do over the coming years. The SDGs, taken together with Health 2020 and the strengthening of public health, provide integrated and value-based approaches to population-based health improvement. Their implementation across the 53 countries of the European Region, alongside the implementation of a comprehensive range of more technically based policies and strategies, has contributed and can continue to contribute to improved health overall, and to the reduction of health inequities, particularly for vulnerable groups.

Some concluding messages

Looking back at the seven strategic action priorities included in my 2010 vision paper, 'Better health for Europe', much has been achieved and learned over these last years. This learning now needs to be disseminated, applied and strengthened by our collective public health communities as we continue to work for better health for Europe in the years ahead.

So, on behalf of all the staff of our Regional and country-based offices in Europe and the many 'witnesses' who helped us tell this story, I end these reflections with some messages drawn from our collective learning in developing and implementing the strategy that has guided our journey over these last 10 years.

Message 1: Never underestimate the power of a common vision

Health 2020, as a value-driven, evidence-informed European health policy framework and a coherent vision for equitable improvement in health and well-being, created new scientific information on the social determinants of health, governance for health, and the economics of health intervention. It provided a strategic approach to health and well-being, dealing with all determinants through national health policies, strategies and plans and, most particularly, the social and political determinants. It saw investment in health as a means of accelerating development, using economic alongside health arguments to promote investment in public health, the benefits of health promotion and disease prevention, and the value of reducing copayment percentages for the provision of health services.

Health 2020 was developed through a broad co-production exercise to engage the widest possible range of internal and external stakeholders concerned with public health in Europe and beyond. We quickly learned that the process was not just about making sure that we put the right words in the document but that we truly engaged people in both policy development and implementation.

We needed not only to get those involved in public health on board to express their views and provide their inputs but also, and more importantly, all the diverse stakeholders in communities. The main goal was to create a sense of unity among the different sectors of society, a feeling of a common cause and ownership shared by all. To accomplish this, we knew we needed to put these principles into practice ourselves. We needed all our staff to reframe our work around Health 2020 values and approaches; to look at our own governance approaches, intersectoral working patterns, partnerships, life course approaches, etc.; to model the behaviours and approaches we were proposing; to take action not just in words but to really, truly, passionately and honestly embrace, nourish, champion and live the vision ourselves.

This catalysed a major change process internally in all our offices. There were evidence gaps, around, for example, the social determinants of health, governance and economics, and new research and evidence gathering was needed. So, we used our practical collective experiences to inform our research agendas. We learned also that our behaviours could reinforce and strengthen the reception and application of our technical norms and standards.

Health 2020 has had significant impact. Within the Regional Office all work has been reframed and aligned with Health 2020 objectives and priorities. Most positively, our Health 2020 approaches were consistent with, and to some extent anticipated, global developments, most notably the United Nations 2030 Agenda for Sustainable Development and the Sustainable Development Goals and helped prepare us to take leadership roles in this area.

An important added value has been that Health 2020 provided an entry window with political decision-makers at all levels and from different sectors. When new ministers come into the picture and when we have opportunities to visit with presidents, prime ministers, and parliamentarians, we can remind them that their countries have adopted this approac. We can also help them frame any health challenges they are concerned about with Health 2020 consistent values of equity, participation and solidarity over, for example, tobacco taxation, migration, copayments, etc. In doing so we can cement the commitment of the country on issues that could be difficult to talk about, let alone do something about.

Message 2: Complex problems need congruent 'joined up' solutions

We learned a lot about governance for health in the WHO European Region and in the Regional Office, through supporting and publishing research on governance, making the concept of governance mainstream, and retraining frontline staff in country offices and others in health diplomacy. In addition, transparency and involvement in the internal governance of the Region has improved through staff training and the strengthening of Standing Committee and Regional Committee processes. Our new narrative is helping to catalyse a transformational shift, away from health and health service dominated governance to whole-of-government, whole-of-society and health-in-all-policies approaches.

Most importantly it has changed the way our staff think, work, plan and address the health challenges we confront. We have also learned a lot about the new skill mix and capabilities that today's public health leaders need to meet their current health challenges and achieve change. These include:

1. initiating and informing policy debates;
2. advocating for polices for health;
3. assessing health needs and capacity for health gain;
4. creating innovative networks for change;
5. stimulating change in complex systems where change often comes from relationship-building, advocacy and negotiation, rather than direct control; and,
6. acknowledging the newly important role of health diplomacy.

Message 3: Relevance and leadership are earned qualities

Both myself as Regional Director and our staff have learned to reflect developmentally on how to achieve progress under the very different circumstances of our Member States, and how to engage with them by strengthening our technical skills in areas where they have expressed a need, (e.g. economic impact data concerning out-of-pocket payments, anticipating health needs, in migration and health, men's health, etc.) and by enhancing our resources through partnerships, networks and new geographically dispersed offices.

In this way we have been able to demonstrate our relevance and leadership in many new and established areas not only for our Region, but also globally. Areas worth highlighting here include:

1. strengthening a more evidence-informed focus on equity;
2. re-emphasizing and reinvigorating public health through delivery of the European Action Plan for Strengthening Public Health Capacities and Services, and a new vision for advancing public health for sustainable development in the WHO European Region as agreed at the Regional Committee in 2018;
3. establishing the Regional Office as a European centre of public health excellence and guidance;
4. energizing the life course approach;
5. investing in people, e.g. through summer schools on health financing and migration and health; and,
6. delivering several public health related European strategies, e.g. on mental health, sexual and reproductive health and men's health.

Message 4: Collaboration beats competition

We have learned that we can enhance resources, policy coherence and impact through partnerships. The Regional Office has actively engaged in forming strategic partnerships with many other stakeholders to jointly improve health and well-being in Europe and beyond.

This has involved establishing new and strengthening existing partnerships and networks, e.g. the Small Countries Initiative and the South-eastern Europe Health Network; enhancing collaboration with the EU and institutions such as the European Centre for Disease Prevention and Control, the Organisation for Economic Co-operation and Development, GAVI and the Global Fund; extending collaboration and joint working with United Nations partners; establishing new ways of collaborating with partners; and moving beyond competition and finding truly mutually beneficial collaborative practices based on sharing information and resources.

Message 5: Think Globally act Regionally

In strengthening the European contribution to global health, the Regional Office has been repositioned as an initiator, tester, and driver of global health approaches. Examples include: health and development; the social determinants of health; Health 2020; governance; catching the moment and taking quick action when required (e.g. on migration and health); addressing difficult issues (e.g. developing strategies for sexual and reproductive health, child abuse and maltreatment, and mental health in institutions).

Message 6: Put evidence-informed health information within the reach of everyone in our Region and beyond

We have learned a lot over these 10 years about ways to put accessible, understandable and useful evidence-informed health information within the reach of everyone in our Region and beyond. This has involved a better understanding of increasing health literacy in the population; making evidence and information more accessible and easier to understand for all; amplifying and broadening the reach of our communication messages through enhanced web and social media feeds; active partnerships with NGOs, universities, cities, networks, regions etc.; the role of ambassadors (e.g. HRH Crown Princess Mary, Patron of WHO/Regional Office for Europe) and high-level advocacy with presidents, prime ministers, ministers of finance and other sectoral leaders (e.g. during country visits and meetings).

Message 7: Invest in people

We have invested a lot in promoting a positive working environment in the Regional Office and ensuring that we have sustainable funding for our work. We have learned a lot from the feedback of our staff and others whose lives have been influenced by our work.

The Regional Office has been transformed through various initiatives taken over the last 10 years, including:

1. developing and implementing the Health 2020 common policy framework;
2. strengthening our country offices with internationally appointed WHO representatives working collaboratively with United Nations Country Teams;
3. raising morale through positive engagement with all Member States;
4. establishing the Regional Office as an important 'go to' centre of excellence in public health in Europe, including the creation of a new 'vision for public health for the 21st century' agreed by the Regional Committee in 2018 *(51)*;
5. securing funding;
6. improving internal management and financial procedures and accountability; and,
7. motivating and retaining staff.

We have also put a lot of energy into gender balancing our staff, our intern programmes and in recruiting younger and highly motivated staff who can lead the Organization into the future.

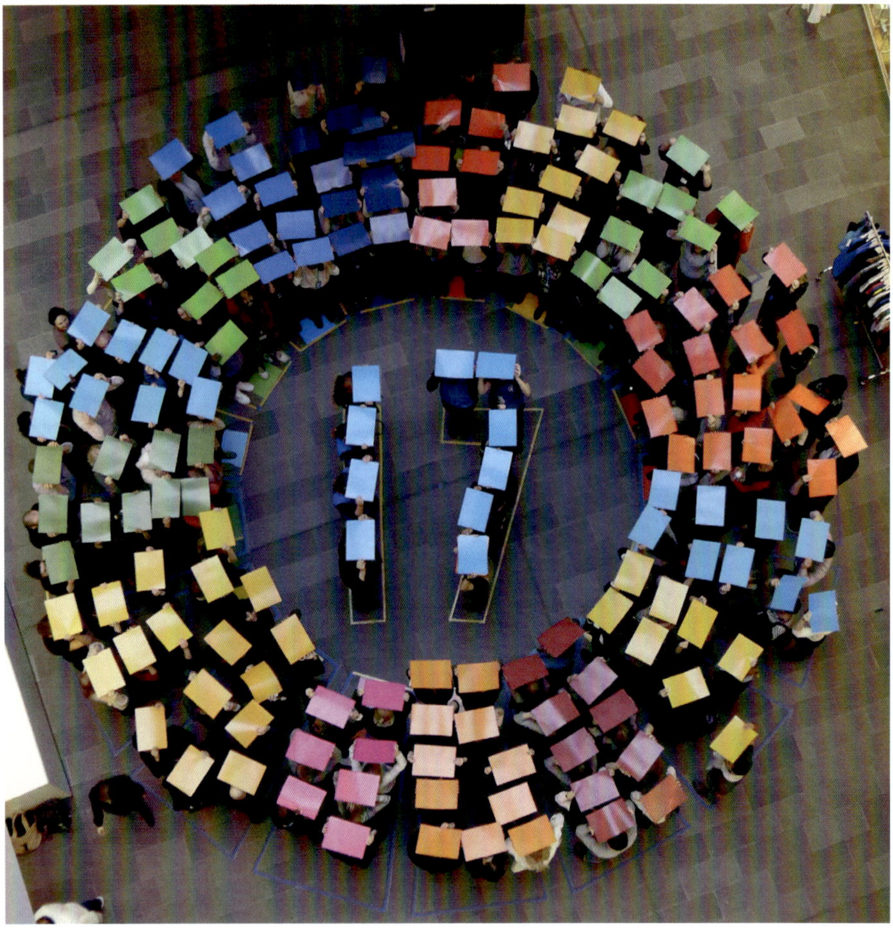

Participants at a seminar for UN employees holding colourful cardboards to recreate the SGDs wheel. UN City, Copenhagen, Denmark, 16 December, 2016. © Line Sigh

The challenges beyond 2020

In 2010 dynamic challenges to global health, together with new scientific knowledge about the origins of health and opportunities created by technology, required a comprehensive response. The Health 2020 health policy framework, supported by new thinking and capacities in public health, was designed to respond to the situation at the time in terms of knowledge and opportunity, and to present politicians and decision-makers with a comprehensive and integrated approach to health improvement for all, with an emphasis on the disadvantaged and those left behind. These issues are intricately linked to the so-called political determinants of health.

Health 2020 will soon reach the end of its time, yet the approaches it introduced are supported by, and to some extend anticipated, new innovations such as the global SDGs and WHO's own Thirteenth General Programme of Work with its 'triple billion' targets. In this sense the WHO Regional Office for Europe can be said to have provided global as well as regional leadership. Implementing these global policies in the European Region in the future may require the elaboration of a new policy framework, yet in a context that will share some old with some new demands.

What has been achieved over the last decade? Certainly, health has improved overall, as has health policy and practice, across the European Region, although wide variations remain in health and well-being both between and within countries. The improvements that have been achieved through the development and implementation of health policies and practices, including advancements in public health capacities, have met 21st century challenges. Yet we can easily identify where we need to do more.

We need more political commitment to health, to give substance to the point that 'health is a political choice'. Future health strategies need to change the political dynamic and debate to see health as a major political objective and health improvement as a marker of political success. We need new organizational and institutional forms that find it easier to elaborate, implement and fund multisectoral actions for health, as we have not found it easy so far to really implement the whole-of-government, whole-of-society and health-in-all-policies approaches that we know we need. We also need new public health and health system capacities, which we often struggle to deliver. Perhaps above all we need people committed to equitable health improvement with new skills and expertise, which are easier to describe than to develop.

Any new health policy framework beyond 2020 will need to consider all these lessons of the last decade, as well as new and accelerating scientific knowledge and advances in health technologies. Perhaps the most important of these is the new understanding concerning the interplay of genetic expression and the environment across the life course, opening the possibility of predictive and personal approaches to disease prevention and management. The accelerating use of information technology, 'big data' and artificial intelligence will also be transformational. These technologies offer many potential benefits, such as improved health outcomes; reduced risk to patients; reduced need for hospitalization; faster communication; integrated management of patient data; better access for patients to health services; and improved screening and diagnostic services. However, the technologies also raise profound issues in areas such as ownership, storage, and confidentiality, to which societies must respond.

Today health and health policy also face a daunting external environment. Dominant here is a change globally in the political environment, towards more divisive and less consensus-based policy thinking. More politicization can be anticipated even in the short run. Diverse Member States may find it difficult to reach consensus on sensitive issues such as sexual and reproductive health, environmental health, migrant health and making the ever-increasing pharmacopeia more affordable for all.

Other challenges are more familiar, including ageing, urbanization, modern media, new forms of work, and the challenges of life-course and multi-determinant policy development, including dealing effectively with the behavioural determinants (tobacco, alcohol, diet, exercise, etc.) The operationalization of multi-determinant health-in-all-policies approaches demands imagination and new evidence. The classical model of health determinants is changing. Many of the current health challenges are related to unsustainable lifestyles and unsustainable production and consumption patterns, for instance the obesity epidemic, the global system of food production, distribution, consumption and waste, and climate change.

All these challenges could dramatically increase public and private spending for health and may not be affordable for health systems on the basis of universality. Health care spending could possibly become the main driver of life expectancy gains, certainly overweighting income effects, education and lifestyle over time. So far, such spending has not outweighed the importance of all-determinant approaches. Yet, over time, it may well be argued by those responsible for the technologies, their development and implementation, that indeed this is the case. On the other hand, effective transformation of our health systems towards promotion and prevention may obviate the need for at least some proportion of such technological interventions. Whatever the future, the political and policy challenges here will be enormous.

For these reasons health systems will receive a more prominent role in strategic thinking. Our current priorities must be extending primary care for all, incorporating health promotion and disease prevention, responding to the shortage of health personnel and implementing more digitalization. Health security and emergency preparedness will also dominate the agenda. Weak health systems anywhere heighten the risk of pathogens everywhere, and accordingly outbreaks will remain a high priority.

Our learning over these last 10 years gives us important pointers to help shape our responses to these new and continuing challenges, both regionally and globally. One thing is very clear: our collective value-driven, evidence-informed health leadership will be needed more than ever as we move into the future.

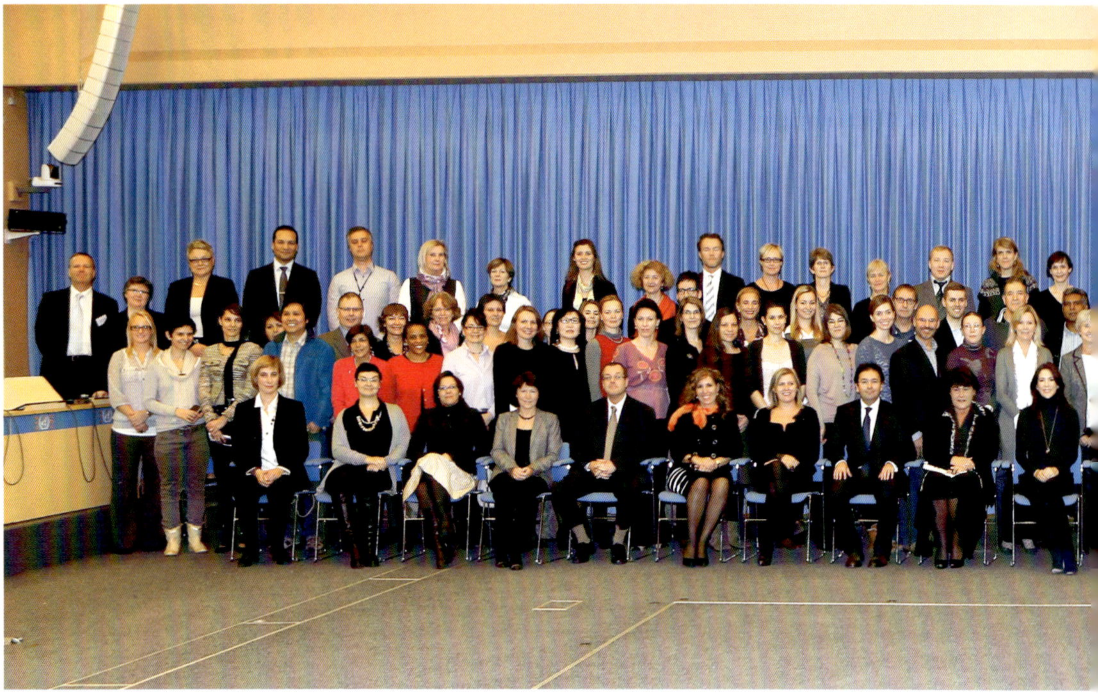

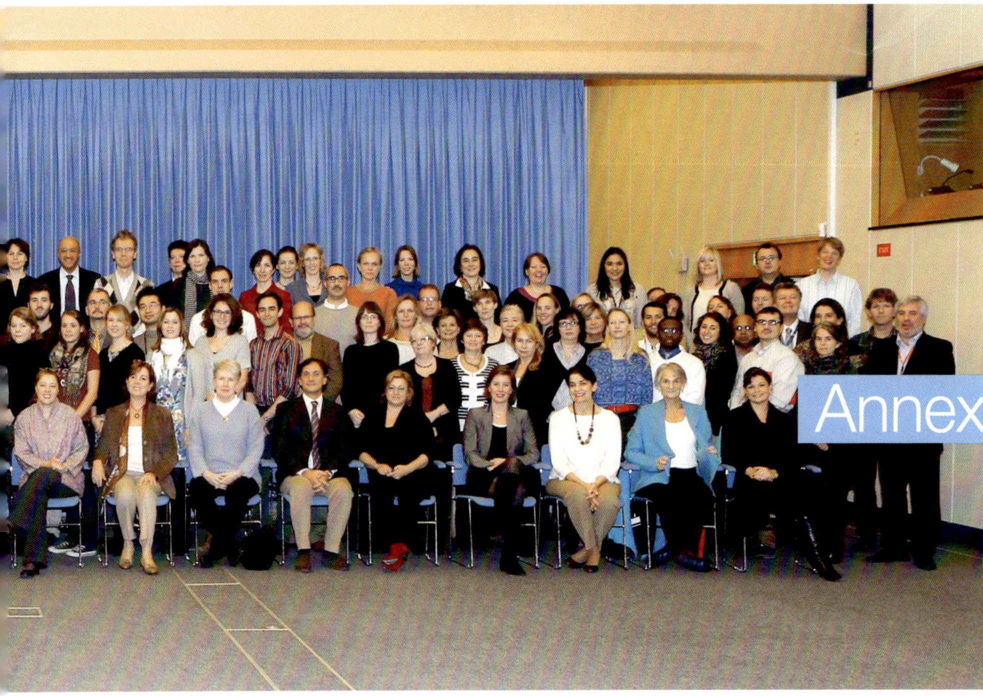

Annexes

WHO Regional Office for Europe staff with HRH Crown Princess Mary, Patron of WHO/Regional Office for Europe, 2012. © WHO/Franz Henriksen

Annex 1 – Witnesses

Róza Ádány

Professor of Public Health, University of Debrecen, Hungary

Sanna Ahonen

Healthy Cities National Network Coordinator, Finland

Recep Akdag

Former Deputy Prime Minister, Former Minister of Health, Turkey

Ayse Akin

Professor of Public Health, Maternal and Child and Reproductive Health, Baskent University, Ankara, Turkey

Olga Algayerova

Executive Secretary, United Nations Economic Commission for Europe (UNECE)

Andrea Ammon

Director, European Centre for Disease Prevention and Control (ECDC)

Vytenis P. Andriukaitis

EU Commissioner for Health and Food Safety

Alanna Armitage

Regional Director, The United Nations Population Fund (UNFPA) Eastern Europe and Central Asia

Jo Eirik Asvall

WHO Regional Director for Europe, 1985–2000

László Attila

Parliamentarian, Romania

Rifat Atun

Professor of Global Health Systems, Harvard University, USA

Clemens Martin Auer

Special Envoy for Health, Austria

Tom Auwers

Secretary General, Federal Ministry of Health, Food Safety and Environment, Belgium

Natasha Azzopardi Muscat

President of the European Public Health Association (EUPHA), Malta

Ran Balicer

Founding Director, Clalit Research Institute and Director of Health Policy Planning at Clalit Health Services, Israel

Ioannis Baskozos

Secretary General of Public Health, Ministry of Health, Greece

Roberto Bertollini

Former WHO Representative to the EU in Brussels and Former Chief Scientist of the WHO Regional Office for Europe

Yelzhan Birtanov

Minister of Healthcare, Kazakhstan

Dragan Bogdanic

Former Minister of Health and Social Welfare, Republika Srpska, Bosnia and Herzegovina

Søren Brostrøm

Director General, Danish Health Authority, Denmark

Hans Bruyninckx

Executive Director, European Environment Agency (EEA)

Ray Busuttil

Former Director General, Public Health Regulation Department, Ministry for Health, the Elderly and Community Care, Malta

Margaret Chan

WHO Director-General, 2006–2017

Marc Danzon

WHO Regional Director for Europe, 2000–2010

Fiona Donovan

WHO Healthy Cities and Counties Coordinator, Ireland

Victor Everhardt

Deputy Mayor for Health, Utrecht, Netherlands

Josep Figueras

Director of the European Observatory on Health Systems and Policies

Christian Friis-Bach

Former Executive Secretary, United Nations Economic Commission for Europe (UNECE)

Amiran Gamkrelidze

Director General of the National Center for Disease Control and Public Health, Georgia

Cees Goos

Former WHO acting Director, Chair European Alcohol Policy Network (APN)

Bjørn Dagfinn Guldvog

Director General of Health and Chief Medical Officer, Norway

Heli Hätönen

Ministerial Adviser at Ministry of Social Affairs and Health, Finland

HRH Crown Princess Mary, Patron of WHO/Regional Office for Europe

Vilborg Ingólfsdóttir

Former WHO National technical focal point, Former Director of Department, Ministry of Welfare, Iceland

Klaus Iohannis

President, Romania

Elena Jablonicka

WHO national counterpart, Ministry of Health, Slovakia

Maris Jesse

Director of Estonian National Institute for Health Development, Estonia

Leo A. Kaprio

WHO Regional Director for Europe, 1966–1985

Afstan Khan

Regional Director for Europe and Central Asia (ECA), Special Coordinator for the Refugee and Migrant Response in Europe, UNICEF

Ilona Kickbusch

Director of the Global Health Centre, The Graduate Institute Geneva, Switzerland

Maria Kirova

Department Head, Asia, Europe, Latin America and the Caribbean, The Global Fund to Fight AIDS, Tuberculosis and Malaria

Taru Koivisto

Director of the Department for Wellbeing and Services, Ministry of Social Affairs and Health, Finland

Mihály Kökény

Former Minister of Health, Hungary

Milojka Kolar-Celarc

Former Minister of Health, Slovenia

Outi Kuivasniemi

Chair of the Regional Evaluation Group 2014, Finland

Maksut Kulzhanov

Professor, Kazakhstan Medical University - Higher School of Public Health (KSPH), Almaty, Kazakhstan

Oleg Kuvshinnikov

Governor of the Vologda Region, Russian Federation, Chairman of the Russian Association of Healthy Cities, Districts and Villages

Sveinn Magnússon

Former Director General for Health, Iceland

Charlotte Marchandise

Deputy Mayor for Health, Rennes, France

Sir Michael Marmot

Director, University College London, Institute of Health Equity, United Kingdom

Rebecca Martin

Director, Center for Global Health at the US Centers for Disease Control and Prevention (CDC), USA

Martin McKee

Professor of European Public Health, London School of Hygiene and Tropical Medicine (LSHTM), United Kingdom

Zuzana Foldesova Motajova

Director, Department of health insurance and macroeconomics, Ministry of Health Slovakia

Carolyn Murphy

Former Director of Administration and Finance at the WHO Regional Office for Europe

Haik Nikogosian

Senior Fellow, Global Health Centre, The Graduate Institute Geneva; Former Minister of Health, Armenia; Former Head of the FCTC Secretariat, Former Special Representative of the WHO Regional Director of Europe

Ellen Trane Nørby

Minister for Health, Denmark

Adil Osmanovic

Minister of Civil Affairs, Bosnia and Herzegovina

Robert Otok

Director, Association of Schools of Public Health in the European Region (ASPHER), Belgium

Yana Panfilova

Founder and Head of the Board of Teenergizer, Ukraine

Stefania Pascut

WHO Healthy Cities Network Coordinator, Udine, Italy

Vesna-Kerstin Petrič

Head, Division for Health Promotion and Prevention of Noncommunicable Diseases, Ministry of Health, Slovenia

Alexandru Rafila

Ministerial Adviser, Romania

Dagmar Reitenbach

Head of Division Global Health, Federal Ministry of Health, Germany

Daniel Reynders

Chair ECDC Management Board, Head of International Relations Unit, Belgian Federal Public Service (FPS) of Health, Food Chain Safety and Environment, Belgium

Franco Santi

Minister of Health and Social Security, Equal Opportunities, National Insurance and Social Affairs, San Marino

David Sergeenko

Minister of Internally Displaced Persons from the Occupied Territories, Labour, Health and Social Affairs, Georgia

Toregeldy Sharmanov

Minister of Health, Kazakh Soviet Socialist Republic, USSR, 1978

Young-soo Shin

Regional Director, WHO Regional Office for the Western Pacific, 2009–2019

Päivi Sillanaukee

Permanent Secretary, Ministry of Social Affairs and Health, Finland

Veronika Skvortsova

Minister of Health, Russian Federation

Selma Sogoric

National Network Coordinator Croatian Healthy Cities Network
Andrija Stampar School of Public Health, Croatia

Ivan Solovic

Director, WHO TB Collaborating Centre, Slovakia

Jozef Suvada

Head of Projects, Standard preventive, diagnostic, therapeutic procedures, Ministry of Health, Slovakia

Istvan Szilard

Co-chair, WHO Collaborating Centre for Migration Health Training and Research, Pécs, Hungary

Tedros Adhanom Ghebreyesus

WHO Director-General

Göran Tomson

Member of the WHO European Advisory Committee on Health Research, Sweden

Agis Tsouros

Former Director, Policy and Governance for Health and Well-being, WHO Regional Office for Europe

Tomris Turmen

Chair of the European Advisory Committee on Health Research (EACHR), Turkey

Annemiek Van Bolhius

Director of Public Health and Health Services, National Institute of Public Health and the Environment (RIVM), Netherlands

Andre van der Zande

President of the International Association of National Public Health Institutes (IANPHI)

Aurelijus Veryga

Minister of Health, Lithuania

Miriam Weber

WHO Healthy City Network Coordinator, Utrecht, Netherlands

Olivia Wigzell

Director General, National Board for Health and Welfare, Sweden

Anne Marie Worning

Former Chief of Cabinet, WHO headquarters in Geneva

Salomudin Jabbor Yusufi

Head of the Department of Medical and Pharmaceutical Education, Health Personnel Policy and Science, Ministry of Health and Social Protection, Republic of Tajikistan

Dineke Zeegers

Director, European Public Health Association (EUPHA), Netherlands

Erio Ziglio

Former Head, WHO European Office for Investment for Health and Development, Venice, Italy

Annex 2 – Executive Summary

Better Health for Europe: more equitable and sustainable, tells the story of how all the people who work in the WHO Regional Office for Europe in Copenhagen, the geographically dispersed offices (GDOs) and the country offices of the WHO European Region have sought, over the last 10 years, to make a reality of this goal. Zsuzsanna Jakab, WHO Regional Director for Europe from 2010 until 2020, narrates the story on behalf of the staff and describes the vision, strategic thinking and processes followed, as well as the impact achieved.

Political leaders, public health managers, health practitioners and advocates from across the WHO European Region and beyond were invited to enrich the narrative with their observations. Extracts from interviews with these witnesses that reflect upon the relevance and utility of the work of the Regional Office are included throughout the book.

The book has three parts:

Part I – Better Health for Europe: the seven strategic action priorities, presents the systematic process the Regional Office has followed in developing the policy frameworks, evidence base, capacities, relationships, partnerships, networks and skills needed to transform and enhance action for better, more equitable and sustainable health and well-being in Europe and beyond.

Part II – Better Health for Europe: achievements, describes the outcomes and impacts of the work of the Regional Office on the two objectives and four priority actions of the Health 2020 European policy framework.

Part III – Better Health for Europe: conclusions and messages, summarizes reflections and looks at challenges beyond 2020.

Part I – Better Health for Europe: the seven strategic action priorities

Building on WHO values, historical developments and an assessment of regional health challenges and assets, seven strategic action priorities were identified with input from stakeholders from across the WHO European Region. They were adopted by the WHO Regional Committee in 2010 and have guided the work of the Regional Office over the last 10 years.

They consisted of:

1. Developing a European health policy framework as a coherent framework for equitable improvements in health and well-being – Health 2020.

   Health 2020 was created as a value-driven, evidence-informed European health policy framework with a wide range of internal and external stakeholders concerned with public health in Europe and beyond. It saw investment in health as a major contributor to development overall and used economic as well as health arguments to promote investment in public health and advocate for all-determinants approaches, the benefits of health promotion and disease prevention, and the value of reducing out-of-pocket copayment percentages for the provision of health services.

   It was informed by newly commissioned scientific research on the social determinants of health, governance for health, and the economics of health intervention. It provided a strategic approach to improving health and well-being, dealing particularly with the political, social, environmental, commercial and cultural determinants, through the creation and implementation of national health policies, implemented through whole-of-government, whole-of-society and health-in-all-policies approaches.

   Health 2020 has had significant impact. By 2016, 93% of 42 responding countries indicated that they had a national health policy aligned with Health 2020, and 88% of countries reported that they had defined Health 2020 related targets or indicators. Within the Regional Office, all work was reframed and aligned with Health 2020 objectives and priorities. Health 2020 had the added value of providing an opening for dialogue, advocacy and influence with political decision-makers at all levels and from different sectors.

2. Improving governance in the WHO European Region and in the Regional Office.

   To mainstream the concept of governance, the Regional Office supported and published research and retrained frontline staff in country offices and others in health diplomacy. Transparency and involvement in the internal governance of the Region was improved through staff training, and strengthening the processes of the Standing Committee of the WHO Regional Committee for Europe and of the Regional Committee itself.

3. Further strengthening of collaboration with Member States.

   The Regional Office was able to demonstrate relevance and leadership in many new and established areas, including,

   - strengthening country offices with internationally appointed WHO representatives working collaboratively with United Nations Resident Coordinators and Country Teams;

- enhancing resources through partnerships, networks and new geographically dispersed offices;
- strengthening technical skills in areas where countries had expressed a need, e.g. economic impact data concerning out-of-pocket payments, anticipating health needs, migration and health, men's health;
- delivering more evidence-informed action options to address inequities;
- re-emphasizing and reinvigorating public health through delivery of the European Action Plan for Strengthening Public Health Capacities and Services and a new vision for advancing public health for sustainable development in the WHO European Region;
- energizing the life-course approach;
- investing in people, e.g. through summer schools on health financing and migration and health;
- delivering many new Health 2020- informed public health- related European strategies, e.g. on mental health, sexual and reproductive health and men's health; and,
- being creatively proactive, rapidly responsive and following through on all commitments.

4. Engaging in strategic partnerships with other stakeholders to jointly improve health and policy coherence in Europe. Strategic partnerships have enhanced resources, policy coherence and impact. Achievement include:
   - establishing new and strengthening existing partnerships and networks, e.g. the Small Countries Initiative and the South-eastern Europe Health Network;
   - enhancing collaboration with the the European Union, the Organisation for Economic Co-operation and Development, the European Centre for Disease Prevention and Control and the Global Fund;
   - extending collaboration with partners in the United Nations System and civil society;
   - establishing new ways of collaborating with partners; and,
   - moving beyond competition and finding mutually beneficial collaborative practices by sharing information and resources.
5. Strengthening the European contribution to global health.

   The Regional Office has been an initiator, tester, and driver of global health approaches. Examples include:
   - health and development;

- the social determinants of health;
- delivering Health 2020;
- governance;
- 'catching the moment' and taking quick action when required, e.g. on migration and health; and,
- addressing difficult issues e.g. developing strategies for sexual and reproductive health, child abuse and maltreatment, and mental health in institutions.

6. Reaching out through an information and communication strategy.

   Much has been learned over the 10 years about ways to put accessible, understandable and useful health information within reach of everyone in the Region and beyond. This has involved:

   - a better understanding of increasing health literacy in the population;
   - making evidence and information more accessible and easier to understand for all;
   - amplifying and broadening the reach of the Regional Office through enhanced web and social media feeds;
   - active partnerships with NGOs, universities, cities, networks, regions etc.; and,
   - the role of ambassadors (e.g. HRH Crown Princess Mary, Patron of WHO/Regional Office for Europe) and high-level advocacy with presidents, prime ministers, ministers of finance and other sectoral leaders (e.g. during country visits and meetings).

7. Promoting the Regional Office as an organization with a positive working environment and sustainable funding for its work.

   The Regional Office has been transformed over the last10 years, through:

   - active involvement of all staff in developing and implementing the Health 2020 policy framework;
   - raising morale through positive engagement with all Member States;
   - establishing the Regional Office as the 'go to' centre of excellence in public health in Europe;
   - improving internal management and financial procedures and accountabilities;
   - motivating and retaining staff;
   - enhancing gender balance among our staff; and
   - strengthening the intern programme and recruiting motivated staff who can lead the Organization into the future.

Part II – Better Health for Europe: achievements

All of the technical work of the Regional Office has been reframed around helping Member States make health a political choice. The principal vehicles for change have been the two objectives of Health 2020:

- improve health for all and reduce the health divide;
- strengthen leadership and participatory governance for health;

and its four priority action areas:

- invest in a life-course approach and empower people;
- tackle Europe's major health challenges;
- strengthen people-centred health systems, public health capacity and emergency preparedness, surveillance and response; and,
- create resilient communities and supportive environments.

Targets, indicators and a monitoring process agreed by all Member States have included:

- reduce premature mortality in the Region;
- increase life expectancy in the Region;
- reduce inequalities in health in the Region;
- enhance the well-being of the population in the Region;
- ensure universal coverage and the 'right to health'; and,
- set national goals and targets related to health.

Significant progress has been made across the Region in addressing all these targets and their various indicators.

Results reported in 2018, include the following:

- life expectancy in the Region is increasing, while the gaps in life expectancy, both between the sexes and between countries, are narrowing.
- significant inequities in health remain between and within countries.
- the Region is on track to achieve the Sustainable Development Goal target to reduce premature mortality from the four major noncommunicable diseases by 1.5% annually until 2030, although gaps within and between countries remain.
- overall, the differences between Member States in the indicators related to social determinants of health – infant mortality, life expectancy, primary school enrolment and unemployment – have narrowed.

The Regional Office has supported countries in these challenges and achievements with a wide variety of tools, research, programmatic initiatives, seminars, training and policy dialogues, expert advisory groups, high-level meetings, action resolutions, outcome monitoring and reporting, network and partnership strengthening and direct advocacy with political leaders and senior public officials.

Part III – Better Health for Europe: conclusions and messages

Two key achievements stand out and now help shape future developments. The first builds on the changed global development narrative, as expressed the United Nations 2030 Agenda for Sustainable Development and the Sustainable Development Goals. These include a wider set of development outcomes than solely economic gain. Health 2020 presented an early example of this thinking and prepared the European Member States to take leadership roles in maintaining health at the centre of the development agenda as well as advocating for UHC.

The second transformative change relates to people and public health leadership. The collaborative work and collective experience in developing and implementing Health 2020 and the European Action Plan for Strengthening Public Health Capacities and Services at all levels has strengthened the voice and work of public health leaders in all 53 Member States and beyond, as well as helping to create new public health leaders for the 21st century. Public health advocates have been empowered with new tools, skills and competencies to champion the new narrative.

Nonetheless, health and health policy still face daunting challenges, notably from a global change in the political environment towards more divisive and less consensus-based policy thinking. More politicization can be expected even in the short run and some Member States may find it more difficult to reach consensus on sensitive issues.

Our learning over the last decade gives us important pointers to help shape responses to these new challenges, both regionally and globally. One thing is clear, our collective value-driven, evidence-informed health leadership will be needed more than ever in the future.

References

1. Kaprio L. A., Forty years of WHO in Europe: the development of a common health policy. Copenhagen: WHO Regional Office for Europe; 1991 (European series, No.40; https://apps.who.int/iris/handle/10665/260455, accessed 1 July 2019).

2. Sixty years of WHO in Europe. Copenhagen: WHO Regional Office for Europe; 2010 (https://apps.who.int/iris/handle/10665/107273, accessed 1 July 2019).

3. European health report 2018: more than numbers – evidence for all. Copenhagen: WHO Regional Office for Europe; 2018 (https://apps.who.int/iris/handle/10665/279904, accessed 1 July 2019).

4. World Bank Country and Lending Group. In: The World Bank/Data [website]. Washington DC: World Bank; 2018 (https://datahelpdesk.worldbank.org/knowledgebase/articles/906519-world-bank-country-and-lending-groups, accessed 1 July 2019).

5. European Health Information Gateway [online database]. Life expectancy at birth. Copenhagen: WHO Regional Office for Europe; 2019 (https://gateway.euro.who.int/en/hfa-explorer/#zURZMYFwEM, accessed 1 July 2019).

6. European Health Information Gateway [online database]. SDR, major noncommunicable diseases, 30-69 years, both sexes. Copenhagen: WHO Regional Office for Europe; 2019 (https://gateway.euro.who.int/en/indicators/hfa_299-1990-sdr-major-noncommunicable-diseases-30-69-years-both-sexes/, accessed 1 July 2019).

7. Review of social determinants and the health divide in the WHO European Region, Updated reprint 2014. Copenhagen: WHO Regional Office for Europe. (https://apps.who.int/iris/handle/10665/108636, accessed 1 July 2019).

8. Javier, J.R., Brumberg, H.L., Sanders, L., Hannon, T.S. and Shah, S. How gaps in policy implementation cause public health malpractice. *The Lancet*. 2018; *391*(10138), p.2414. doi:10.1016/S0140-6736(18)31038-9

9. Haines, A., Kuruvilla, S. & Borchert, M. Bridging the implementation gap between knowledge and action for health. *Bulletin of the World Health Organization: the International Journal of Public Health 2004; 82(10): 724-731 (*https://apps.who.int/iris/handle/10665/72583, accessed 1 July 2019).

10. Healthy Environments for Healthier People. Copenhagen: WHO Regional Office for Europe; 2018 (http://www.euro.who.int/en/health-topics/environment-and-health/noise/publications/2018/healthy-environments-for-healthier-people-2018, accessed 1 July 2019).

11. High-level meeting: HSS respond to NCDs. Outcome statement. Copenhagen: WHO Regional Office for Europe; 2018 (http://www.euro.who.int/en/media-centre/events/events/2018/04/high-level-regional-meeting-health-systems-respond-to-ncds-experience-in-the-european-region/documentation/working-documents/outcome-statement, accessed 1 July 2019).

12. Action plan for the prevention and control of noncommunicable diseases in the WHO European Region. Copenhagen: WHO Regional Office for Europe (EUR/RC66/11: http://www.euro.who.int/en/about-us/governance/regional-committee-for-europe/past-sessions/66th-session/documentation/working-documents/eurrc6611-action-plan-for-the-prevention-and-control-of-noncommunicable-diseases-in-the-who-european-region, accessed 1 July 2019).

13. Fact sheet: Mental health [website]. Copenhagen: WHO Regional Office for Europe; 2019 (http://www.euro.who.int/en/health-topics/noncommunicable-diseases/mental-health/data-and-resources/fact-sheet-mental-health-2019, accessed 1 July 2019).

14. Data and resources: Mental Health [website]. Copenhagen: WHO Regional Office for Europe; 2019 (http://www.euro.who.int/en/health-topics/noncommunicable-diseases/mental-health/data-and-resources, accessed 1 July 2019).

15. Report on the health of refugees and migrants in the WHO European Region: no public health without refugee and migrant health (2018). Copenhagen: WHO Regional Office for Europe; 2019 (http://www.euro.who.int/en/publications/abstracts/report-on-the-health-of-refugees-and-migrants-in-the-who-european-region-no-public-health-without-refugee-and-migrant-health-2018, accessed 1 July 2019).

16. Strategy and action plan for refugee and migrant health in the WHO European Region. Copenhagen: WHO Regional Office for Europe; 2016 (EUR/RC66/8; http://www.euro.who.int/en/health-topics/health-determinants/migration-and-health/publications/2016/strategy-and-action-plan-for-refugee-and-migrant-health-in-the-who-european-region, accessed 1 July 2019).

17. Jo Eirik Asvall's memorial guide: 1931–2010. Copenhagen: WHO Regional Office for Europe; 2010 (http://www.euro.who.int/en/publications/abstracts/jo-eirik-asvalls-memorial-guide-19312010, accessed 1 July 2019).

18. Basic documents, 46th ed. Geneva: World Health Organization; 2007 (https://apps.who.int/iris/handle/10665/43637, accessed 1 July 2019).

19. Where WHO works [website]. Geneva: World Health Organization; 2019 (https://www.who.int/country-cooperation/where-who-works/en/, accessed 1 July 2019).

20. The Alma-Ata Declaration [website]. Geneva: World Health Organization; 1978 (https://www.who.int/social_determinants/tools/multimedia/alma_ata/en/, accessed 1 July 2019).

21. Targets for Health for All: Targets in support of the European regional strategy for Health for All. Copenhagen: WHO Regional Office for Europe; 1986 (https://apps.who.int/iris/handle/10665/325996, accessed 1 July 2019).

22. The Ottawa Charter for Health Promotion: First International Conference on Health Promotion, Ottawa, 21 November 1986 [website]. Geneva: World Health Organization; 1986 (https://www.who.int/healthpromotion/conferences/previous/ottawa/en/, 1 accessed 1 July 2019).

23. Regional Cooperation Council (former Stability Pact for South East Europe) [website]. Rome: Farnesina Ministero degli affari esteri e della cooperazione internazionale; 2008 (https://www.esteri.it/mae/en/politica_estera/aree_geografiche/europa/ooii/patto_di_stabilit_dei_balcani.html, accessed 1 July 2019) (in Italian).

24. The Tallinn Charter: Health Systems for Health and Wealth [website]. Copenhagen: WHO Regional Office for Europe; 2008 (http://www.euro.who.int/en/publications/policy-documents/tallinn-charter-health-systems-for-health-and-wealth, accessed 1 July 2019).

25. Fact Sheets. Universal health coverage (UHC) [website]. Geneva: World Health Organization; 2019 (http://www.who.int/universal_health_coverage/en/, accessed 1 July 2019).

26. Health 2020. A European policy framework and strategy for the 21st century. Copenhagen: WHO Regional Office for Europe; 2013 (https://apps.who.int/iris/handle/10665/131303, accessed 1 July 2019).

27. European Action Plan for Strengthening Public Health Capacities and Services. Copenhagen: WHO Regional Office for Europe; 2012 (EUR/RC62/12 Rev.1 http://www.euro.who.int/en/health-topics/Health-systems/public-health-services/publications/2012/european-action-plan-for-strengthening-public-health-capacities-and-services, accessed 1 July 2019).

28. Targets and indicators for Health 2020. Version 3. Copenhagen: WHO Regional Office for Europe; 2016 (http://www.euro.who.int/en/health-topics/health-policy/health-2020-the-european-policy-for-health-and-well-being/publications/2016/targets-and-indicators-for-health-2020.-version-3-2016, accessed 1 July 2019).

29. European Health Information Initiative. Copenhagen: WHO Regional Office for Europe; 2019 (http://www.euro.who.int/en/data-and-evidence/european-health-information-initiative-ehii/european-health-information-initiative, accessed 1 July 2019).

30. Commission on Social Determinants of Health. Closing the gap in a generation: health equity through action on the social determinants of health: final report of the commission on social determinants of health. Geneva: World Health Organization; 2008 (https://apps.who.int/iris/handle/10665/43943, accessed 1 July 2019).

31. Marmot, M., Allen, J., Goldblatt, P., Boyce, T., McNeish, D., Grady, M. and Geddes, I. The Marmot review: Fair society, healthy lives. The Strategic Review of Health Inequalities in England Post-2010; 2010 (http://www.instituteofhealthequity.org/resources-reports/fair-society-healthy-lives-the-marmot-review, accessed 1 July 2019).

32. Implementing a Health 2020 vision: governance for health in the 21st century. Making it happen. Copenhagen: WHO Regional Office for Europe; 2013 (http://www.euro.who.int/en/publications/abstracts/implementing-a-health-2020-vision-governance-for-health-in-the-21st-century.-making-it-happen, accessed 1 July 2019).

33. OECD, WHO Regional Office for Europe, European Observatory on Health Systems and Policies. Promoting Health, Preventing Disease: The Economic Case. Maidenhead: Open University Press; 2015 (https://www.oecd-ilibrary.org/economics/promoting-health-preventing-disease_9780335262274-en;jsessionid=pSd7olYeUHcEC0hS4oUTMhjd.ip-10-240-5-9, accessed 1 July 2019).

34. The Case For Investing In Public Health. A public health summary report for EPHO 8. Copenhagen: WHO Regional Office for Europe; 2014 (https://apps.who.int/iris/handle/10665/170471, accessed 1 July 2019).

35. World Health Organization and World Economic Forum. From Burden to "Best Buys": Reducing the Economic Impact of Non-Communicable Diseases in Low- and Middle-Income Countries. Cologny/Geneva: World Economic Forum; 2011 (https://apps.who.int/medicinedocs/en/m/abstract/Js18804en/, accessed 1 July 2019).

36. Which are the most effective and cost-effective interventions for tobacco control? Copenhagen: WHO Regional Office for Europe; 2003 (http://www.euro.who.int/en/data-and-evidence/evidence-informed-policy-making/publications/pre2009/which-are-the-most-effective-and-cost-effective-interventions-for-tobacco-control, accessed 1 July 2019).

37. Saving lives, spending less: a strategic response to noncommunicable diseases. Geneva: World Health Organization; 2018 (https://apps.who.int/iris/handle/10665/272534, accessed 1 July 2019).

38. Prevention and control of noncommunicable diseases in Kyrgyzstan. The case for investment (2017). Copenhagen: WHO Regional Office for Europe; 2017 (http://www.euro.who.int/en/countries/kyrgyzstan/publications/prevention-and-control-of-noncommunicable-diseases-in-kyrgyzstan.-the-case-for-investment-2017, accessed 1 July 2019)

39. Prevention and control of NCDs in Belarus: The case for investment (2018). Copenhagen: WHO Regional Office for Europe; 2018 (http://www.euro.who.int/en/countries/belarus/publications/prevention-and-control-of-ncds-in-belarus-the-case-for-investment-2018, accessed 1 July 2019)

40. Turner, D.A., Khioe, R.F.S., Shepstone, L., Lenaghan, E., et al. The Cost Effectiveness of Screening in the Community to Reduce Osteoporotic Fractures in Older Women in the UK: Economic Evaluation of the SCOOP Study. *Journal of Bone and Mineral Research*, 2018; *33*(5), pp.845-851. doi:*10.1002/jbmr.3381.*

41. Ding, D., Lawson, K.D., Kolbe-Alexander, T.L., Finkelstein, E.A., et al. The economic burden of physical inactivity: a global analysis of major non-communicable diseases. *The Lancet*, 2016; *388*(10051), pp.1311-1324. doi:10.1016/S0140-6736(16)30383-X.

42. Asaria, M., Doran, T., Cookson, R. The costs of inequality: whole-population modelling study of lifetime inpatient hospital costs in the English National Health Service by level of neighbourhood deprivation. *Journal of Epidemiology and Community Health*. 2016;70(10):990-6. doi:10.1136/jech-2016-207447.

43. Grimm, MM. Does inequality in health impede growth? International Institute of Social Studies of Erasmus University Rotterdam (ISS).*Working Paper Series/General Series*. 2010;501:1-31.

44. Mackenbach JP, Meerding WJ, Kunst AE. Economic costs of health inequalities in the European Union. *Journal of Epidemiology & Community Health*. 2011;65(5):412-9. doi: 10.1136/jech.2010.112680.

45. Chemical safety: Publications [website]. Copenhagen: WHO Regional Office for Europe; 2019 (http://www.euro.who.int/en/health-topics/environment-and-health/chemical-safety/publications, accessed 1 July 2019)

46. Climate change: Publications [website]. Copenhagen: WHO Regional Office for Europe; 2019 (http://www.euro.who.int/en/health-topics/environment-and-health/Climate-change/publications, accessed 1 July 2019)

47. Strengthening resilience: a priority shared by Health 2020 and the Sustainable Development Goals. Copenhagen: WHO Regional Office for Europe; 2017 (http://www.euro.who.int/en/countries/monaco/publications/strengthening-resilience-a-priority-shared-by-health-2020-and-the-sustainable-development-goals-2017, accessed 1 July 2019)

48. Public Health, Environmental and Social Determinants of Health (PHE). NTDs: WHO launches toolkit to optimize water, sanitation and hygiene interventions [website]. Geneva: World Health Organization; 2019 (https://www.who.int/phe/news/toolkit-water-sanitation-hygiene/en/, accessed 1 July 2019)

49. Environment and health for European cities in the 21st century: making a difference. Copenhagen: WHO Regional Office for Europe; 2016 (http://www.euro.who.int/en/health-topics/environment-and-health/urban-health/publications/2017/environment-and-health-for-european-cities-in-the-21st-century-making-a-difference-2017, accessed 1 July 2019).

50. Embedding a cultural context of health approach across the WHO European Region. Copenhagen: WHO Regional Office for Europe; 2018 (http://www.euro.who.int/en/publications/abstracts/embedding-a-cultural-contexts-of-health-approach-across-the-who-european-region-2018, accessed 1 July 2019).

51. Advancing public health for sustainable development in the WHO European Region. Copenhagen: WHO Regional Office for Europe; 2018 (EUR/RC68/17 http://www.euro.who.int/en/about-us/governance/regional-committee-for-europe/past-sessions/68th-session/documentation/working-documents/eurrc6817, accessed 1 July 2019).

52. Public Health Services: The 10 Essential Public Health Operations [website]. Copenhagen: WHO Regional Office for Europe; 2012 (http://www.euro.who.int/en/health-topics/Health-systems/public-health-services/policy/the-10-essential-public-health-operations, accessed 1 July 2019).

53. Ádany R, Villerusa A, Bislimovska J, Kulzhanov M. Public health education in Central and Eastern Europe, and Central Asia. *Public Health Reviews*. 2011;33(1):105. doi: 10.1007/BF03391623.

54. On the road to Health 2020 policy targets: Monitoring qualitative indicators. An update. (2017). Copenhagen: WHO Regional Office for Europe; 2017 (http://www.euro.who.int/en/health-topics/health-policy/health-2020-the-european-policy-for-health-and-well-being/publications/2017/on-the-road-to-health-2020-policy-targets-monitoring-qualitative-indicators.-an-update.-2017, accessed 1 July 2019).

55. Joint Action Plan: Organization for Economic Co-operation and Development (OECD) and WHO/Europe. Copenhagen: WHO Regional Office for Europe; 2012 (http://www.euro.who.int/en/about-us/partners/organisation-for-economic-co-operation-and-development-oecd/joint-action-plan-organization-for-economic-co-operation-and-development-oecd-and-whoeurope, accessed 1 July 2019).

56. Organization and financing of public health services in Europe: country reports (2018). Copenhagen: WHO Regional Office for Europe; 2018 (http://www.euro.who.int/en/publications/abstracts/organization-and-financing-of-public-health-services-in-europe-country-reports-2018, accessed 1 July 2019).

57. Health 2020: the European policy for health and well-being. Health 2020 Implementation Package [website]. Copenhagen: WHO Regional Office for Europe; 2012 (http://www.euro.who.int/en/health-topics/health-policy/health-2020-the-european-policy-for-health-and-well-being/implementation-package, accessed 1 July 2019).

58. Promoting intersectoral action for health and well-being in the WHO European Region: health is a political choice. Copenhagen: WHO Regional Office for Europe; 2015 (EUR/RC65/16 http://www.euro.who.int/en/about-us/governance/regional-committee-for-europe/past-sessions/65th-session/documentation/working-documents/eurrc6516-promoting-intersectoral-action-for-health-and-well-being-in-the-who-european-region-health-is-a-political-choice, accessed 1 July 2019).

59. Laboratory services: Better Labs for Better Health [website]. Copenhagen: WHO Regional Office for Europe; 2018 (http://www.euro.who.int/en/health-topics/Health-systems/laboratory-services/better-labs-for-better-health, accessed 1 July 2019).

60. Developing national action plans on transport, health and environment. A step-by-step manual for policy-makers and planners. Copenhagen: WHO Regional Office for Europe; 2014 (http://www.euro.who.int/en/publications/abstracts/developing-national-action-plans-on-transport,-health-and-environment.-a-step-by-step-manual-for-policy-makers-and-planners, accessed 1 July 2019).

61. Violence and injuries: Road traffic injuries [website]. Copenhagen: WHO Regional Office for Europe; 2015 (http://www.euro.who.int/en/health-topics/disease-prevention/violence-and-injuries/areas-of-work/road-traffic-injuries, accessed 1 July 2019).

62. Environmental policy. About the protocol on Water and Health [website]. Geneva: UNECE; 1999 (http://www.unece.org/?id=2975, accessed 1 July 2019).

63. The Portuguese National Health Plan, Interim Report on the National Health Plan: Revision and Extension to 2020 (The NRP-Revision), Comments from WHO Europe. Copenhagen: WHO Regional Office for Europe; 2015 (http://1nj5ms2lli5hdggbe3mm7ms5.wpengine.netdna-cdn.com/files/2015/07/2015_OMS_Interim-Report-on-the-National-Health-Plan_revision-and-extension-to.pdf, accessed 1 July 2019).

64. Healthy Ireland. A framework for improved health and wellbeing 2013–2025. Dublin: Government of Ireland; 2013 (https://health.gov.ie/blog/publications/healthy-ireland-a-framework-for-improved-health-and-wellbeing-2013-2025/, accessed 1 July 2019).

65. The Minsk Declaration: The Life-course Approach in the Context of Health 2020. Copenhagen: WHO Regional Office for Europe; 2015 (http://www.euro.who.int/en/publications/policy-documents/the-minsk-declaration, accessed 1 July 2019).

66. Strategy on women's health and well-being in the WHO European Region. Copenhagen: WHO Regional Office for Europe; 2016 (http://www.euro.who.int/en/health-topics/health-determinants/gender/publications/2016/strategy-on-womens-health-and-well-being-in-the-who-european-region-2016, accessed 1 July 2019).

67. Strategy on the health and well-being of men in the WHO European Region. Copenhagen: WHO Regional Office for Europe; 2018 (http://www.euro.who.int/en/health-topics/health-determinants/gender/publications/2018/strategy-on-the-health-and-well-being-of-men-in-the-who-european-region-2018, accessed 1 July 2019).

68. High Level Political Forum on Sustainable Development 2017 [website]. New York: United Nations; 2017 (https://sustainabledevelopment.un.org/hlpf/2017, accessed 1 July 2019).

69. Ashgabat Declaration on the Prevention and Control of Noncommunicable Diseases in the Context of Health 2020. Copenhagen: WHO Regional Office for Europe; 2013 (http://www.euro.who.int/en/health-topics/noncommunicable-diseases/ncd-background-information/ashgabat-declaration-on-the-prevention-and-control-of-noncommunicable-diseases-in-the-context-of-health-2020, accessed 1 July 2019).

70. Vienna Declaration on Nutrition and Noncommunicable Diseases in the Context of Health 2020. Copenhagen: WHO Regional Office for Europe; 2013 (http://www.euro.who.int/en/media-centre/events/events/2013/07/vienna-conference-on-nutrition-and-noncommunicable-diseases/documentation/vienna-declaration-on-nutrition-and-noncommunicable-diseases-in-the-context-of-health-2020-2013, accessed 1 July 2019).

71. Strategy and action plan for healthy ageing in Europe, 2012–2020. Copenhagen: WHO Regional Office for Europe; 2012 (EUR/RC62/10 Rev.1 http://www.euro.who.int/en/health-topics/Life-stages/healthy-ageing/publications/2012/strategy-and-action-plan-for-healthy-ageing-in-europe,-20122020, accessed 1 July 2019).

72. Investing in children: the European child and adolescent health strategy 2015–2020. Copenhagen: WHO Regional Office for Europe; 2014 (EUR/RC64/12 http://www.euro.who.int/en/health-topics/Life-stages/child-and-adolescent-health/policy/investing-in-children-the-european-child-and-adolescent-health-strategy-20152020, accessed 1 July 2019).

73. Investing in children: the European child maltreatment prevention action plan 2015–2020. Copenhagen: WHO Regional Office for Europe; 2014 ((EUR/RC64/13; http://www.euro.who.int/en/about-us/governance/regional-committee-for-europe/past-sessions/64th-session/documentation/working-documents/eurrc6413-investing-in-children-the-european-child-maltreatment-prevention-action-plan-20152020, accessed 8 August 2019).

74. Action Plan for Sexual and Reproductive Health: towards achieving the 2030 Agenda for Sustainable Development in Europe – leaving no one behind (2016). Copenhagen: WHO Regional Office for Europe; 2016 (http://www.euro.who.int/en/health-topics/Life-stages/sexual-and-reproductive-health/publications/2016/action-plan-for-sexual-and-reproductive-health-towards-achieving-the-2030-agenda-for-sustainable-development-in-europe-leaving-no-one-behind-2016, accessed 1 July 2019).

75. European Vaccine Action Plan 2015–2020. Copenhagen: WHO Regional Office for Europe; 2014 (http://www.euro.who.int/en/health-topics/disease-prevention/vaccines-and-immunization/publications/2014/european-vaccine-action-plan-20152020-2014, accessed 1 July 2019).

76. European strategic action plan on antibiotic resistance. Copenhagen: WHO Regional Office for Europe; 2011 (http://www.euro.who.int/en/about-us/governance/regional-committee-for-europe/past-sessions/sixty-first-session/documentation/working-documents/wd14-european-strategic-action-plan-on-antibiotic-resistance, accessed 1 July 2019).

77. Advancing food safety initiatives: strategic plan for food safety including foodborne zoonoses 2013–2022. Geneva: World Health Organization; 2014 (http://www.who.int/foodsafety/strategic-plan/en, accessed 1 July 2019).

78. European strategic directions for strengthening nursing and midwifery towards Health 2020 goals. Copenhagen: WHO Regional Office for Europe; 2015 (http://www.euro.who.int/en/health-topics/Health-systems/nursing-and-midwifery/publications/2015/european-strategic-directions-for-strengthening-nursing-and-midwifery-towards-health-2020-goals, accessed 1 July 2019).

79. Action plan for the health sector response to HIV in the WHO European Region (2017). Copenhagen: WHO Regional Office for Europe; 2017 (http://www.euro.who.int/en/health-topics/communicable-diseases/hivaids/publications/2017/action-plan-for-the-health-sector-response-to-hiv-in-the-who-european-region-2017, accessed 1 July 2019).

80. Action plan for the health sector response to viral hepatitis in the WHO European Region. Copenhagen: WHO Regional Office for Europe; 2017 (EUR/RC66/10 http://www.euro.who.int/en/about-us/governance/regional-committee-for-europe/past-sessions/66th-session/documentation/working-documents/eurrc6610-action-plan-for-the-health-sector-response-to-viral-hepatitis-in-the-who-european-region accessed 1 July 2019).

81. Framework for control and prevention of soil-transmitted helminthiases in the WHO European Region 2016–2020. Copenhagen: WHO Regional Office for Europe; 2016 (http://www.euro.who.int/en/publications/abstracts/framework-for-control-and-prevention-of-soil-transmitted-helminthiases-in-the-who-european-region-20162020-2016, accessed 1 July 2019).

82. Roadmap to implement the 2030 Agenda for Sustainable Development, building on Health 2020, the European policy for health and well-being. Copenhagen: WHO Regional Office for Europe; 2017 (EUR/RC67/9 http://www.euro.who.int/en/about-us/governance/regional-committee-for-europe/past-sessions/67th-session/documentation/working-documents/eurrc679-roadmap-to-implement-the-2030-agenda-for-sustainable-development,-building-on-health-2020,-the-european-policy-for-health-and-well-being, accessed 1 July 2019).

83. Governance for health in the 21st century. Copenhagen: WHO Regional Office for Europe; 2012 (http://www.euro.who.int/en/publications/abstracts/governance-for-health-in-the-21st-century, accessed 1 July 2019).

84. Organization. Collaborating centres [website]. Copenhagen: WHO Regional Office for Europe; 2019 (http://www.euro.who.int/en/about-us/organization/collaborating-centres, accessed 1 July 2019).

85. Financing dialogue. Session 3: Promoting Coordinated Resource Mobilization [PowerPoint Presentation]. Geneva: World Health Organization; 2015 (https://www.who.int/about/finances-accountability/funding/financing-dialogue/Presentation-on-promoting-Coordinated-Resource-Mobilization.pdf, accessed 1 July 2019).

86. Strengthening the role of the Regional Office's geographically dispersed offices (GDOs): a renewed GDO strategy for Europe. Copenhagen: WHO Regional Office for Europe; 2012 (EUR/RC62/11 http://www.euro.who.int/en/about-us/governance/regional-committee-for-europe/past-sessions/sixty-second-session/documentation/working-documents/eurrc6211-strengthening-the-role-of-the-regional-offices-geographically-dispersed-offices-gdos-a-renewed-gdo-strategy-for-europe, accessed 1 July 2019).

87. United Nations Development Group and UN Regional Coordination Mechanism. Regional UN System Meetings for Europe and Central Asia. Note for Record and Conclusions. 11–12 May, 2016. Geneva: ILO; 2016 (http://www.un-rcm-europecentralasia.org/fileadmin/DAM/RCM_Website/home/Regional-UN-System-Meetings_Note-for-Record-and-Conclusions.pdf, accessed 1 July 2019).

88. Sustainable Development Goals. Coalition for health and well-being in Europe and central Asia [website]. Copenhagen: WHO Regional Office for Europe; 2016 (http://www.euro.who.int/en/health-topics/health-policy/sustainable-development-goals/partnerships-and-intersectoral-action/coalition-for-health-and-well-being-in-europe-and-central-asia, accessed 1 July 2019).

89. Air quality guidelines - global update 2005 [website]. Geneva: World Health Organization; 2005 (https://www.who.int/phe/health_topics/outdoorair/outdoorair_aqg/en/, accessed 1 July 2019).

90. Framework of engagement with non-State actors. Geneva: World Health Organization; 2016 (WHA69.10. Agenda item 11.3. http://apps.who.int/gb/ebwha/pdf_files/wha69/a69_r10-en.pdf, accessed 1 July 2019).

91. Small countries of the WHO European Region exchange ideas and experiences of equity, sustainable development [website]. Copenhagen: WHO Regional Office for Europe; 2019 (http://www.euro.who.int/en/countries/iceland/news/news/2019/4/small-countries-of-the-who-european-region-exchange-ideas-and-experiences-of-equity,-sustainable-development, accessed 1 July 2019).

92. Implementation of the 2030 Agenda for Sustainable Development: Report by the Director-General. Geneva: World Health Organization; 2017 (EB144/11 Rev.1 https://apps.who.int/gb/ebwha/pdf_files/EB144/B144_11Rev1-en.pdf, accessed 1 July 2019).

93. Health and Sustainable Development Goals - Team meeting (2018). Copenhagen: WHO Regional Office for Europe; 2018 (http://www.euro.who.int/en/health-topics/health-policy/sustainable-development-goals/publications/2018/health-and-sustainable-development-goals-team-meeting-2018, accessed 1 July 2019).

94. United Nations Refugees and Migrants. Global Compact for Migration [website]. New York: United Nations; 2018 (https://refugeesmigrants.un.org/migration-compact, accessed 1 July 2019).

95. Global Health Partners. GAVI Alliance [website] Copenhagen: WHO Regional Office for Europe; 2016 (http://www.euro.who.int/en/about-us/partners/global-health-partnerships/gavi-alliance, accessed 1 July 2019).

96. Promoting the health of refugees and migrants: Framework of priorities and guiding principles to promote the health of refugees and migrants. Geneva: World Health Organization; 2016 (https://www.who.int/migrants/about/framework_refugees-migrants.pdf, accessed 1 July 2019).

97. Promoting the health of refugees and migrants. Draft global action plan, 2019–2023. Geneva: World Health Organization; 2019 (A72/25 https://apps.who.int/gb/ebwha/pdf_files/WHA72/A72_25-en.pdf, accessed 1 July 2019).

98. Migration and Health. Public Health Aspects of Migration in Europe (PHAME) newsletter 2014-2019. Copenhagen: WHO Regional Office for Europe; 2014 (http://www.euro.who.int/en/health-topics/health-determinants/migration-and-health/resources/phame-newsletter, accessed 1 July 2019).

99. Toolkit for assessing health system capacity to manage large influxes of refugees, asylum-seekers and migrants. Copenhagen: WHO Regional Office for Europe; 2016 (http://www.euro.who.int/en/publications/abstracts/toolkit-for-assessing-health-system-capacity-to-manage-large-influxes-of-refugees,-asylum-seekers-and-migrants-2016, accessed 1 July 2019).

100. Media Centre. WHO and European Commission adopt joint declaration [website]. Copenhagen: WHO Regional Office for Europe; 2010 (http://www.euro.who.int/en/media-centre/sections/press-releases/2010/09/who-and-european-commission-adopt-joint-declaration, accessed 1 July 2019).

101. European Health Information Initiative: European policy-makers need answers. Copenhagen: WHO Regional Office for Europe; 2015 (http://www.euro.who.int/en/data-and-evidence/european-health-information-initiative-ehii/european-health-information-initiative, accessed 1 July 2019).

102. European Health Information Gateway [online database]. A wealth of information at your fingertips. Copenhagen: WHO Regional Office for Europe; 2015 (https://gateway.euro.who.int/en/, accessed 1 July 2019).

103. European Health Information Gateway [online database]. A wealth of information at your fingertips. Health for All explorer. Copenhagen: WHO Regional Office for Europe; 2015 (https://gateway.euro.who.int/en/hfa-explorer/, accessed 1 July 2019).

104. Facilitating health reporting in the WHO European Region: A comparative analysis of indicators across Health 2020,the Sustainable Development Goals and the Global Action Plan for the Prevention and Control of Noncommunicable Diseases 2013–2020. Copenhagen: WHO Regional Office for Europe; 2013–2020 (http://www.euro.who.int/__data/assets/pdf_file/0005/322718/Facilitating-health-reporting.pdf, accessed 1 July 2019).

105. Migration and Health. Health Evidence Network (HEN) synthesis reports [website]. Copenhagen: WHO Regional Office for Europe; 2016–2018 (http://www.euro.who.int/en/health-topics/health-determinants/migration-and-health/publications/health-evidence-network-hen-synthesis-reports, accessed 1 July 2019).

106. Evidence-informed policy-making. Evidence-informed Policy Network (EVIPNet) website]. Copenhagen: WHO Regional Office for Europe; 2012 (http://www.euro.who.int/en/data-and-evidence/evidence-informed-policy-making/evidence-informed-policy-network-evipnet, accessed 1 July 2019).

107. McFarlane J. How fake medical news is seriously damaging our health: From vaccines and heart pills to cancer drugs and diets, as experts report a rise in misinformation online, a special investigation tackles the dangerous myths threatening our health. The Daily Mail. 25 November 2018 (https://www.dailymail.co.uk/health/article-6424819/How-fake-news-SERIOUSLY-damaging-health.html, accessed 1 July 2019).

108. Evidence-Informed Policy Network: EVIPNet in action: 10 years, 10 stories. Geneva: World Health Organization; 2016 (https://www.who.int/evidence/resources/publication/en/, accessed 1 July 2019).

109. Media Centre. Newsletters [website]. Copenhagen: WHO Regional Office for Europe; 2019 (http://www.euro.who.int/en/media-centre/newsletters, accessed 1 July 2019).

110. Media Centre. WHO/Europe news highlights [website]. Copenhagen: WHO Regional Office for Europe; 2018–2019 (http://www.euro.who.int/en/media-centre/newsletters/whoeurope-news-highlights-archive, accessed 1 July 2019).

111. Media Centre. European Environment and Health Process Newsletter [website]. Copenhagen: WHO Regional Office for Europe; 2014-2017 (http://www.euro.who.int/en/media-centre/newsletters/european-environment-and-health-process-newsletter, accessed 1 July 2019).

112. Media Centre. Flu Focus [website]. Copenhagen: WHO Regional Office for Europe; 2010–2014 (http://www.euro.who.int/en/media-centre/newsletters/flu-focus, accessed 1 July 2019).

113. Media Centre. Health systems newsletter [website]. Copenhagen: WHO Regional Office for Europe; 2015–2019 (http://www.euro.who.int/en/media-centre/newsletters/health-systems-newsletter, accessed 1 July 2019).

114. Media Centre. HEN News [website]. Copenhagen: WHO Regional Office for Europe; 2015–2019 (http://www.euro.who.int/en/media-centre/newsletters/hen-news, accessed 1 July 2019).

115. Media Centre. Joint TB, HIV and viral Hepatitis (JTH) newsletter [website]. Copenhagen: WHO Regional Office for Europe; 2017–2019 (http://www.euro.who.int/en/media-centre/newsletters/joint-tb,-hiv-and-viral-hepatitis-jth-newsletter, accessed 1 July 2019).

116. Media Centre. Noncommunicable diseases newsletter [website]. Copenhagen: WHO Regional Office for Europe; 2015–2019 (http://www.euro.who.int/en/media-centre/newsletters/noncommunicable-diseases-newsletter, accessed 1 July 2019).

117. Media Centre. Observatory e-Bulletin [website]. Copenhagen: WHO Regional Office for Europe; 2018–2019 (http://www.euro.who.int/en/media-centre/newsletters/observatory-e-bulletin, accessed 1 July 2019).

118. Media Centre. Publications news [website]. Copenhagen: WHO Regional Office for Europe; 2015–2017 (http://www.euro.who.int/en/media-centre/newsletters/publications-news, accessed 1 July 2019).

119. Media Centre. Public Health Panorama. Copenhagen: WHO Regional Office for Europe; 2019 (http://www.euro.who.int/en/media-centre/newsletters/public-health-panorama, accessed 1 July 2019).

120. Media Centre. Regions for Health Network newsletter [website]. Copenhagen: WHO Regional Office for Europe; 2017–2019 (http://www.euro.who.int/en/media-centre/newsletters/newsletter, accessed 1 July 2019).

121. Media Centre. Roma inclusion newsletter [website]. Copenhagen: WHO Regional Office for Europe; 2016–2019 (http://www.euro.who.int/en/media-centre/newsletters/roma-inclusion-newsletter, accessed 1 July 2019).

122. Media Centre. Vaccine-preventable diseases and immunization (VPI) news [website]. Copenhagen: WHO Regional Office for Europe; 2018-2019 (http://www.euro.who.int/en/media-centre/newsletters/vaccine-preventable-diseases-and-immunization-vpi-news, accessed 1 July 2019).

123. 68th session. WHO/Europe RC68 app. Copenhagen: WHO Regional Office for Europe; 2019 (http://www.euro.who.int/en/about-us/governance/regional-committee-for-europe/68th-session/whoeurope-rc68-app, accessed 1 July 2019).

124. Google Fit. Coaching you to a healthier and more active life [website]. Mountain View, California: Google; 2019 (https://www.google.com/fit/, accessed 1 July 2019).

125. International Health Regulations: Emergency risk communication package pioneered by WHO/Europe rolls out globally. Copenhagen: WHO Regional Office for Europe; 2018 (http://www.euro.who.int/en/health-topics/emergencies/international-health-regulations/news/news/2019/5/emergency-risk-communication-package-pioneered-by-whoeurope-rolls-out-globally, accessed 1 July 2019).

126. Technical briefing on the upcoming WHO European Health Equity Status Report Initiative. Copenhagen: WHO Regional Office for Europe; 2018 (EUR/RC68/TD/4 http://www.euro.who.int/__data/assets/pdf_file/0020/380513/68td04e_TechnicalBriefing4_180597.pdf?ua=1, accessed 1 July 2019).

127. Equity in health project [website]. Copenhagen: WHO Regional Office for Europe; 2012 (http://www.euro.who.int/en/data-and-evidence/equity-in-health-project, accessed 1 July 2019).

128. High-level Conference on Health Equity. About the High-level Conference on Health Equity [website]. Copenhagen: WHO Regional Office for Europe; 2019 (http://www.euro.who.int/en/media-centre/events/events/2019/06/high-level-conference-on-health-equity/about, accessed 1 July 2019).

129. Health Equity Policy Tool: A framework to track policies for increasing health equity in the WHO European Region. Copenhagen: WHO Regional Office for Europe; 2019 (http://www.euro.who.int/en/media-centre/events/events/2019/06/healthy,-prosperous-lives-for-all-in-the-european-region-high-level-conference-on-health-equity/publications/health-equity-policy-tool.-a-framework-to-track-policies-for-increasing-health-equity-in-the-who-european-region-working-document-2019, accessed 1 July 2019).

130. Global action plan for the prevention and control of noncommunicable diseases 2013-2020. Geneva: World Health Organization; 2013 (https://apps.who.int/iris/handle/10665/94384, accessed 1 July 2019).

131. Health diplomacy: European perspectives. Copenhagen: WHO Regional Office for Europe; 2017 (http://www.euro.who.int/en/publications/abstracts/health-diplomacy-european-perspectives-2017, accessed 1 July 2019).

132. Thirteenth General Programme of work 2019–2023 [website]. Geneva: World Health Organization; 2018 (https://www.who.int/about/what-we-do/thirteenth-general-programme-of-work-2019-2023, accessed 1 July 2019).

133. Concept Note. Assessment Tool for Governance for Health and Well-being. Copenhagen: WHO Regional Office for Europe; 2019 (http://www.euro.who.int/en/health-topics/health-policy/health-2020-the-european-policy-for-health-and-well-being/publications/2018/concept-note-assessment-tool-for-governance-for-health-and-well-being-2018, accessed 1 July 2019).

134. Tool for mapping governance for health and well-being: the organigraph method. Copenhagen: WHO Regional Office for Europe; 2018 (http://www.euro.who.int/en/publications/abstracts/tool-for-mapping-governance-for-health-and-well-being-the-organigraph-method-2018, accessed 1 July 2019).

135. Multisectoral and intersectoral action for improved health and well-being for all: mapping of the WHO European Region. Copenhagen: WHO Regional Office for Europe; 2018 (http://www.euro.who.int/en/health-topics/health-policy/health-2020-the-european-policy-for-health-and-well-being/publications/2018/multisectoral-and-intersectoral-action-for-improved-health-and-well-being-for-all-mapping-of-the-who-european-region-governance-for-a-sustainable-future-improving-health-and-well-being-for-all-2018, accessed 1 July 2019).

136. Preconception care to reduce maternal and childhood mortality and morbidity

Meeting report and packages of interventions: WHO HQ, February 2012. Geneva: World Health Organization; 2013 (https://www.who.int/maternal_child_adolescent/documents/concensus_preconception_care/en/, accessed 1 July 2019).

137. WHO Regional strategy on sexual and reproductive health: Reproductive Health/Pregnancy Programme. Copenhagen: WHO Regional Office for Europe; 2001 (EUR/01/5022130 http://www.euro.who.int/data/assets/pdf_file/0004/69529/e74558.pdf, accessed 1 July 2019).

138. World Health Report. Executive Summary. Achieving Health for all [website]. Geneva: World Health Organization; 1998 (https://www.who.int/whr/1998/media_centre/executive_summary6/en/, accessed 1 July 2019).

139. Commission on Ending Childhood Obesity. Report of the Commission on Ending Childhood Obesity Geneva: World Health Organization; 2016 https://www.who.int/end-childhood-obesity/publications/echo-report/en/, accessed 1 July 2019).

140. Better health, better lives: children and young people with intellectual disabilities and their families. Copenhagen: WHO Regional Office for Europe; 2010 (EUR/51298/17/5 http://www.euro.who.int/en/health-topics/noncommunicable-diseases/mental-health/publications/2010/european-declaration-on-the-health-of-children-and-young-people-with-intellectual-disabilities-and-their-families2, accessed 1 July 2019).

141. Ageing and life-course: The Global strategy and action plan on ageing and health. Copenhagen: WHO Regional Office for Europe; 2017 (http://www.who.int/ageing/global-strategy/en/, accessed 1 July 2019).

142. Age-friendly environments in Europe. A handbook of domains for policy action. Copenhagen: WHO Regional Office for Europe; 2017 (http://www.euro.who.int/en/publications/abstracts/age-friendly-environments-in-europe.-a-handbook-of-domains-for-policy-action-2017, accessed 1 July 2019).

143. Ageing and life-course: WHO Global Network for Age-friendly Cities and Communities. Copenhagen: WHO Regional Office for Europe; 2017 (https://www.who.int/ageing/projects/age_friendly_cities_network/en/, accessed 1 July 2019).

144. Evidence-informed policy-making. Estonia tackles obesity with tax on sugar-sweetened beverages [website]. Copenhagen: WHO Regional Office for Europe; 2016 (http://www.euro.who.int/en/data-and-evidence/evidence-informed-policy-making/news/news/2016/22/estonia-tackles-obesity-with-tax-on-sugar-sweetened-beverages, accessed 1 July 2019).

145. Noncommunicable diseases and mental health: NCD Global Monitoring Framework. Geneva: World Health Organization; 2011 (http://www.who.int/nmh/global_monitoring_framework/en/, accessed 1 July 2019).

146. United Nations. A/RES/68/300. Agenda item 118. Resolution adopted by the General Assembly on 10 July 2014. New York: United Nations; 2014 (https://www.who.int/nmh/events/2014/a-res-68-300.pdf, accessed 1 July 2019).

147. Noncommunicable diseases and their risk factors: STEPwise approach to surveillance (STEPS) [website]. Geneva: World Health Organization; 2017 (https://www.who.int/ncds/surveillance/steps/en/, accessed 1 July 2019).

148. Pharmaceutical Pricing and Reimbursement Information (PPRI) network for countries of the Commonwealth of Independent States (CIS) [website]. Vienna: WHO Collaborating Centre for Pharmaceutical Pricing and Reimbursement Policies; 2017 (https://ppri.goeg.at/Regional_PPRI_networks, accessed 1 July 2019).

149. Tobacco control can save billions of dollars and millions of lives. Geneva: World Health Organization; 2017 (http://www.who.int/news-room/detail/10-01-2017-tobacco-control-can-save-billions-of-dollars-and-millions-of-lives, accessed 1 July 2019).

150. Tobacco. Data and statistics [website]. Copenhagen: WHO Regional Office for Europe; 2013 (http://www.euro.who.int/en/health-topics/disease-prevention/tobacco/data-and-statistics, accessed 1 July 2019).

151. WHO Framework Convention on Tobacco Control. Geneva: World Health Organization; 2003 (http://www.who.int/fctc/text_download/en/, accessed 1 July 2019).

152. Tobacco Free Initiative (TFI). WHO report on the global tobacco epidemic. Geneva: World Health Organization; 2017 (http://www.who.int/tobacco/mpower/en/, accessed 1 July 2019).

153. United Nations. A/RES/66/2. Agenda item 117. Political Declaration of the High-level Meeting of the General Assembly on the Prevention and Control of Non-communicable Diseases. New York: United Nations; 2011 (http://www.who.int/nmh/events/un_ncd_summit2011/political_declaration_en.pdf, accessed 1 July 2019).

154. Framework for alcohol policy in the WHO European Region. Copenhagen: WHO Regional Office for Europe; 2006 (http://www.euro.who.int/en/publications/abstracts/framework-for-alcohol-policy-in-the-who-european-region, accessed 1 July 2019).

155. Management of substance abuse. Global strategy to reduce harmful use of alcohol. Geneva: World Health Organization; 2010 (http://www.who.int/substance_abuse/activities/gsrhua/en/, accessed 1 July 2019).

156. Better food and nutrition in Europe – Progress report (2018). Copenhagen: WHO Regional Office for Europe; 2018 (http://www.euro.who.int/en/health-topics/disease-prevention/nutrition/publications/2018/better-food-and-nutrition-in-europe-progress-report-2018, accessed 1 July 2019).

157. European Food and Nutrition Action Plan 2015–2020. Copenhagen: WHO Regional Office for Europe; 2014 (http://www.euro.who.int/en/publications/abstracts/european-food-and-nutrition-action-plan-20152020-2014, accessed 1 July 2019).

158. HBSC: Health behaviour in school-aged children. World Health Organization collaborative cross-national survey [website]. St Andrews: University of St Andrews; http://www.hbsc.org/about/index.html, accessed 1 July 2019).

159. Physical activity strategy for the WHO European Region 2016–2025. Copenhagen: WHO Regional Office for Europe; 2015 (http://www.euro.who.int/en/publications/abstracts/physical-activity-strategy-for-the-who-european-region-20162025, accessed 1 July 2019).

160. The European Mental Health Action Plan 2013–2020. Copenhagen: WHO Regional Office for Europe; 2015 (https://apps.who.int/iris/handle/10665/175672, accessed 1 July 2019).

161. Tuberculosis (TB). UN General Assembly high-level meeting on ending TB. Geneva: World Health Organization; 2018 (https://www.who.int/tb/features_archive/UNGA_HLM_ending_TB/en/, accessed 1 July 2019).

162. Tuberculosis action plan for the WHO European Region 2016–2020. Copenhagen: WHO Regional Office for Europe; 2015 (EUR/RC65/17 Rev.1 http://www.euro.who.int/en/about-us/governance/regional-committee-for-europe/past-sessions/65th-session/documentation/working-documents/eurrc6517-rev.1-tuberculosis-action-plan-for-the-who-european-region-20162020, accessed 1 July 2019).

163. Teenergizer [website]. Kyiv, Ukraine: Teenergizeer 2019 (http://teenergizer.org/t/en/about , accessed 1 July 2019).

164. Central Asian and Eastern European Surveillance of Antimicrobial Resistance Annual report 2018. Copenhagen: WHO Regional Office for Europe; 2018 (http://www.euro.who.int/en/health-topics/disease-prevention/antimicrobial-resistance/publications/2018/central-asian-and-eastern-european-surveillance-of-antimicrobial-resistance-annualreport-2018-2018, accessed 8 August 2019).

165. Antimicrobial resistance: Global action plan on antimicrobial resistance [website]. Geneva: World Health Organization; 2015 (https://www.who.int/antimicrobial-resistance/global-action-plan/en/, accessed 1 July 2019).

166. Immunization, Vaccines and Biologicals. Addressing Vaccine Hesitancy. Report of the SAGE working group on vaccine hesitancy. Geneva: World Health Organization; 2014 (https://www.who.int/immunization/programmes_systems/vaccine_hesitancy/en/, accessed 1 July 2019).

167. Guide to tailoring immunization programmes. Copenhagen: WHO Regional Office for Europe; 2013 (http://www.euro.who.int/en/health-topics/communicable-diseases/poliomyelitis/publications/2013/guide-to-tailoring-immunization-programmes, accessed 8 August 2019).

168. The Tashkent declaration: the move from malaria control to elimination in the WHO European Region – a commitment to action. Copenhagen: WHO Regional Office for Europe; 2006 (https://apps.who.int/iris/handle/10665/107789, accessed 1 July 2019).

169. Regional framework for prevention of malaria reintroduction and certification of malaria elimination 2014–2020. Copenhagen: WHO Regional Office for Europe; 2014 (http://www.euro.who.int/en/publications/abstracts/regional-framework-for-prevention-of-malaria-reintroduction-and-certification-of-malaria-elimination-20142020-2014, accessed 1 July 2019).

170. Regional framework for surveillance and control of invasive mosquito vectors and re-emerging vector-borne diseases 2014–2020. Copenhagen: WHO Regional Office for Europe; 2013 (http://www.euro.who.int/en/publications/abstracts/regional-framework-for-surveillance-and-control-of-invasive-mosquito-vectors-and-re-emerging-vector-borne-diseases,-20142020-2013, accessed 1 July 2019).

171. Health services delivery: Framework for Action towards Coordinated/Integrated Health Services Delivery (CIHSD) launched [website]. Copenhagen: WHO Regional Office for Europe; 2013 (http://www.euro.who.int/en/health-topics/Health-systems/health-services-delivery/news/news/2013/10/framework-for-action-towards-coordinatedintegrated-health-services-delivery-cihsd-launched, accessed 1 July 2019).

172. Health systems in times of global economic crisis: an update of the situation in the WHO European Region. Copenhagen: WHO Regional Office for Europe; 2013 (http://www.euro.who.int/en/media-centre/events/events/2013/04/oslo-conference-on-health-systems-and-the-economic-crisis/documentation/working-documents/health-systems-in-times-of-global-economic-crisis-an-update-of-the-situation-in-the-who-european-region, accessed 1 July 2019).

173. WHO Regional Office for Europe, European Observatory on Health Systems and Policies. Using economic evidence to help make the case for investing in health promotion and disease prevention. Copenhagen: WHO Regional Office for Europe; 2018 (http://www.euro.who.int/data/assets/pdf_file/0003/380730/pb-tallinn-02-eng.pdf?ua=1, accessed 1 July 2019).

174. Thomson, S., Evetovits, T., Cylus, J., Jakab, M. Monitoring financial protection to assess progress towards universal health coverage in Europe. *Public Health Panorama*. 2016;2(03):357-66 (https://apps.who.int/iris/handle/10665/325385, accessed 1 July 2019).

175. Jakab M, Farrington J, Borgermans L, Mantingh F, editors. Health systems respond to noncommunicable diseases: time for ambition. Copenhagen: WHO Regional Office for Europe; 2018 (http://www.euro.who.int/en/publications/abstracts/health-systems-respond-to-noncommunicable-diseases-time-for-ambition-2018, accessed 1 July 2019).

176. Public health services. Web-based version of self-assessment tool to evaluate essential public health operations (EPHOs) now available [website]. Copenhagen: WHO Regional Office for Europe; 2016 (http://www.euro.who.int/en/health-topics/Health-systems/public-health-services/news/news/2016/06/web-based-version-of-self-assessment-tool-to-evaluate-essential-public-health-operations-ephos-now-available, accessed 1 July 2019).

177. Public health services. Coalition of Partners [website]. Copenhagen: WHO Regional Office for Europe; 2018 (http://www.euro.who.int/en/health-topics/Health-systems/public-health-services/coalition-of-partners, accessed 1 July 2019).

178. Global Capacities Alert and Response (GCR). IHR (2005) Monitoring and Evaluation framework: Joint External Evaluation tool (JEE tool) first edition. Geneva: World Health Organization; 2016 (https://www.who.int/ihr/publications/WHO_HSE_GCR_2016_2/en/, accessed 1 July 2019).

179. WHO's new Health Emergencies Programme. Geneva: World Health Organization; 2016 (https://www.who.int/features/qa/health-emergencies-programme/en/, accessed 1 July 2019).

180. European Health Information gateway. Life Expectancy [online database]. Copenhagen: WHO Regional Office for Europe; 2015 (https://gateway.euro.who.int/en/hfa-explorer/#jkVjff4fYb, accessed 1 July 2019).

181. Bachmaha, M. Vaccination Crisis in Ukraine: Its Origins and Consequences. *Krytyka*. October 2016 (https://krytyka.com/en/ukraines-public-health-challenge/articles/vaccination-crisis-ukraine-its-origins-and-consequences, accessed 1 July 2019).

182. Commission on Social Determinants of Health. Closing the gap in a generation: health equity through action on the social determinants of health: final report: executive summary. Geneva: World Health Organization; 2008 (https://apps.who.int/iris/handle/10665/69832, accessed 1 July 2019).

183. Building resilience: a key pillar of Health 2020 and the Sustainable Development Goals Examples from the WHO Small Countries Initiative. Copenhagen: WHO Regional Office for Europe; 2019 (http://www.euro.who.int/en/publications/abstracts/building-resilience-a-key-pillar-of-health-2020-and-the-sustainable-development-goals-examples-from-the-who-small-countries-initiative-2017, accessed 1 July 2019).

184. Health 2020 priority area four: creating supportive environments and resilient communities. A compendium of inspirational examples (2018). Copenhagen: WHO Regional Office for Europe; 2018 (http://www.euro.who.int/en/about-us/networks/small-countries-initiative/key-resources/health-2020-priority-area-four-creating-supportive-environments-and-resilient-communities.-a-compendium-of-inspirational-examples-2018, accessed 1 July 2019).

185. Health and the environment in the WHO European Region: Creating resilient communities and supportive environments. Copenhagen: WHO Regional Office for Europe; 2013 (http://www.euro.who.int/__data/assets/pdf_file/0005/215645/HEALTH-AND-THE-ENVIRONMENT-IN-THE-WHO-EUROPEAN-REGION-Creating-resilient-communities-and-supportive-environments.pdf, accessed 1 July 2019).

186. United Nations SDG. United Nations Conference on Sustainable Development, Rio+20 [website]. New York: United Nations; 2012 (https://sustainabledevelopment.un.org/rio20.html, accessed 1 July 2019).

187. Development of the health economic assessment tools (HEAT) for walking and cycling. Meeting report of the consensus workshop in Bonn, Germany, 1–2 October 2013. Copenhagen: WHO Regional Office for Europe; 2013 (http://www.euro.who.int/__data/assets/pdf_file/0005/248900/Development-of-the-health-economic-assessment-tools-HEAT-for-walking-and-cycling.pdf, accessed 1 July 2019).

188. Water sanitation hygiene. Water safety planning [website]. Geneva: World Health Organization; 2019 (https://www.who.int/water_sanitation_health/water-quality/safety-planning/en/, accessed 1 July 2019).

189. Parma Declaration on Environment and Health. Copenhagen: WHO Regional Office for Europe; 2010 (EUR/55934/5.1 Rev. 2 http://www.euro.who.int/en/publications/policy-documents/parma-declaration-on-environment-and-health, accessed 1 July 2019).

190. Emergency risk communication (ERC) 5-step capacity-building package. Copenhagen: WHO Regional Office for Europe; 2017 (http://www.euro.who.int/en/health-topics/emergencies/international-health-regulations/emergency-risk-communications/emergency-risk-communications-tools/national-health-emergency-risk-communication-training-package, accessed 1 July 2019).

191. WHO Report on Surveillance of Antibiotic Consumption. Geneva: World Health Organization; 2018 (https://www.who.int/medicines/areas/rational_use/oms-amr-amc-report-2016-2018/en/, accessed 1 July 2019).

192. Antimicrobial Stewardship: A competency-based approach [online course]. Geneva: World Health Organization; 2018 (https://openwho.org/courses/AMR-competency, accessed 1 July 2019).

193. WHO EpiData [online data]. Copenhagen: WHO Regional Office for Europe; 2019 (http://www.euro.who.int/en/health-topics/disease-prevention/vaccines-and-immunization/publications/surveillance-and-data/who-epidata, accessed 1 July 2019).

194. Vaccines and immunization. Data and statistics [online data]. Copenhagen: WHO Regional Office for Europe; 2019 (http://www.euro.who.int/en/health-topics/disease-prevention/vaccines-and-immunization/data-and-statistics, accessed 1 July 2019).

195. The Ashgabat Statement: Europe commits to being malaria free. Copenhagen: WHO Regional Office for Europe; 2017 (http://www.euro.who.int/en/health-topics/communicable-diseases/pages/news/news/2017/09/the-ashgabat-statement-europe-commits-to-staying-malaria-free, accessed 1 July 2019).

196. Strategic framework for leishmaniasis control in the WHO European Region 2014–2020. Copenhagen: WHO Regional Office for Europe; 2014 (http://www.euro.who.int/en/health-topics/communicable-diseases/vector-borne-and-parasitic-diseases/publications/2014/strategic-framework-for-leishmaniasis-control-in-the-who-european-region-20142020-2014, accessed 1 July 2019).

197. Environmental Noise Guidelines for the European Region. Copenhagen: WHO Regional Office for Europe; 2018 (http://www.euro.who.int/en/publications/abstracts/environmental-noise-guidelines-for-the-european-region-2018, accessed 1 July 2019).

198. Barbazza, E., Pedersen, H. B., Birtanov, Y., Huber, M., Immonen, K., Jakab, M., et al. Ten evidence-based policy accelerators for transforming primary health care in the WHO European Region. Public Health Panorama, December 2018, vol.4, issue 4, 507-514 (https://apps.who.int/iris/handle/10665/324844, accessed 1 July 2019).

199. Health emergency response to the crisis in the Syrian Arab Republic Annual Report 2018. Copenhagen: WHO Regional Office for Europe; 2018 (http://www.euro.who.int/en/countries/turkey/publications/health-emergency-response-to-the-crisis-in-the-syrian-arab-republic-annual-report-2018-2019, accessed 1 July 2019).

200. Media Centre. Over 100 000 people sick with measles in 14 months: with measles cases at an alarming level in the European Region, WHO scales up response. Copenhagen: WHO Regional Office for Europe; 2019 (http://www.euro.who.int/en/media-centre/sections/press-releases/2019/over-100-000-people-sick-with-measles-in-14-months-with-measles-cases-at-an-alarming-level-in-the-european-region,-who-scales-up-response, accessed 1 July 2019).

201. The Global Compact on Refugees [website]. Geneva: UNHCR The UN Refugee Agency; 2019 (https://www.unhcr.org/the-global-compact-on-refugees.html, accessed 1 July 2019).

202. Tuberculosis Regional Eastern European and Central Asian Project (TB-REP) mid-term update (2017) Copenhagen: WHO Regional Office for Europe; 2017 (http://www.euro.who.int/en/health-topics/communicable-diseases/tuberculosis/publications/2017/tuberculosis-regional-eastern-european-and-central-asian-project-tb-rep-mid-term-update-2017, accessed 1 July 2019).

203. News. Non-State actors accredited in 2018 and applications now open for 2019 [website]. Copenhagen: WHO Regional Office for Europe; 2018 (http://www.euro.who.int/en/about-us/partners/news/news/2018/12/non-state-actors-accredited-in-2018-and-applications-now-open-for-2019, accessed 1 July 2019).

204. European Observatory on Health Systems and Policies. About us [website]. Copenhagen: WHO Regional Office for Europe; 2019 (http://www.euro.who.int/en/about-us/partners/observatory/about-us, accessed 1 July 2019).

205. Human resources update, including on the global internship programme. Geneva; World Health Organization; 2018 (EB144/47 https://apps.who.int/gb/ebwha/pdf_files/EB144/B144_47-en.pdf, accessed 1 July 2019).

206. Monitoring noncommunicable disease commitments in Europe. Theme in focus: progress monitor indicators. Copenhagen: WHO Regional Office for Europe; 2017 (http://www.euro.who.int/en/health-topics/noncommunicable-diseases/pages/news/news/2017/10/european-region-makes-huge-gains-in-ncd-response,-but-needs-faster-progress, accessed 1 July 2019).

207. Newsroom. Alcohol. Key facts [website]. Geneva: World Health Organization; 2018 (https://www.who.int/news-room/fact-sheets/detail/alcohol, accessed 1 July 2019).

208. Media Centre. Press release. WHO calls on countries to reduce sugars intake among adults and children. [website]. Geneva: World Health Organization; 2015 (https://www.who.int/mediacentre/news/releases/2015/sugar-guideline/en/, accessed 1 July 2019).

209. Tuberculosis surveillance and monitoring report in Europe. Copenhagen: WHO Regional Office for Europe; 2019 (http://www.euro.who.int/en/health-topics/communicable-diseases/tuberculosis/publications/2019/tuberculosis-surveillance-and-monitoring-report-in-europe-2019, accessed 1 July 2019).

210. HIV/AIDS surveillance in Europe 2018. Copenhagen: WHO Regional Office for Europe; 2018 (http://www.euro.who.int/en/health-topics/communicable-diseases/hivaids/publications/2018/hivaids-surveillance-in-europe-2018-2018, accessed 1 July 2019).

211. MPOWER measures. Copenhagen: WHO Regional Office for Europe; 2007 (http://www.euro.who.int/en/health-topics/disease-prevention/tobacco/publications/key-policy-documents/who-framework-convention-on-tobacco-control-who-fctc/mpower, accessed 1 July 2019).

212. Return on investment of treating depression in the WHO European Region [Infographic]. Copenhagen: WHO Regional Office for Europe; 2017 (http://www.euro.who.int/en/media-centre/events/events/2017/04/world-health-day-2017-depression-lets-talk/infographics-on-depression-world-health-day-2017/infographic-return-on-investment-of-treating-depression-in-the-who-european-region-2017, accessed 8 August 2019).

213. Global Antimicrobial Resistance Surveillance System (GLASS) [website]. Geneva: World Health Organization; 2015 (https://www.who.int/glass/en/, accessed 8 August 2019).

214. European Action Plan for Strengthening Public Health Capacities and Services. Copenhagen: WHO Regional Office for Europe; 2012 (EUR/RC62/12 Rev.1; http://www.euro.who.int/en/health-topics/Health-systems/public-health-services/publications/2012/european-action-plan-for-strengthening-public-health-capacities-and-services, accessed 11 August 2019).

215. European action plan to reduce the harmful use of alcohol 2012–2020. Copenhagen: WHO Regional Office for Europe; 2012 (http://www.euro.who.int/en/health-topics/disease-prevention/alcohol-use/publications/2012/european-action-plan-to-reduce-the-harmful-use-of-alcohol-20122021, accessed 8 August 2019).

216. Action plan to improve public health preparedness and response in the WHO European Region 2018–2023. Copenhagen: WHO Regional Office for Europe; 2019 (http://www.euro.who.int/en/publications/abstracts/action-plan-to-improve-public-health-preparedness-and-response-in-the-who-european-region-20182023, accessed 8 August 2019).

217. Protocol on Water and Health [website]. Copenhagen: WHO Regional Office for Europe; 2017 (http://www.euro.who.int/en/health-topics/environment-and-health/water-and-sanitation/protocol-on-water-and-health, accessed 9 August 2019).

218. Health 2020 implementation package [website]. Copenhagen: WHO Regional Office for Europe; 2012 (http://www.euro.who.int/en/health-topics/health-policy/health-2020-the-european-policy-for-health-and-well-being/implementation-package, accessed 21 August 2019).

219. The European health report 2012: charting the way to well-being. Copenhagen: WHO Regional Office for Europe; 2013 (http://www.euro.who.int/en/publications/abstracts/european-health-report-2012, accessed 21 August 2019).

220. The European health report 2015. Targets and beyond – Reaching new frontiers in evidence. Copenhagen: WHO Regional Office for Europe; 2015 (http://www.euro.who.int/en/publications/abstracts/european-health-report-2015-the.-targets-and-beyond-reaching-new-frontiers-in-evidence, accessed 21 August 2019).

221. Fact sheets on sustainable development goals: health targets. Copenhagen: WHO Regional Office for Europe; 2017 (http://www.euro.who.int/en/health-topics/health-policy/sustainable-development-goals/publications/2017/fact-sheets-on-sustainable-development-goals-health-targets, accessed 21 August 2019).

222. Progress report on the roadmap to implement the 2030 Agenda for Sustainable Development, building on Health 2020, the European policy for health and well-being. Copenhagen: WHO Regional Office for Europe; 2019 (http://www.euro.who.int/en/about-us/governance/regional-committee-for-europe/69th-session/documentation/working-documents/eurrc698e-progress-report-on-the-roadmap-to-implement-the-2030-agenda-for-sustainable-development,-building-on-health-2020,-the-european-policy-for-health-and-well-being, accessed 21 August 2019).

223. EUR/RC69/14 Draft WHO European roadmap for implementation of health literacy initiatives through the life course. Copenhagen; WHO Regional Office for Europe, 2019 (http://www.euro.who.int/en/about-us/governance/regional-committee-for-europe/69th-session/documentation/working-documents/eurrc6914-draft-who-european-roadmap-for-implementation-of-health-literacy-initiatives-through-the-life-course, accessed 21 August, 2019)

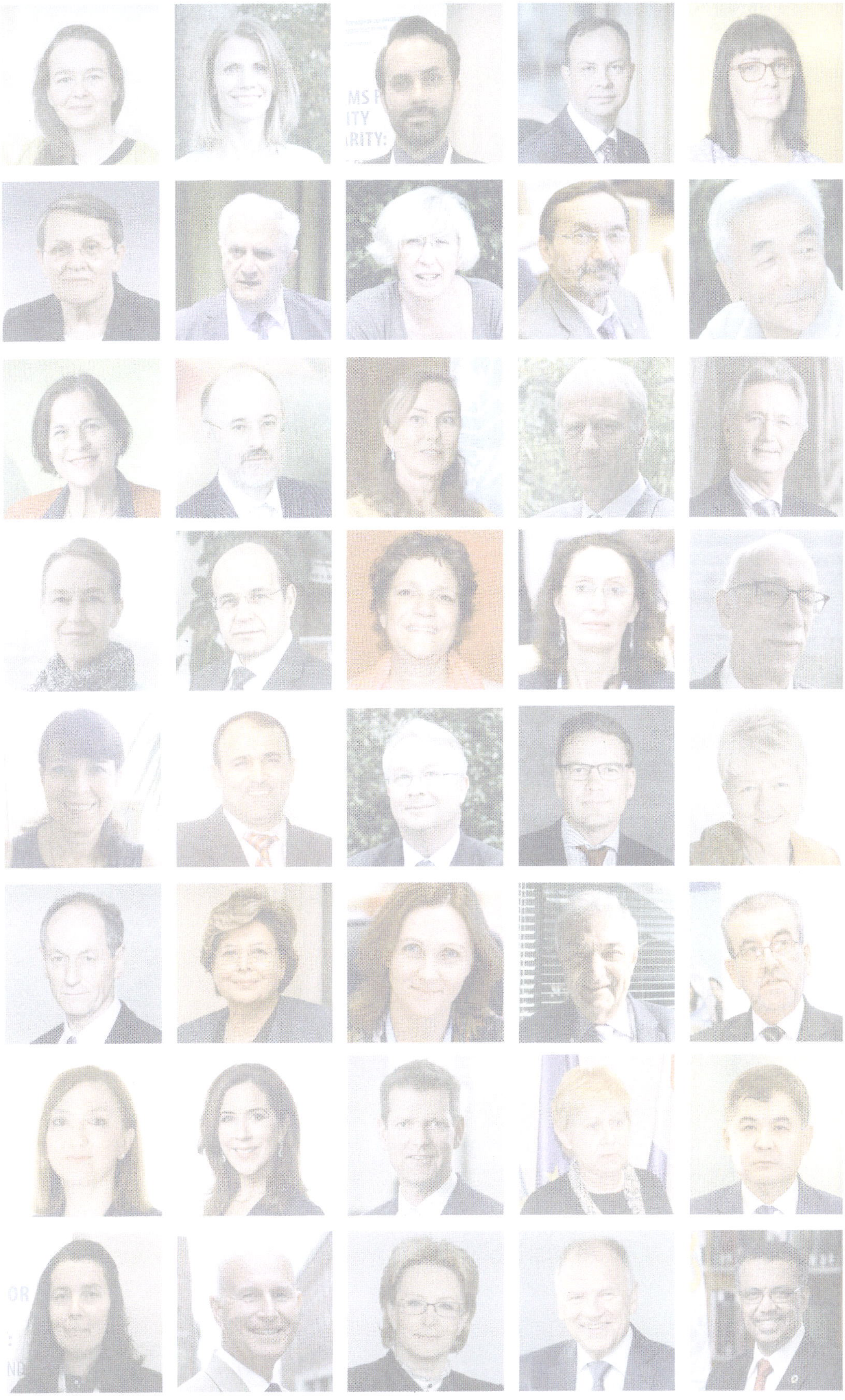

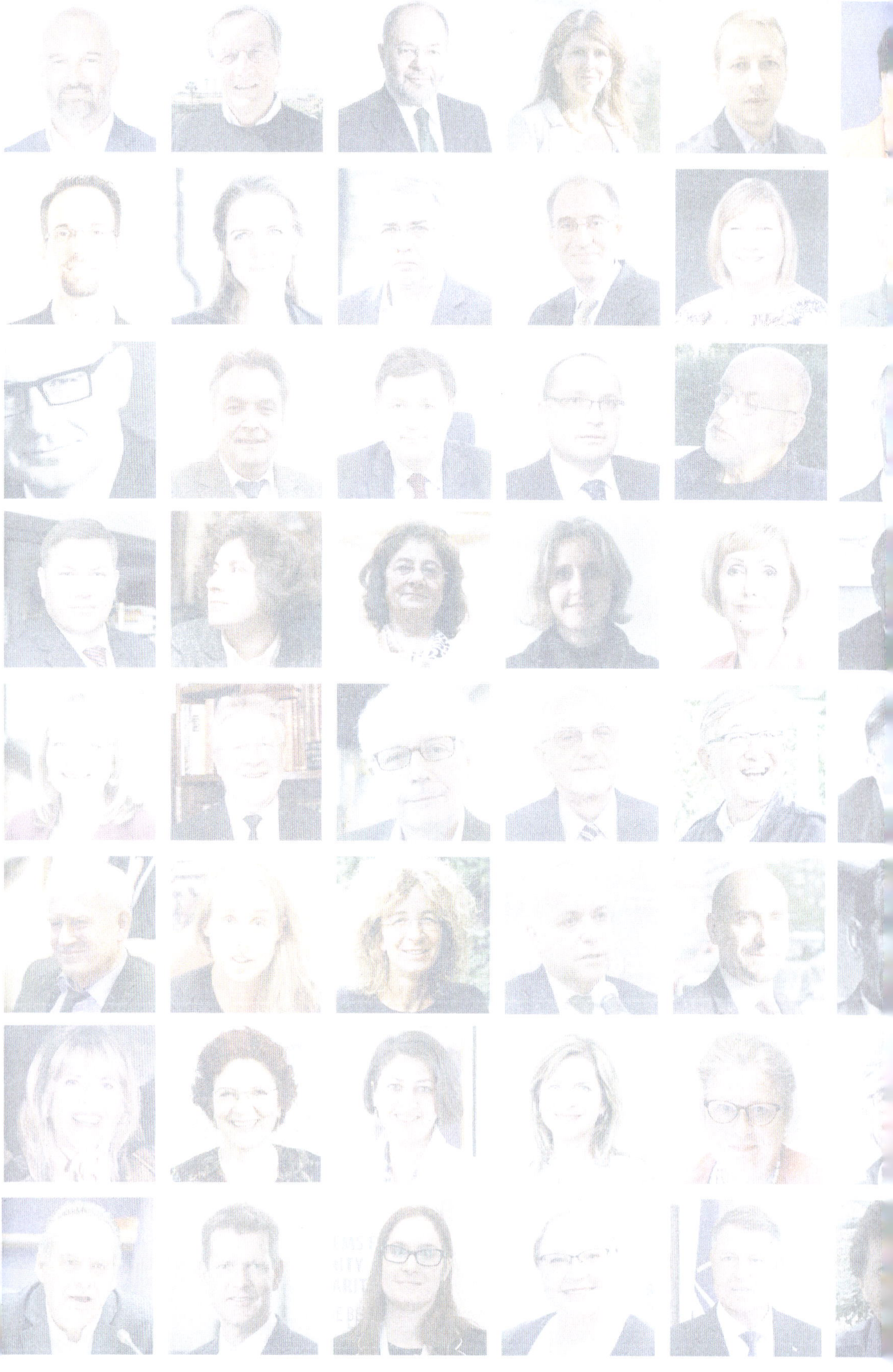